WY 21 DAL 1

Contexts of nursing:
an introduction

Contexts of nursing: an introduction

Second edition

Edited by

John Daly

Sandra Speedy

Debra Jackson

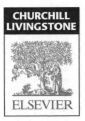

CHURCHILL
LIVINGSTONE

ELSEVIER

Sydney Edinburgh London New York Philadelphia St Louis Toronto

ELSEVIER

Churchill Livingstone
is an imprint of Elsevier

Elsevier Australia
(a division of Reed International Books Australia Pty Ltd)
30–52 Smidmore Street, Marrickville, NSW 2204
ACN 001 002 357

This edition © 2006 Elsevier Australia

First edition © 2000. Reprinted 2000 (twice), 2001 (twice), 2003, 2004

National Library of Australia Cataloguing-in-Publication Data

Contexts of nursing : an introduction.

2nd ed.
Bibliography.
Includes index.

ISBN–13: 978–0–7295–3746–9
ISBN–10: 0–7295–3746–3

1. Nursing — Australia. 2. Nursing — Social aspects — Australia. 3. Nursing — Study
and teaching — Australia. 4. Nursing ethics. 5. Medical care — Australia. I. Daly, John.
II. Speedy, Sandra. III. Jackson, Debra.

610.730994

Publishing Director: Vaughn Curtis
Developmental Editor: Suzanne Hall
Publishing Services Manager: Helena Klijn
Edited by Ruth Matheson
Proofread by Jon Forsyth
Cover design by Trina McDonald
Internal design and typesetting by Egan-Reid Ltd
Index by Jon Forsyth
Printed in Australia by Southwood Press

CONTENTS

CONTENTS

CONTRIBUTORS

Alan Barnard RN BA MA PhD
  Senior Lecturer, School of Nursing, Queensland University of Technology

Sally Borbasi RN BEd(Nurs) MA(Educ) PhD
  Professor of Nursing, School of Nursing and Midwifery, Griffith University

Esther Chang RN PhD
  Director of Research, School of Nursing, Family and Community Health, College of Social and Health Sciences, University of Western Sydney

Judith Clare RN MA(Hons) PhD FRCNA
  Professor of Nursing, School of Nursing, Midwifery and Health, Flinders University of South Australia

Moya Conrick RN, RM DippApSc BN MClEd PhD
  School of Nursing, Griffith University

Jane Conway RN BHSc GradCertHRM GradDipFET DEd
  Manager, Pre and Post Registration Nursing and Midwifery Education, CCH Professional Development Service, Conjoint Senior Lecturer, School of Nursing and Midwifery, University of Newcastle

Debra K Creedy RN BA(Hons) MEd(Research) PhD
  Dean of Health, Griffith University

Patrick Crookes RN RNT Cert Ed BSc(Nursing) PhD
  Interim Dean, Faculty of Health and Behavioural Science, Professor and Head Department of Nursing, University of Wollongong

John Daly RN BA BHSc(Nurs) MEd(Hons) PhD FCN(NSW) FRCNA FINE
  Professor and Head, School of Nursing, Family and Community Health, College of Social & Health Sciences, University of Western Sydney, NSW

Philip Darbyshire RNMH RSCN DipN(Lond) RNT MN PhD
  Chair of Nursing and Head of Department, Department of Nursing and Midwifery Research & Practice Development, Children, Youth & Women's Health Service, Flinders University of South Australia

Gay Edgecombe RN RM CHN BApplSc MS PhD FRCNA
  Clinical Chair, Community Child Health Nursing, RMIT University, Division of Nursing and Midwifery, Melbourne

Doug Elliott RN PhD
  Professor of Nursing, Faculty of Nursing, University of Sydney

Mary FitzGerald RN PhD
  Professor of Nursing, University of Newcastle, and Central Coast Health, Teaching and Research Unit, New South Wales

Jean Gilmour RGON BA PhD DipSocSci CertTchg
Senior Lecturer, School of Health Sciences, Massey University, New Zealand

Madonna Greehan RN RM GrDipHealthEthics
School of Nursing, University of Melbourne

Rhonda Griffiths RN PhD
Director, Centre for Applied Nursing Research, School of Nursing, Family and Community Health, College of Social and Health Sciences, University of Western Sydney

Desley Hegney RN RM COHN CNNN DNE BA(Hons) PhD FRCNA FCN FAIM
Professor of Rural and Remote Area Nursing, Director, Centre for Rural and Remote Area Health, University of Southern Queensland and University of Queensland, Toowoomba

Amanda Henderson RN RM ICU(Certificate) BSc GradDipNurs(Education) MScSoc PhD
Nursing Director Education, Princess Alexandra Hospital, Queensland; Adjunct Associate Professor, Griffith University, Queensland

Colin Holmes RN PhD
Professor, School of Nursing Sciences, James Cook University, Townsville

Annette Huntington RGON CertTchg PhD
Associate Professor and Colonel Commandant of the Royal New Zealand Nursing Corps, School of Health Sciences, Massey University, New Zealand

Debra Jackson RN CommNursCert BHSc(Nurs) MNurs PhD
Professorial Fellow, School of Nursing, Family and Community Health, College of Social and Health Sciences, University of Western Sydney, NSW

Megan-Jane Johnstone RN BA PhD FRCNA
Professor of Nursing, Director of Research, Division of Nursing and Midwifery, RMIT University, Melbourne

Judy Lumby RN ICN PhD MHPEd BA MAICD
Executive Director of the College of Nursing, Emeritus Professor at the University of Technology Sydney, Honorary Professor at the University of Sydney, and Adjunct Professor with the University of Western Sydney

Judith Mair PhD LLB DNE RN RM
Legal Educator

Margaret McMillan RN BA MCurrSt(Hons) DNE PhD GradCertMgt FRCNA
Deputy Executive Dean, Faculty of Health, University of Newcastle

Sioban Nelson RN PhD
School of Nursing, University of Melbourne

Akram Omeri RN PhD CTN MCN FRCNA
Transcultural Nurse Consultant, Adjunct A/Professor, School of Nursing, Family & Community Nursing, University of Western Sydney

Tracey Osmond RN Cert Orth GradCert Experiential Learning MEd(Adult) FCN AFACHSE
Director, Education Services, College of Nursing, Sydney

Judith M Parker AM, RN BA(Hons) PhD
Visiting Professor, Department of Nursing Studies, University of Hong Kong

Steve Parker RN RMHN NDipT(Nursing) BEd PhD
Senior Lecturer, School of Nursing and Midwifery, Flinders University of South Australia

Sandra Speedy RN BA(Hons) DipEd MURP EdN MAPS FANZCMHN
Consultant Psychologist, Emeritus Professor, Southern Cross University, Lismore, NSW

Kim Usher DNE DHS BA MNursS PhD RN RPN RMRN
Head, School of Nursing Sciences, James Cook University, Townsville

Kim Walker RN PhD
Clinical Associate Professor, Practice Development and Research Coordinator, St Vincent's Private Hospital, Sydney

Sarah Winch RN BA(Hons) PhD
Nursing Director Research, Princess Alexandra Hospital, Queensland, and Adjunct Senior Lecturer, School of Social Science, University of Queensland

PREFACE

Welcome to the second edition of *Contexts of nursing*! Five years have passed since we published the very successful first edition of this work. Since the publication of that first edition, we have published versions of this book in the United Kingdom and the United States. Nursing as a discipline has matured and developed in many ways since the year 2000, within Australia and New Zealand and globally, and this new edition reflects that development.

As with the first edition, this volume introduces students to the theory, language and scholarship of nursing. Our major objective has been (and remains) to provide a comprehensive coverage of key ideas underpinning the practice of contemporary nursing. This book is a collection of views and voices; consequently the chapters are not all identical in nature. This reflects our position that it is important that students/readers engage with various (and sometimes conflicting) views to challenge and extend them.

We have specifically sought out a range of contributors who not only reflect the dynamic nature of nursing scholarship in Australia and New Zealand, but who are helping to shape contemporary nursing in this part of the world. These scholars have been chosen not only because of their expert knowledge, but also because of their professional standing, leadership, and the sometimes controversial stances they take on various contemporary issues. We have not sought to silence the controversies or quieten the debates; rather, we present them to you, the reader, as a stimulus for reflection, discussion and debate, and as a catalyst to further develop your own positions on various issues.

We have explained previously why the notion of 'contexts' has appeal for us in conceptualising nursing knowledge as a fabric comprised of theoretical threads. This knowledge-as-fabric metaphor provides access to a number of other related ideas, such as weaving and tapestry. In this edition we have included some additional chapters on new topics. Some new threads have been woven into the fabric of nursing knowledge presented in this work. Selection of these topics was based on extensive consultation with nurses who found our first edition useful in undergraduate and graduate courses and in their teaching and learning. Of course student evaluations of the work were also considered. In addition, a number of experienced nurse authors and editors provided useful critique and feedback, which has helped us in shaping this new volume. We hope that the new contexts and topics we have included in this edition will make the book truly comprehensive and contemporary.

Though we have updated and added new content to this second edition of *Contexts of nursing*, this edition is based on the same aims and objectives which underpinned the design and development of the first edition of the work. Nursing knowledge and its foundational elements are explored and considered in relation to professional nursing practice. Our emphasis on pedagogic strength and accessibility, and the use of reflective questions and exercises to stimulate critical thinking and learning, has been maintained.

PREFACE

The editors acknowledge Suzanne Hall and Vaughn Curtis, and the rest of the team at Elsevier, for their ongoing encouragement, support and assistance in the preparation and production of this collection. Elsevier Australia joins the editors in thanking Dr Michael Bauer, La Trobe University, Dr Cally Berryman, Victoria University, and Linda Goddard, Charles Sturt University, for their valuable comments provided in the manuscript review process.

Most of all, we thank our contributors, who have risen to the challenge of developing engaging, scholarly and teaching/learning-oriented work to stimulate reflection, discussion and debate.

John Daly
Sandra Speedy
Debra Jackson
Sydney, August 2005

CHAPTER ONE

Presenting nursing . . . a career for life

John Daly, Sandra Speedy & Debra Jackson

LEARNING OBJECTIVES

By reflecting on this chapter, readers will be able to:

▲ list some of the myths, legends and stereotypes that surround nursing;

▲ arrive at a personal beginning definition of nursing;

▲ establish their passion for nursing;

▲ describe the different types of nurse in Australia and New Zealand;

▲ verbalise some of the choices that a nursing degree offers for graduates; and

▲ describe what is the meaning of the term 'professional conduct'.

KEY WORDS
Nursing, stereotypes, critical perspective, career codes of conduct, lifelong learning

WHY NURSING?

Nursing is a unique career choice. It is a curious mix of technology and myth . . . of science and art . . . reality and romance. It blends the concrete and the abstract. It combines thinking and doing . . . 'being with' and 'doing for'. Nurses have privileged access to people's homes and share some of the most precious and highly intimate moments in people's lives—moments that remain hidden from most other people and professions. Nurses witness birth and death, and just about everything in between. Nurses bear witness to suffering and pain, and also share in moments of great joy and happiness. Because of the special place in society that nurses hold, nurses enjoy a high level of community trust. Indeed, in Australia and New Zealand, nurses continually rank very highly in surveys of public confidence.

Nursing can be a career for life. A degree in nursing provides a foundation for lifelong learning. It is the entry requirement to a fulfilling career, to a range of postgraduate courses in areas as diverse as paediatrics, midwifery, cancer care, community nursing, women's health, nurse education and nursing research. Age and experience are valued in nursing. Unlike many other professions and career choices in which people experience increasing difficulty in obtaining work as they get older, nurses can remain productively employed until retirement. Nursing is a career to which one can always return. Career interruption because of family responsibilities (or other reasons) can be extremely disadvantaging in some professions, but many nurses have effectively blended very successful careers with raising families. Nursing opens many doors. Internationally, Australian and New Zealand nurses are well respected and are eligible for registration in many other countries.

In this opening chapter we aim to share what captured us and created our passion and enthusiasm for the career that is nursing—the passion and enthusiasm that has sustained and carried us successfully through our nursing careers. We also describe the different types and levels of nurse in Australia and New Zealand, and aim to introduce you to some of the ideas of interest to nurses and nursing, many of which are discussed in more detail in subsequent chapters of this book.

NURSING: MYTHS, LEGENDS AND STEREOTYPES

Perhaps more than any other professional group, nursing and nurses are the subject of myth and popular belief; there are also many romantic connotations. Certain of these myths and beliefs are almost folkloric, yet they strongly influence the ways in which nurses are perceived by the general public, and also in the ways that nurses see themselves. Through the media, nursing is often portrayed as a dramatic, exciting, glamorous and romantic activity, with nurses frequently represented in the role of handmaiden/helper to doctors.

Several of the almost legendary attributes that surround nursing are derived from myths about Florence Nightingale and her work in the Crimean War. For example, the romantic notion of the 'angel of mercy', the quiet, modest and self-effacing woman who, with a religious-like fervour, would tirelessly and uncomplainingly nurse the ill and injured back to full strength, and the image of the 'lady with the lamp' fearlessly working at the frontline of a war zone, and instilling calm, peace and tranquillity where only chaos and suffering have reigned, have become enduring and mythologised popular images of the nurse.

Because of her continued allure, much of Nightingale's life has been reconstructed and, in the process, subject to various forms of poetic licence. An excellent example of this poetic licence is explored by Jones (1988b) in her critical examination of *The white angel*, a motion picture released in 1936, which purported to be a biographical representation of the life of Florence Nightingale. On its release, this film was widely acclaimed, both within and outside the nursing profession, with influential professional nursing journals promoting the movie as 'a good educational picture', and commending it to the nursing profession, 'especially those concerned with information and education' (Jones 1988b:222). However, although the movie was widely accepted as factual, even by the nursing community, Jones (1988b) proposes that the screenplay contained a series of key errors, which serve to trivialise major events in the life of Nightingale, and reinforce the myth that her decision to become a nurse was made in the manner of a religious calling.

[S]he is dressed in white, thus fulfilling the image of the title [*The white angel*], but the image does more than just show Nightingale in white. Her dress and veil are like a bridal gown and veil in style as well as color. The association of white with virginity and purity is important, as is the bridal association. At the same time she announces her decision to be a nurse, Nightingale announces to her parents that she will never marry. Because she is visually presented as a bride at the same time that she rejects marriage, the subliminal message is that her marriage is to her profession, just as a nun's marriage is to Christ (Jones 1988b:225–6).

However, notwithstanding the influence of myth and legend, nursing does have a noble history, and there are many stories of the fortitude, bravery and courage shown by Australian nurses in wartime and other times of community hardship (e.g. Biedermann 2004). In Chapter 2 of this book, you will find an in-depth discussion of the history of modern nursing and, after reading it, you will have greater insights and understandings of the origins of some of the myths that surround nursing.

Nursing is endlessly fascinating to many people and this is reflected in the number of television shows, novels and movies that feature nursing and nurses as a major component. There is not the same level of interest in bank workers, or bus drivers or beauty therapists for example. Nursing is ripe with imagery. Many of the images associated with nursing are seemingly at odds with one another, yet all may be conjured up by the word 'nurse'. Images of selflessness (Fealy 2004), kindness, compassion and dedication, hard work, long hours, submission and low pay are among the things that come to mind for some people when they think of nursing. But though nursing has current or historical elements of all these things, there is so much more to nursing than these portray.

Nursing and nurses are subject to various entrenched stereotypes, and some of these are at least partly derived from the myth that surrounds nursing. Kalisch et al (1983) identified some major stereotypes of nurses, and though this work was undertaken in the United States, it is relevant to nurses in Australia, as well as nurses in other parts of the world (see also Muff 1988). The media and popular literature also tend to present nurses as having stereotyped personal characteristics such as youth, femaleness, purity and naivety, altruism and idealism, compliance, and diminutive stature and 'good character' (Kalisch et al 1983, De Vries et al 1995, Fealy 2004).

Nurses are also credited with having certain qualities and virtues that are grounded in romanticism. De Vries et al (1995), in their study of images of nurses as portrayed in popular medical romances, found that nurses are almost always represented as youthful, pure, virginal, kind, petite, beautiful, subservient, sensitive, considerate, competent and able females. In addition to these personal characteristics, the heroines of these stories are typically presented as Caucasian, with blonde hair and green or blue eyes. They are also portrayed and represented as being emotional and hence not to be taken seriously (Ceci 2004a).

Darbyshire (1995), in his exploration of the depiction of Nurse Ratched in the popular film *One flew over the cuckoo's nest*, discusses a counter image of nursing— the battleaxe/torturer. Unlike the nurses found in the medical romance genre, Nurse Ratched is not petite or subservient, and nor is she acquiescent or particularly beautiful. Hunter (1988), in her discussion of the book upon which the film is based, proposes that the Nurse Ratched character is but one example of misogynistic literary tendencies which, she argues, frequently satirically portray the battleaxe/torturer/oppressor nurse as female, and the tender, gentle carer nurse figure as male. Hunter (1988) supports this notion by exploring the images evoked in Tolstoy's description of the gentle hero, Gerasim (*The death of Ivan Ilyich*, 1886), and Whitman's poem 'The wound dresser' (*Leaves of grass*, 1891), and comparing them with those evoked by Kesey's Nurse Ratched (*One flew over the cuckoo's nest*, 1962). In Chapter 4 of this book, Philip Darbyshire scrutinises some current and past nursing stereotypes in more detail.

Though we still see nurses portrayed in various stereotypical and sometimes highly sexualised ways, which is exemplified in the myth of 'nurse as whore', these stereotypes coexist with some of the noble and romantic images of nursing. Failure to challenge these stereotypes is dangerous for nurses and nursing: the nurse has the status of a worker rather than a professional (Fealy 2004) and becomes the 'good nurse', a social construction which suits powerbrokers both inside and outside nursing. This perpetuates an anti-intellectual bias against nursing, manifest in the view that good nurses are practical people, rather than highly educated professionals.

Coexisting with the romantic myths and stereotypes surrounding nursing is the reality of nursing. This reality is that which makes contact with the visceral and raw aspects of humanity that are usually hidden from the world, but with which nurses become acquainted because of the illness, the incapacity, the frailty, the disability or other needs of those who are the recipients of nursing care. Nursing provides opportunities for human connectedness and growth that few other careers can offer.

But why is this significant? It is clear, as Fealy states, that it is:

... naive to assume that ideology will not continue to influence the development of nursing, and that factors such as class and gender relationships, power brokerage and economics, will not continue to reside at the heart of commentary on the nurse (Fealy 2004:655).

It is for this reason that nurses need to be aware of the danger lurking in latent meaning and rhetoric, and recognise that a reality is being created on behalf of nursing, a reality that is not necessarily theirs. It is important to recognise that the concept of 'nurse' is socially constructed, and that nurses may want to believe in their power and control, but the broader societal context situates nurses in a much more fragile position. Nursing exists within a male-dominated healthcare system, bound by authority and power of that class. The sense of 'self as nurse' is thus subject to what David (2000) refers to as 'received behaviors', which can result in 'horizontal violence', behaviours of aggression towards other nurses, in order to maintain fragile perceptions of self. These behaviours are self-defeating, as they destroy collegial relationships, and 'limit freedom of thought and action, and preserves nurses' borderline status' (David 2000:84).

HOW TO DEFINE NURSING?

The urge to define nursing has attracted the attention of nurse scholars for a number of years. While defining a nurse is relatively simple, as you will see as you read further in this chapter, nursing itself has proved somewhat more challenging to define. Though you can probably describe what you think nursing is, the nature and breadth of activities that comprise nursing have contributed to the difficulties associated with defining nursing. Some definitions centre on the functions of a nurse, rather than offering an intrinsic definition of nursing. Henderson produced such a definition of nursing:

> The unique function of the nurse is to assist the individual, sick or well, in the performance of those activities contributing to health or its recovery (or to a peaceful death) that he [sic] would perform unaided if he [sic] had the necessary strength, will or knowledge. And to do this in such a way as to help him [sic] gain independence as rapidly as possible (Henderson, cited in Tomey & Alligood 1998:102).

What needs to be noted in passing is the sexist language that continues to be used when referring to nursing. Language is 'not a neutral information-carrying vehicle', but creates meaning; this meaning changes over time, which makes language very powerful (Fealy 2004:650); its importance cannot be underestimated. David (2000) provides a useful analysis of how nurses collude with their oppressors by uncritically accepting outsiders' social construction of nurses and nursing, suggesting that nurses need to socially construct themselves and their context in order to regain their identity and power.

The complexities and difficulties associated with defining nursing means that some definitions may seem cumbersome and quite ambiguous. But remember that this is more a reflection of the complex nature of nursing than any lack of clarity on behalf of those who have proffered a definition. The International Council of Nurses (ICN), a coalition of nurses' associations that represents nurses in more than 120 countries, has captured some of the complexities in its definition:

> Nursing encompasses autonomous and collaborative care of individuals of all ages, families, groups and communities, sick or well and in all settings. Nursing includes the promotion of health, prevention of illness, and the care of ill, disabled and dying people. Advocacy, promotion of a safe environment, research, participation in shaping health policy and in patient and health systems management, and education are also key nursing roles (http://www.icn.ch/definition.htm).

In 2003, the Royal College of Nursing (RCN) published a definition of nursing that was the culmination of 18 months' research, and included extensive consultation. The

RCN proffered a definition and six key characteristics that capture the essence and varied activities of nursing. The six characteristics are quite detailed and cover issues such as values, relationships and interventions. The full statements can be seen at the RCN website at http://www.rcn.org.uk/downloads/definingnursing/definingnursing-a5.pdf. The RCN definition reads as follows:

> Nursing is the use of clinical judgement in the provision of care to enable people to improve, maintain or recover health to cope with health problems and to achieve the best possible quality of life whatever their disease or disability, until death (http://www.rcn.org.uk/downloads/definingnursing/definingnursing-a5.pdf).

So what is it that excited us about becoming nurses? And, more importantly, what has sustained us on our journeys?

CHOOSING NURSING

Nursing was a gender choice given the societal and historical context of the time (early 1960s). It was certainly viewed as an appropriate career choice for females, but also offered potential for achievement, growth and development. But further to that, there was an overriding quest for understanding and caring for people. This was demonstrated in an egalitarian approach that proved to be unacceptable in nursing at the time (1963), when spending time with and caring about patients was viewed as naive and misguided. Such a view denied empathy and concern, and existed through the 1980s and 1990s (McVicar 2003). Currently, the concept of nurses distancing themselves from their patients has been superseded by recognition of the importance of the nurse–patient relationship or the 'therapeutic alliance' (Speedy 1999), which is now characterised as 'emotional labour' (McQueen 2004).

NURSING: WHAT SUSTAINS US

One of the most sustaining things about nursing and being a nurse is the opportunity to contribute a perspective that is informed by feminism. A feminist perspective is 'concerned with gender, power relations, patriarchy and hegemony in society, emphasising gender as a key factor in determining the experiences of women in . . . nursing' (Fealy 2004:650). Feminist theory can be used to examine power relationships in nursing and healthcare, resulting in the exposure of the 'doctor–nurse game', and more recently in the 'health administrator–nurse game' (Dendaas 2004), which elaborates on how nurses can be losers in the power stakes.

The issue of gender is important for nurses because it is critical to the maintenance of power relations, and the formation of an identity in nursing. Nurses are socialised early in their development to adopt 'appropriate' behaviours and beliefs about how to behave as professionals; how to, as women (predominantly), 'look, talk and feel' (Peter 2004). Their age, gender, family and life experiences all contribute to and influence the way they perceive the power structures and dynamics of the world that is nursing work (Roberts 2000). To be unaware of the impact of power relations and the oppression arising from these is to be locked in a cycle of relationships that serve to severely disadvantage nurses and nursing, perpetuating disunity and disempowerment.

It should be noted in passing that many young women of today appear to have an uneasy relationship with feminism; however, the real problem has been identified as: 'can I be who I am and be feminist?' (Baumgardner & Richards 2003:448). This confusion is understandable, since young women are unclear about what feminism requires of them (and does not require of them). For example, can they still like fashion, have boyfriends, and be who they want to be? They 'often think of feminism as telling them what they can't do, rather than as a philosophy that *shows them the potential for what they can do*' (Baumgardner & Richards 2003:448, emphasis added), and hence what they can contribute. This suggests that it is time to assist young women to develop clarity about this situation.

A natural consequence of a feminist perspective was an interest in the theory and practice of feminist research, which demanded refocusing on the experiences of women. This required some fortitude and commitment, because at that time there was scepticism and ridicule directed towards those who advocated its usage, particularly from researchers who promoted a 'hard science' perspective as the only valid and reliable form of research. However, feminist research is now more readily accepted as an appropriate methodology in many (but not all) research camps.

A sustaining factor within a nursing career is the opportunity to provide leadership in as many ways as possible, be it research, management or practice. Effective leadership requires particular attributes, such as high-level communication skills, awareness of one's beliefs, values, attitudes and emotions, respect for others, commitment, passion, flexibility and adaptability.

Transformational leaders are able to create shared visions, act as role models, inspire, motivate, intellectually stimulate and mentor others (Reinhardt 2004). In many ways, 'leadership is a process of drawing out rather than putting in' (Kitson 2004:211). This implicitly suggests that everyone has a responsibility to exercise leadership qualities. Acknowledging that nursing has many talented participants, Kitson implores us to desist from 'eating our young', or cutting our leaders down ('tall poppy syndrome'), and suggests that, as we work with patients, families, colleagues and managers, we:

> . . . draw out our vision, our values and beliefs about nursing; our notion of service; our understanding of our own humanity and our ability to face pain, suffering, anxiety, anger and all the other human emotions that nurses face on a daily basis (Kitson 2004:211).

By developing these understandings, we can understand and accept ourselves, and see beyond to the dysfunctionality of organisations and workplaces in order to reform them. This requires nurse leaders to be political and astute (Antrobus 2004, Dendaas 2004, Donnelly 2003).

Women have specific leadership skills that can be harnessed, although these are typically disparaged. Research literature suggests that, in general, successful women leaders value interconnectedness, inclusivity and relationships, whereas male leaders value competition, dominance, ambition, aggression and decisiveness (Robinson-Walker 1999). Rudan (2003), in focusing on leadership in nursing, identified a warm demeanour, personal and professional interest in followers, nurturing behaviour, promotion of growth in others, and the use of humour and interpersonal talk as some of the characteristics that make for successful nurse leadership. These are all the skills that nurses at every level of the profession have, to a greater or lesser degree, which provides them with opportunities to assume leadership roles whatever the level and location of their work.

Over the years of our own nursing careers we have witnessed many changes—from changes in how students are prepared for registration as nurses, through to changes to the environment in which nurses work. Nurses work in climates of continual change, and are challenged by the demands of ageing and increasingly complex clients, as well as themselves. Elsewhere, Jackson notes:

> As nurses we are facing some of the greatest tests in the history of the discipline. In a climate of persistent international volatility and instability, and with ever diminishing resources, we are challenged to provide increasingly complex care to incredibly diverse and/or fractured communities. We are further challenged to provide inclusive, sensitive, accessible and user friendly services that defy entrenched, cumbersome sometimes inflexible health care cultures (Jackson 2003:347).

In addition to these challenges, nursing is currently making attempts to address an international widespread shortage of experienced nurses, particularly specialist nurses. Recruitment and retention issues have contributed to an ageing nursing workforce, increasing casualisation of that workforce, and increasing international recruitment (Jackson et al 2001). Furthermore, issues including bullying, abuse and violence, professional autonomy, imposed organisational change, occupational health and safety issues, and constant restructuring (Jackson et al 2001) have been associated with difficulties in retaining a viable nursing workforce in that they contribute to a working environment that can be experienced as hostile and difficult (Jackson et al 2002). However, despite these difficulties, nursing still offers the qualifications and skills upon which satisfying and rewarding careers can be built.

TYPES OF NURSE IN AUSTRALIA AND NEW ZEALAND

There are a number of entry points into nursing. In Australia and New Zealand, the title 'nurse' refers to someone who is either registered or enrolled by national or state-registering authorities. Nurses belong to a regulated professional group that is responsible to the community it serves for supplying healthcare to a constantly high standard, through the maintenance of professional standards and personal integrity. Currently, there are three types of nurse who practice in a wide range of health and community settings (see the box below for some examples). These are the assistant in nursing or nurse's aide, the enrolled nurse and the registered nurse. In Australia, enrolled and registered nurses are required to meet national competency standards, as explicated by the Australian Nursing and Midwifery Council. Further details about these types of nurses are given below.

Clinical practice settings for nurses

Nurses practise in a wide range of health and community settings, including:

- acute hospital settings;
- day surgery nursing;
- daycare clinics;

- residential care facilities (such as nursing homes);
- school nursing;
- drug and alcohol nursing;
- general community nursing;
- specialist community nursing (such as mental health nursing);
- occupational health nursing;
- general practice (or practice) nursing;
- justice health (including remand centres, prisons and juvenile justice settings); and
- rural and remote area nursing.

Assistant in nursing or nurse's aide

The *assistant in nursing* (AIN) or *nurse's aid* is a person who carries out some nursing duties under the direct supervision of a registered nurse. Most often the duties are associated with activities of daily living, such as hygiene, feeding and personal care. Many undergraduate students undertake employment as an AIN while they are studying their undergraduate degree at university. In New South Wales, for example, it is estimated that in excess of 60% of graduates in nursing have gained clinical experience through AIN employment while engaged in undergraduate education (Bulter & Garvey 2003).

In recognition of the status of these undergraduate student AINs, provision has been made (in some areas) for them to perform more wide-ranging and advanced duties than those performed by those AINs who are not engaged in undergraduate nurse education (Bulter & Garvey 2003). According to 'New South Wales Health Circular 2001/80', student AINs are able to practise an 'extended role', with permissible duties varying according to the level of undergraduate education the student has achieved. These duties range from the provision of hygiene and comfort measures, and simple observations in the first year, through to more complex procedures in the third year ('New South Wales Health Circular 2001/80').

There are various titles given to persons fulfilling the AIN (or very similar) role, and these various titles are applied in various locations. Some of the other titles are nurse's aide, care worker or personal care assistant. AINs (and similar workers) are known as unregulated health workers, and they do not come under the auspices of nurse-registering authorities. Rather, the registered nurse under whose supervision they are working is accountable in the event of an adverse situation occurring.

Enrolled nurse

The *enrolled nurse* (EN) is one who has completed an approved educational course leading to enrolment with nurse-registering authorities. The EN course is shorter than courses leading to registration as a nurse, usually being of 12–18 months' duration. The model of education also differs, in that trainee ENs are employed by health facilities and work during their training. In New South Wales, trainee ENs experience much of their classroom teaching in the Technical and Further Education (TAFE) sector.

Unlike the registered nurse (whose names appear in a register), the names of enrolled nurses are entered onto a roll. Like the registered nurse, the EN is subject to the regulation and censure of nurse-registering authorities. ENs have responsibility for their actions and are accountable to registering authorities and also to the registered nurse under whose supervision they are working. Unlike the AIN, who must work under the direct supervision of a registered nurse, some registering authorities permit the EN to practise under the direct or indirect supervision of a registered nurse (http://www.nursesboard.sa.gov.au). Furthermore, some registering authorities authorise ENs who are able to meet certain requirements to practise without the supervision of a registered nurse (e.g. http://www.nursesboard.sa.gov.au). However, this practice is strictly monitored.

There are a number of career development opportunities available to ENs and these can include access to professional development courses that permit an extended role, such as medication administration. Some ENs wish to study further to complete qualifications to become registered nurses. Many universities and colleges give some recognition of prior learning to ENs, meaning that they may be able to undertake a shortened version of the Bachelor of Nursing degree.

Registered nurse

The term *registered nurse* (RN) refers to one who has undertaken and completed an approved program leading to nurse registration as a nurse, holds an appropriate qualification, has met all requirements of registering authorities, and whose name appears on a register of nurses in accordance with the relevant state, territory or national Act. The RN is considered to be a first-level nurse and, as such, is permitted to practise without supervision and is accountable and responsible for action taken and decisions made. Nurses who are registered include general nurses, mental health nurses and nurse practitioners (http://www.nursesreg.nsw.gov.au).

RNs have various career progression paths and various titles, depending on where they are located, so as you enter hospitals and community health settings you will encounter RNs with varying degrees of experience and status. These can include clinical nurse consultants (CNCs), clinical nurse specialist (CNSs), nurse managers, nurse educators, nurse researchers and other levels of nurse.

PROFESSIONAL CONDUCT

Nurses are expected to be people of integrity who conduct themselves with a high level of personal honour and veracity. It is important that members of the public feel safe in hospitals, and believe themselves to be in competent hands when in the hands of nurses. If people do not feel safe, they would not be able to feel secure in leaving their loved ones in the care of nurses and healthcare facilities. Nursing authorities act to ensure the safety of the public by holding nurses accountable for their actions and making nurses answerable for their behaviour or any complaints that are made against them. In order to gain initial registration, nursing applicants need to demonstrate they are of 'good character'.

Nurses are answerable to a registering authority that has the power to question nurses, and suspend or remove them from the register. The conduct of nurses is also guided by various codes that inform professional conduct. In 1990, the Australasian

Nurse Registering Authorities (ANRAC) instigated the Code of Professional Conduct for Nurses in Australia in response to a perceived need for a clear statement to guide registered and enrolled nurses. Subsequently, the Australian Nursing Council (now the Australian Nursing and Midwifery Council or ANMC) continued to progress the Code to ensure its continued relevance to contemporary health environments. In order to maintain currency, the Code was reviewed in 1995 and 2003. It is the responsibility of every Australian nurse to be familiar with the Code and use it to guide their everyday practice (http://www.anmc.org.au). The Australian Nursing and Midwifery Council (ANMC) Code of Professional Conduct for Nurses in Australia is available from the ANMC website at http://www.anmc.org.au. The International Council of Nurses (ICN) has a code for nurses and this is considered to provide the basis for ethical international nursing practice. The ICN Code of Ethics for Nurses Australia can be downloaded from the ICN site at http://www.icn.ch/icncode.pdf.

REGULATION OF PRACTICE

In Australia, nurse registration in each state and territory is governed by registration Acts, and administered by state and territory registration authorities. These authorities are charged with regulating nursing practice. Although there has been a lot of discussion in Australia about national registration, the current situation is that nurse registration is obtained on a state-by-state basis. Thus, if nurses are registered in New South Wales and wish to work as nurses in South Australia, they first need to apply to the South Australian Nurses Board for registration. In New Zealand, nurses are registered by a central registering authority, the Nursing Council of New Zealand. However, if nurses are registered in New Zealand and wish to practise in Australia, they need to seek registration in the state or territory in which they wish to practise. Australian and New Zealand nurses have mutual recognition through the *Trans Tasman Mutual Recognition Act 1997*. For more information about this Act in relation to nurses, see http://www.nursesreg.nsw.gov.au/mutual.htm.

When seeking to register in Australia, nurses from some countries receive recognition, while nurses from other countries need to sit exams or complete other education prior to gaining registration. More information about initial registration and registration from state-to-state and country-to-country can be found on relevant websites. A selection of these websites appears below and you may find it interesting to browse through some of these:

▲ Nurses and Midwives Board New South Wales: http://www.nursesreg.nsw.gov.au/howapply.htm

▲ Nurses Board of South Australia: http://www.nursesboard.sa.gov.au/reg_cre.html

▲ Nursing Council of New Zealand: http://www.nursingcouncil.org.nz/reg.html

▲ Nursing Board of Tasmania: http://www.nursingboardtas.org.au/nbtonline.nsf/$LookupDocName/FEES

▲ Nurses Board of Victoria: http://www.nbv.org.au/nbv/nbvonlinev1.nsf/$LookupDocName/registration_&_practice_standards

CONCLUSION

Nursing attracts people from all walks of life. Many readers of this text will be entering nursing as school leavers, but others will be mature-aged students who come to nursing with a variety of life experiences. Welcome to nursing, and congratulations on making a choice that will open many doors for you and provide you with a career for life. You may find it challenging and, possibly, not quite what you expected. But, go with your passion, and believe in yourself—because you can create your life. The road you have chosen is not an easy one, but you need to believe in yourself, as we do, to succeed. We may have had a more facilitative environment, so for that we are grateful, and we need to be. What a blessed life we have had, on behalf of nursing.

REFLECTIVE QUESTIONS

1   What are the main reasons you have chosen a career in nursing?

2   Why do you think nursing has proved difficult to define?

3   What do you see as essential personal qualities for nurses?

4   Consider the nursing stereotypes identified by Kalisch et al (1983). Can you identify some examples of these stereotypes from your own experiences?

5   What has been your experience of nursing? What motivated you to go there? What now sustains you?

RECOMMENDED READINGS

Chang E, Hancock K, Johnson A, Daly J, Jackson D 2005 Role stress in nurses: a review of related factors and strategies for moving forward. *Nursing and Health Sciences* 7(1):57–65.

Cooper C 2001 *The art of nursing: a practical introduction*. W B Saunders, Philadelphia.

Daly J, Speedy S, Jackson D, Lambert V, Lambert C eds 2005 *Professional nursing: concepts, contexts and challenges*. Springer Corporation, New York.

Jackson D, Daly J 2004 Current challenges and issues facing nursing in Australia. *Nursing Science Quarterly* 17(4):352–5.

Jackson D, Mannix J, Daly J 2001 Retaining a viable workforce: a critical challenge for nursing. *Contemporary Nurse* 11(2/3):163–72.

CHAPTER TWO

Visioning the future by knowing the past

Sioban Nelson & Madonna Greehan

LEARNING OBJECTIVES

After reading this chapter, readers should be able to:

- ▲ develop a critical understanding of the commonly accepted history of nursing;

- ▲ understand the benefits of knowing about nursing's past;

- ▲ identify the lineage of nursing and its occupational relatives;

- ▲ identify significant events that have influenced nursing's evolution in Australia; and

- ▲ describe aspects in nursing and midwifery that warrant historical research.

KEY WORDS
History, nursing, midwifery, regulation, education, hospitals

WHAT IS THE PAST?

The past naturally means different things to different people. It is sometimes referred to as history, heritage, tradition, or even the 'background' to a specific subject. If we reflect specifically about a vision of nursing's past, the Australian imagination might stretch to visions of a neatly frocked Miss Florence Nightingale sporting a burning lamp in the military wards of Scutari in the Crimean War in the mid-nineteenth century, to a military nurse soothing the brow of an injured soldier in World War I, or perhaps to an image of the authoritative Sister Kenny, the controversial Australian nurse who revolutionised polio management in the mid-twentieth century. But are these images really reflective of the past in nursing?

When we recall 'the past', there are two relevant issues worth considering. One is to think about what 'the past' means to us as individuals and to contemplate how we arrived at this particular understanding of 'the past'. It is often the case that most of us rarely give the past a second thought. For example, we have tended to accept one or more of these three images of nurses described above without ever really questioning whether they are realistic interpretations of the past. A second point is to realise that when we do think about the past, we do so from our present perspective, simply because it is not possible to travel back in time. We think about, and interpret, the past with the influence of our twenty-first century values and our present understanding of what we believe nursing and healthcare to be. This naturally gives us a 'contemporary' view of the past. Similarly, the language and terms that we use to describe aspects of the past through this chapter, such as 'health', 'care', 'healthcare', 'nurse', 'midwife', or even 'hospital', have a natural affinity with our contemporary understanding of the terms, but were likely to convey vastly different meanings at different stages in the past.

With these two issues in mind (that the past means something to us and that we see this image of the past from our present perspective), we can see, for instance, that the three rather romantic images of nursing we described are shaped to construct a past that we all can imagine or comfortably associate with. Let us examine these 'comfortable' notions of nursing's past a little more closely.

Traditional views of the past

During the early twentieth century, nursing scholarship readily accepted that 'real' nursing, as we know it to be today, began during the time of Miss Florence Nightingale (1820–1910). Published histories of nursing by American luminaries such as Isabel Stewart and Lavinia Dock extolled the virtues of bringing nursing out of the dark ages into the light of modern times under the reforms advocated by Nightingale and her contemporaries (Dock & Stewart 1920). These populist narratives have tended to focus on the glorious achievements of individual leaders without much attention given to those people doing the day-to-day nursing work. It is also true that many aspects of women's work have largely escaped attention in conventional histories because women's work constituted ordinary and mundane activities. For instance, midwifery, a traditional role of women, has received even less attention than nursing, but recent histories of midwifery practice have sought to highlight the role of women who did everyday midwifery in Australia (Gaff-Smith 2003, 2004).

14

Traditional histories about the exploits of nursing leaders and the more recent biographical narratives about pioneering women have a fundamental connection. Both approach their subject with a degree of nostalgia, which makes for comfortable storytelling of romantic proportions—stories that never challenge our comfortable view of the past in any way. Commonly, writers of these popular histories have 'cherry-picked' their past to tell glorious tales about their respective subjects. In the case of nursing histories, they recall the triumph of 'reformed' nursing over all other forms of attention; in the case of recent midwifery histories, they can seductively convey a sense that there was a 'golden age' in midwifery when the lore of wise women was the natural order of things. Golden ages and triumphs are rarities in any realistic history, but their resonance is unsurprising. In constructing a past based on these recollections, the American historian, Laurel Thatcher Ulrich, urges a note of caution on the cover of her book *The age of homespun* when she remarks that today, '[i]n an age when even meals are rarely made from scratch, homespun easily acquires the glow of nostalgia' (Ulrich 2002).

Apart from relying on nostalgia and past glories, one drawback of these 'cherry-picked' histories is that in examining nursing or midwifery, neither approach considers the place of these occupations in relation to the broader society in which they were practised. Their historical subjects are distanced from relationships with other people, with society, and from the political times in which they lived and worked. In the same way that popular culture in the guise of history emphatically declared that Florence Nightingale was the leading light of nursing in the nineteenth century, some twentieth century popular culture claiming to be history can be used to seductively reinterpret the past for us and use these uncritical approaches to advocate returning to a past time when all was well. This is perhaps one of the most salient reasons to advocate for an awareness of a bigger picture of nursing's and midwifery's developmental path. As the Australian historian Graeme Davison suggests, 'changing history is often first among the political objectives of those who seek to change the future' (Davison 2000:260).

An enlightened view of the past

Recent scholarship in nursing history uses the discipline of historiography to explore new ways of thinking about the past in midwifery and nursing. Historiography challenges 'received', or commonly accepted, history by critically examining the past from a broader perspective, one which recognises that nurses and nursing, midwives and midwifery have existed, and always will exist, as part of a broader society. The discipline of historiography does not pick and choose the most triumphant phases in the past, nor does it glorify past events or ideologies; instead, an historiographical approach focuses a critical eye on how things came to be as they are. It throws a wider net than the more traditional forms of history can, and it is a systematic way to apply knowledge about the past to shed light on current issues and perhaps those in the future.

One example is the current shortage of nurses and midwives affecting most parts of Australia. Using historical inquiry to examine when and why shortages occurred in the past, what solutions were posed, and what the outcomes were, we can use this information to explore this same issue in Australia's contemporary healthcare workforce. We can identify specific factors outside nursing and midwifery per se that contributed to past workforce shortages, including political and social processes, such as changing treatments for illness, which meant that more people were capable of surviving grave illnesses, but that more nursing care was needed for them to do so. We can nominate other factors contributing to workforce shortages such as: the effect of war; the transition of women's sphere from the home to the workplace; developments of technology, science and education; and new opportunities in other work spheres. We can propose reasons for trends, phases, consistencies and nuances in the ways that shortages of nurses and midwives have been managed in the past. Armed with this historical perspective of the problem, we can compare the present with the past to shed light on current workforce shortages and perhaps plan future workforces more effectively.

Historiographical approaches have other benefits over traditional histories. They consider those who have been excluded from conventional histories, such as the Aboriginal people of the Australian nation or migrants. They explore why these people have been invisible in received history. For example, one of the deficits of conventional histories about healthcare in Australia is an absence of references to indigenous healthcare practices or practitioners. Here we do not mean the Aboriginal witch-doctor, but the stories of the many female nurses who were sent from mission stations to train as nurses in the mid-twentieth century. We rarely hear about the contributions to healthcare from Aboriginal people like Sadie Corner and Lowitja (Lois) O'Donohue who, despite the odds, trained as nurses in Australia's white healthcare system. To explore this fascinating and instructive aspect of nursing history in Australia would entail a story of politics, race, policy, social attitudes, geography, and of gender. It is one of many in Australian nursing history waiting to be told.

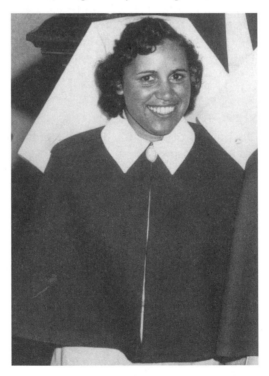

Sadie Corner. Reproduced with the permission of the Salvation Army Australia, Southern Territory Archives and Museum, Melbourne.

Using an historiographical approach to Australian nursing's past, we begin our discussion with a lineage of nursing and consider some of its descendants. We will then explore the nature of healthcare in Australia since European colonisation, and consider the historical influences on nursing and outline milestones in its evolution. Finally, we will discuss the concept that midwifery and nursing have separate histories.

THE ROOTS OF MODERN NURSING

To begin at a beginning in nursing defies logic because the act of nursing is as old as the human race. But we need to start somewhere in historical terms to advance our discussion. If we start with the premise that the way that nurses and midwives work in the twenty-first century is 'modern', then we can attempt to visualise what 'premodern' nursing was.

Premodern nursing

Until the recent decentralisation of healthcare in the twentieth century, nurses in the English-speaking world have predominantly worked in modern hospitals and institutions, but before the introduction of this kind of systematic care, familial attention was the most common form of nursing provided. The medically derived, institutional approach to care emerged in the late nineteenth century with the rise of the modern hospital (Rosenberg 1987). This ordered style of caregiving has been hailed as a modern innovation, but scholars of nursing and health history have recently argued that it was not 'new'; rather, it constituted new ways of doing old things in which structure, and standards, were replicated, but were evangelised as modern innovations (Nelson 1999).

The roots of 'modern nursing' lie in the domain of religious communities such as nuns whose lives constituted a religious devotion to the care of strangers, which was seen as emulating the work of Jesus Christ (Nelson 2000, Rosenberg 1987, MacGinley 1996). Rewards for living out this life of earthly devotion were expected in heaven. This was a sphere of nursing where the quiet achievements of tending to the infirm, by providing a place of refuge, giving nourishment, and perhaps applying palliative treatments, have largely been overlooked in the more traditional histories of the nursing profession.

Like their overseas counterparts, traditional histories of nursing in Australia such as Muriel Doherty's history of Sydney's Royal Prince Alfred Hospital have tended to begin their lineage of nursing with the work of secular (ostensibly non-religious) institutions (Doherty & Russell 1996). This is perhaps unsurprising because more records pertaining to this era of institutional development have survived. Establishments such as asylums, orphanages, industrial schools and hospitals emerged as a form of containment of poverty and other social ills that flourished in England after the Industrial Revolution. Many attendants at this time were also inmates of the establishments who gained experience in 'nursing', as they attended their fellow patients. But by the mid-nineteenth century, these attendants became the subject of fierce criticism from social commentators. Through one of his serialised novels, the famous writer, Charles Dickens, brought to the imagination of the reading public two memorable caricatures who came to symbolise all that was perceived to be wrong with nurses, and nursing (Dickens 1843). Dickens' attention was focused on women as institutional nurses.

17

The 'old style' nurse

In *The life and adventures of Martin Chuzzlewit*, which first appeared in 1843, Dickens introduced Mrs Gamp, a nurse and midwife in London, and her friend Betsy Prig, a hospital nurse who occasionally worked as a 'private' nurse in people's homes. Gamp and Prig were depicted as middle-aged, uncouth, drunken, ignorant and untrustworthy attendants to childbearing women and the sick. These women lacked education, refinement and morals, earning the contempt of all who read of their exploits. Dickens' unflattering portrayal of the nineteenth century nurse is exaggerated according to some scholars in this field (Summers 1989), but the graphic pen and ink sketches of Mrs Gamp that accompanied Charles Dickens' texts left little to the imagination of the reader. In an age when printed material was the most influential form of media, these narratives helped to create or 'construct' an image of nurses as unclean, and unsuited to the important duty of caring for the sick and childbearing women. It was this ignorant type of nurse, according to many, who needed to be driven out of the business of caring for their fellow human beings by the emerging nursing reform movement.

The 'modern' nurse

By the mid-nineteenth century, there were alternatives to the type of attendant symbolised by Mrs Gamp and her counterparts. Exemplars of the new style of nurse were female followers of Christianity who formed 'sisterhoods'. English sisterhoods fostered a religious communal life in the same way that nuns lived with their work focusing on 'nursing' the poor. Women such as Elizabeth Fry, Agnes Jones and Sister Dora represented the future potential of nursing—what it could be if the old, unclean and unscientific nurse characterised by Mrs Gamp could be driven out. The reform of nursing was closely associated with a more general movement based on the notion of 'humanism', which had great influence throughout the English-speaking world. This movement linked improvements in sanitation and hygiene with the alleviation of poverty, and consequent improvements in a regulated social order; logically, improved social order led to other desirable effects for broader society, such as a reduction in crime and responsible parenthood (Walkowitz 1992).

At the same time as the humanist movement emerged, other confluent developments were to shape the future of nursing and midwifery in Australia and other parts of the English-speaking world. Australia had been colonised for almost 60 years when two significant medical advancements impacted on nursing. These were the use of anaesthetic for operations such as amputation, and new ideas about the transmission of infection. Each of these progressions meant that treatment for previously untreated infirmities could be effected, but like many new modes of treatment, there were consequences of these advances. They necessitated more complex systems in the form of hospitals and supporting nursing staff to accommodate their success. The nursing staff needed to be cooperative, literate and capable of understanding medical and scientific developments, especially means of managing infection and complicated postoperative care. For nursing, these consequences translated into reforms centring on rigorous control of staff in institutions, more emphasis on the literacy level of potential pupils, and attracting a better class of woman as nurse. To understand why this reform was perceived to be so essential, we turn now to a brief examination of nursing in Australia since colonisation.

HEALTHCARE IN EARLY AUSTRALIA

Modern nursing in Australia bears little resemblance to 'nursing' in nineteenth and twentieth century Australia. In the twenty-first century, we are accustomed to concepts of illness prevention, readily available treatment, and a healthcare environment under-pinned by regulatory controls. It can be quite an unfamiliar experience to cast our minds back to a time in the past when sanitation did not exist, when access to running water meant the existence of a nearby stream, when 'watching' the patient at night was done by candlelight, and when an understanding of the transmission of infection was in its infancy. What is important to think about here is a history of nursing in the context of the life of the colonies *as they existed at the time*, and the associated expec-tations of settlers about nurses *at that time*, rather than simply concentrating on the gulf between nursing then and our present-day perspectives, ideals and advances.

For most of Australia's nineteenth century populace, the care of the sick was undertaken at home by the most able member of a family; sometimes 'help' was obtained if the family could afford it. Hospitals, as we know them, were in their infancy and excluded all kinds of cases from admission including smallpox and forms of cancer. Pregnant women too were excluded from admission, but this 'rule' was for their own protection as hospitals were thought to house contaminants known as 'miasmas' or 'vapours' circulating in the air, which were thought to cause sickness. Disease entities as we know them did not exist and the pregnant woman's home continued to be the preferred place for birth until well into the 1940s, with the exception of female factories (jails) for incarcerants and the early nineteenth century benevolent asylums.

Care provided in the community

We know from records such as private diaries, letters and administrative documents that a variety of people were consulted by the infirm and childbearing women during the colonial period. Who they chose depended on who was available, what the purchaser expected of his or her care, and what they could afford to pay (Martyr 2002). Men and women worked in the capacities of doctor, nurse, midwife, herbalist, oculist, druggist and dentist. 'Care' given by any of these attendants in the colonial community could be bought and sold as services or goods in the same way that a conventional 'marketplace' operates, but importantly, the Australian colonial marketplace of health in the nineteenth century was devoid of the legal restrictions and control that govern the provision of healthcare today.

Rural areas and poorer suburbs of large towns did not always attract doctors (who also tended to charge higher fees). Often local women filled the gap by attending midwifery cases in a neighbourly capacity. Many held no formal education in nursing or midwifery, but their experience of having their own families constituted their 'training'. Because many simply adopted this kind of work for reasons of changed family circumstance, they were termed 'handywomen' in the same way that a handyman is known today for performing a multitude of tasks around a house. Handywomen tended the sick, prepared the dead for burial, assisted childbearing women, and sometimes ran the local postal service. The Australian historian, Glenda Strachan, has analysed attendances in the rural district of Dungog in New South Wales where, between 1856 and 1896, a variety of women attended at almost half of the registered births (Strachan 2001).

Numerous other examples of handywomen acting as nurse or midwife to others can be found in the histories of Australian local communities. For instance, one local history of the western district of Victoria nominates seven women who worked in this capacity (Forth et al 1998). Similarly, the Australian nurse historian, Joan Durdin, writes that, in South Australia, Mrs Elizabeth Knight was a well-respected Mount Gambier midwife who reportedly began working at the age of 70 after the death of her husband (Durdin 1991). This traditional role for women was available until the early part of the twentieth century.

Institutional care

By the middle of the nineteenth century, there was a proliferation of institutional forms of charitable care. The organisation and delivery of institutional healthcare (using the term loosely), from the time of white colonisation until the early twentieth century, was not a primary concern of colonial governments, although they did contain a small proportion of the population including prisoners and those deemed to be lunatics. The new colonies of Australia instead embraced philanthropically driven institutional care, as did other parts of the English-speaking world, but, in Australia, their development was rather haphazard. Where colonists expanded the white frontier, hospitals were established in response to industrial catastrophes such as mining disasters (Collins 1999). These institutions usually had little or no government support, but were financed and managed by local committees. The attendants were often a married couple who could provide food, do the laundry and attend to the patients. Other establishments employed men as nurses (Collins & Kippen 2003).

Exactly what institutional care was available depended on the geographic locality and the size of the population. Many early charitable institutions such as benevolent asylums, hospitals and refuges were formed as cooperative ventures between local medical practitioners who had identified a need in the community and local philanthropists who hoped for spiritual redemption in heaven in exchange for their good works on earth. Admission to an institution was a complicated process controlled by those in charge of the local management committee who could refuse a person's admission simply on the basis of the individual's bad character. Usually, the person seeking assistance presented themselves to a financial supporter (a subscriber) of the institution. The subscriber signed an admission 'ticket' to vouch for the person's character and, on presenting at the institution, the applicant was subjected to an interview to ascertain their status as deserving of the charity being sought.

Institutional nurses

Female applicants for pupil nurse positions in hospitals were frequently subject to similar requirements. They needed a testimonial or letter of support from a minister of religion or medical practitioner to recommend them for the position, and then the hospital's management committee interviewed them in person in an attempt to weed out potential troublemakers. Even with these attempts at control, nurses were occasionally reprimanded for their behaviour, for their bad language, for being drunk on duty, or for being cruel to the patients.

It is hard to know exactly what nurses' duties entailed on a day-to-day basis in charitable institutions, as very few records exist that explain the details of their work. A substantial amount of a pupil nurse's work involved some form of cleaning: scrubbing floors; brushing carpets; dusting; polishing brassware and furniture;

washing the patients; and providing nourishments for those who could not do it for themselves. This level of household work seems onerous today because we imagine nurses to be 'attending' to the sick, rather than working in a domestic capacity. But this period in the evolution of healthcare was famous for its concern for fresh air evidenced by rigorous ventilation and airing practices; the nurse's role in maintaining the cleanest possible environment was of paramount importance.

Hospitals were often not sewered until the late nineteenth century, and bodily wastes (faeces, urine, other fluids, amputated limbs) were placed in buckets stored at the end of wards and, later, thrown out into the hospital's refuse pit located within the hospital grounds. Smells were everywhere. When someone was discharged from the institution or died, the nurse cleaned and fumigated straw mattresses known as palliasses in special airing rooms. The nurse also carried soiled linen to the laundry for washing. In the mid-nineteenth century hospital, domestic chores were integral to keeping the environment as pleasant as possible.

There was little time for learning about disease and how to manage it. By the late nineteenth century, most hospitals were employing women as nurses in preference to men. Many hospitals instituted structured training schemes for nurses in which a series of lectures was given by medical practitioners, which pupil nurses attended if they could absent themselves from their ward work. Each hospital trained its own nurses for the specific requirements of the hospital; these were usually organised around the institution's associated medical speciality. For example, a hospital established for people with tuberculosis trained its nurses in 'tubercular' nursing only; an infectious diseases hospital trained nurses to work in this field. After completing their training, if either of these nurses wanted subsequently to work in another hospital (e.g. in a hospital for women where pregnancy or gynaecology was the specialty), those nurses' previous training was often regarded as inadequate. Nurses were sometimes rejected for positions on this basis or were required to undertake more training at individual institutions.

Nineteenth century nursing was a rather domesticated job, and certainly extremely hard work for little reward, so it is little wonder that, at times, few people were attracted to the position of 'hospital nurse'. There were, however, some benefits in becoming a hospital nurse. The occupation offered an ideal opportunity for women to take on paid work as an alternative to 'service' in a household. There was usually some form of education offered, which was otherwise not easily available. A position as a hospital nurse usually meant that the nurse was required to live on the premises. A guaranteed roof over her head afforded a degree of safety for a woman, and the growing numbers of nurses 'living in' offered a degree of camaraderie.

Nightingale-trained nurses

Considering the lack of a 'system' of healthcare in the colonies, it is perhaps unsurprising then that Australian society was considerably taken by the writings and ideas of Florence Nightingale in the mid-nineteenth century. Miss Nightingale developed a reputation for establishing training schools for nurses, which the Australian newspapers applauded.

To commemorate her work in the Crimean War, a group of social reformers in Britain, not Miss Nightingale herself, established what became known as the 'Nightingale Fund for Nursing' to support 'the training of nurses and matrons for the sick poor, and especially for hospitals including those in the colonies' (Doherty

& Russell 1996:11). The Nightingale Fund was an extremely effective public relations machine, which portrayed nursing as dangerous and in need of urgent reform. The central, enduring message of the Nightingale Fund was that nursing needed to rid itself of old and ignorant women (represented by the image of Mrs Gamp) by opening it up as a profession for educated 'ladies' of good character (in the image of Florence Nightingale) who could act as role models for the nurses around them (Baly 1987).

Led by Miss Lucy Osburn, the first group of Nightingale nurses arrived in Sydney in 1868 following a request from Sir Henry Parkes, then Colonial Secretary of New South Wales, for assistance in improving conditions at the Sydney Hospital (Doherty & Russell 1996). Traditional histories of nursing in Australia have accorded these Nightingale nurses with remarkable achievements (e.g. instituting reforms to raise standards in colonial nursing, introducing structured nurse training where none existed, and changing the image of nurses from the old Mrs Gamp to a young, educated female (Godden 1997)). The Australian historian, Judith Godden, argues that nursing by women was successfully imbued with overtones of devotion to duty, which helped to remake nursing's image as 'a religiously-inspired philanthropic vocation' (Godden 1997:185). An adherence to the persona of the dutiful nurse had significant implications for nursing throughout the twentieth century, as professional nursing associations that advocated this vocational approach resisted attempts to agitate for better conditions of work for nurses across the nation.

Despite the rhetoric of traditional nursing histories, Nightingale nursing was not immediately embraced by all of the Australian colonies, nor was it adopted in its English format of bonding successful trainees to parishes, but, by the last decade of the nineteenth century, Tasmania, South Australia and Victoria welcomed the gradual arrival of Nightingale-trained nurses.

Religious nurses

On the basis of received Australian nursing history, we can be forgiven for accepting that little happened before the arrival of Lucy Osburn and her Nightingales. Yet in August 1838, well in advance of Miss Osburn, a party of five religious nurses arrived on Australia's colonial shores from Dublin (MacGinley 1996). This small group of Catholic Sisters of Charity began their ministering work at Parramatta's female factory, the women's jail, and visited the sick poor in their own homes. The sisters opened the first St Vincent's Hospital at Sydney's Pott's Point in 1857, and from this enterprise a network of hospitals administered by the Sisters of Charity developed across Australia. Today the St Vincent's hospitals provide a considerable proportion of public health services.

The Australian Inland Mission nurses

Other religious groups harnessed the vocational image of nursing made popular through depictions of the Nightingale nurse. The Australian Inland Mission (AIM), an offshoot of the Presbyterian Church largely orchestrated by the Reverend John Flynn of the Flying Doctor fame (National Archives of Australia 2000), established a network of centres in the early twentieth century, which were staffed by trained Christian nurses known as 'deaconesses'.

In the style of other charitable organisations, the AIM proposed to provide healthcare to those living in the Australian outback, and by happy coincidence, evangelise the Christian message through its activities. The AIM employed trained

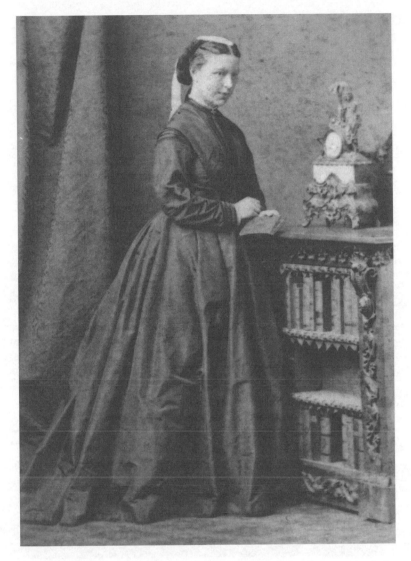

Lucy Osburn. Reproduced with the permission of The Sydney Hospital.

nurses for their deaconess positions, but most deaconess nurses were not educated in midwifery. In isolated places, some knowledge of maternity care was invaluable and the Women's Hospital in Melbourne accommodated requests from the Presbyterian Church for short terms of midwifery training, like the one month offered to deaconess Nurse Bett in 1909 prior to taking up her position as Deaconess Nurse at Oodnadatta in South Australia (Women's Hospital Ladies Committee of Management Meeting Minutes 1909). A Melbourne woman, Sister Jean Finlayson, was an AIM deaconess who also worked at Oodnadatta. Jean, pictured below on a mode of transport suitable for outback conditions, was subsequently the first appointed nurse to the Northern Territory's Alice Springs AIM Centre in 1915, which later became the Alice Springs Hospital (Cockrill 1999).

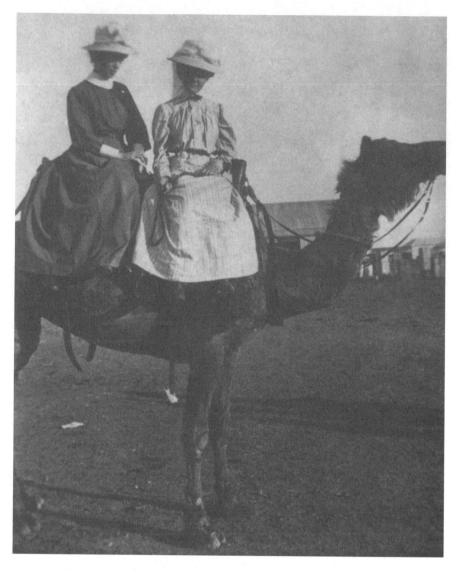

Jean Finlayson (right) and fellow deaconness at Alice Springs, c1915. Reproduced with the permission of Adelaide House Museum, Alice Springs.

Aboriginal nurses

The Salvation Army (SA), too, adopted a role in providing healthcare and training nurses. Like the Catholic hospitals, the SA built a network of hospitals around Australia, which were big enough to become training schools for nurses, and formed their own district nursing services. According to SA records, the SA's Melbourne hospital, Bethesda, became home to many young Aboriginal girls in the 1950s who travelled from Mount Margaret Mission in Western Australia and Colebrook in South Australia to undertake training either as nurses' aides or as general nurses because many mainstream hospitals would not accept Aboriginal pupils for training (Salvation

Army Archives). A graduate of the Bethesda scheme, Sadie Corner (now Canning), was the first Aboriginal woman to work as a trained nurse and hospital matron in Western Australia. Sadie was later awarded an MBE and Queen's Jubilee Medal for her contribution to the health needs of the community of Leonora and surrounding district (Australian Legal Information Institute 2000).

Lowitja (Lois) O'Donohue CBE, AM, was one Aboriginal woman who graduated from the Royal Adelaide Hospital in 1954 as a trained general nurse, but she was not initially accepted as a trainee on the basis of her race. Overcoming this opposition, Lois worked in Adelaide as a charge sister and later spent time in India with a missionary society before taking up positions in Aboriginal affairs (State Library of South Australia 2001).

The modern hospital as preferred place for healthcare delivery

A combination of institutional and community nursing and midwifery has formed the basis of care in Australia since European colonisation. By the early twentieth century, the modern hospital secured a position as the preferred place for the delivery of healthcare underpinned by expanding staffs of nurses. Our brief discussion of the evolution of nursing and midwifery represents a glimpse of Australia's health landscape since European settlement. In expanding a vision of nursing's past, it is critical to throw a wide net to think broadly about the past, because nursing and nurses do not exist in isolation from society. We do this in the next section by examining some examples of external pressures that have shaped the profession in Australia.

HISTORICAL INFLUENCES ON NURSING

No profession or occupation can escape outside influences. These influences are sometimes referred to as 'accidents of history' or 'windows of opportunity', which we are usually not even aware of at the time that influence is upon us. Through a critical study of our occupational backgrounds, we can reflect on how these influences have shaped nursing as we know it today, and help us to understand why some issues concerning nursing and midwifery appear complicated (e.g. why national standards in nursing and midwifery do not exist in Australia). In this section we focus specifically on two historical influences that have contributed to the evolution of nursing and midwifery in a significant way. They are: the lack of government interest in nursing and midwifery and the attendant consequences arising from an unregulated healthcare environment; and the organisation of government, first as colonies, and from 1901 as a federation of states and territories.

These two major influences stem from Australia's past status as a colony of Britain and its natural affinity to the customs and conventions of the British government, administration and way of life. As an outpost of Britain, Australia was susceptible to the worldwide trends and influences of the rest of the English-speaking world. Aspects of healthcare and, logically, the evolution of nursing and midwifery in the young colonies were no exception. To facilitate our discussion here, we consider these two nominated influences on nursing individually, but in doing so we do not mean to convey that these events or processes were isolated or predictable; rather, they were confluent with, and contingent on, other events. We begin with the lack of government interest in nursing.

The effect of the unregulated marketplace and subsequent regulation

Mirroring the lack of government interest in matters of nursing and midwifery in England, there were no restrictions on nurses, midwives or healers or their practice in Australia until the early twentieth century. Without a system to regulate practice and practitioners, anyone could claim to have skills learnt through personal experience, working as an apprentice, or by attending public lectures given by doctors on 'nursing' and 'midwifery nursing'. The unfortunate public had no way of knowing if an individual's qualifications were adequate, or if a nurse or midwife who claimed skills actually possessed them. In this unregulated environment, the movement to reform nursing already underway in the English-speaking world gained momentum, implementing voluntary professional regulation as a strategy to raise standards in nursing and midwifery.

Support for regulation

Agitations for voluntary regulation occurred worldwide in concert with other developments, including the rise of the modern hospital and the parallel ascendency of medicine. The concept of the modern hospital emerged in the late nineteenth century from the charitable institutional model, the main difference being that the charitable hospital had been organised and administered by committees of laypersons, whereas the modern hospital became the domain of the medical practitioner, buttressed by a staff of female nurses. As we have alluded to, modern medical science offered advances in treatment that were possible only with the cooperation of a dedicated hospital staff who were able to intelligently obey orders, and contributed to the smooth running of the institution. In this environment, the voluntary regulation of nursing and midwifery was championed by trained nurses and doctors who recognised the benefits that regulation would bring to their hospital worlds.

Advocates of voluntary professional regulation claimed that it would do two things. First, it would provide the public with a recognised practitioner who, having completed recognised training and education, could legitimately call herself a trained nurse, thereby permitting the public to differentiate the trained from the untrained nurse; second, it would protect the status of the legitimate practitioner from untrained 'imposters' who, it was claimed, falsely used the title 'qualified nurse'.

An early attempt at introducing voluntary regulation for nurses and midwives in 1892 under the auspices of the Nurses Association of Australasia was spectacularly unsuccessful (Grehan 2004). Subsequent attempts at voluntary regulation were more effective with New South Wales setting the pace in the form of the Australian Trained Nurses Association, followed shortly after by Victoria which declined to join the 'national' organisation, setting up its own association, the Victorian Trained Nurses Association. This deviation had one significant drawback. Only national nursing organisations were admitted as members of the International Council of Nurses, which had been established in 1899 to promote issues relating to the nursing profession throughout the world. The lack of a national group led by nurses prevented Australia's nurses and midwives from joining the fledgling international community of professional nurses.

At local Australian levels, regulation was advanced by an elite group of hospital matrons, hospital-trained nurses and doctors who set benchmarks in nursing training and education, and approved specific hospitals as future training schools for nurses.

The associations occasionally refused registration to individuals whose training was deemed to be inadequate, but they had little control over who was actually employed as a nurse or midwife because hospital committees were still responsible for engaging their own staff, and private nursing in people's homes was still the norm for many episodes of illness. For nurses and midwives in rural areas, registration under the auspices of the trained nurses associations made little difference to employment prospects.

Voluntary regulation set a pattern that was continued with subsequent legislation in Australia for nurses and midwives across Australia. Voluntary, and parliamentary, regulation aimed to *contain* certain types of practice and practitioner, rather than endorse a particular discipline. Government regulation of nursing and midwifery was enacted in different states at different times, and historically there has been enormous variation in how regulations were set. This diversity of regulations brings us to the second significant historical influence on nursing and midwifery, the make-up of Australia's parliaments.

The Commonwealth/state divide

Australia began its parliamentary history with the formation of colonies under British rule. Each colony developed distinct regulatory requirements for aspects of commerce, trade and legal matters under its own constitution. The colonies were protective of their own borders and interests, but, in 1901, they overcame their territorial differences to form a federation of states with a national government. Critically they retained the ability to set state-specific regulations. The variations in nursing and midwifery regulations across Australia are a legacy of this political landscape, initially marked out by the formation of the Australian colonies.

State regulation of occupations

Under the 1901 Australian Constitution, the federal government adopted some controls over the states, especially in relation to financial matters, but this top tier of government has no power to make national regulations over occupations, nor does it have the ability to enforce the states to cooperate with each other by standardising regulations. The regulation of midwifery state by state provides a good example of why this can present as a problem. In the 1980s, to register as a midwife in Queensland, a student midwife was required to have conducted 20 births over 12 months of training. In larger cities, where medical students and student midwives competed for practical experience, a student midwife was sometimes short of the set target, and the hospitals had to devise ways that would permit the student midwife to achieve registration under the state regulations. At the same time, in another state, regulations may have deemed that a target of 10 births permitted registration as a midwife because there were fewer births happening in that state.

These fundamental differences often precluded nurses and midwives from registering in other states, and state governments have successfully protected their nursing and midwifery workforces by ignoring requests to institute uniform national standards in education for nurses and midwives. A resolution of this issue means that the states must agree on education and training benchmarks.

Moves to nationalise regulations

The globalisation of workforces and the development of trade agreements have also added some urgency to the introduction of national regulations for nurses and midwives in Australia. In 1992, the Australian and New Zealand national governments signed a *Mutual Recognition Agreement*, extending it more recently to include the Australian state governments under the *Trans-Tasman Mutual Recognition Arrangement* (Council of Australian Governments, undated). These cooperative measures were designed to 'promote economic integration and increased trade' by freeing up restrictions on business and the organisation of occupations. Bringing this agreement to fruition in the nursing and midwifery workforce has proved to be a complex issue, because New Zealand's national government already sets national standards of nurses' and midwives' regulation, yet diverse regulations in Australia are set by the states. More recently, shortages of nurses and midwives all over Australia, rather than free trade requirements, have provided the impetus to examine ways to free up regulatory restrictions on nurses and midwives.

The consequences of a political path arising from colonial settlement and its administration resonate today as the Australian Nursing and Midwifery Council pursues ways to effect national standards of nursing and midwifery education and regulation (Australian Nursing and Midwifery Council 2005). The political landscape, the unregulated healthcare arena and the consequent regulation issues are examples of many historical influences, which deserve consideration in developing a vision of nursing's past in Australia. Tumultuous events, which we explore in the next section as milestones in nursing, could also be seen as historical influences on the profession because of their broad impact.

MILESTONES IN AUSTRALIAN NURSING

Even in the relatively short history of Australian nursing, there have been notable events or momentous occasions that constitute milestones. Here we concentrate on two milestones and their sequelae. The first of these notable events is the role of war in the story of Australian nursing history, and the second is the transition of nursing and midwifery education from the apprentice system into tertiary education.

War

Conflicts have been a significant theme in Australian nursing history. Notable and some conventional nursing histories have given attention to the work of nurses during war service and the effect on the workforce at home. The pattern of Australian nurses volunteering to serve overseas commenced with the Boer War, continued during World Wars I and II, and later during the conflicts in Korea, Vietnam and the Pacific. For many of us unaccustomed to what war services meant for nurses, it may seem surprising that nurses enthusiastically stepped up for duty, as Sister Evelyn Davies did, saying that she was 'glad to be taking part in the great adventure' (Barker, cited in Reid et al 1999:26).

The Boer War, World Wars I and II

Nurses from each state in Australia joined volunteer troops who served in the 1899–1902 Boer War. The nurses themselves served either with the British nursing forces or as private contingents, but there are few surviving records to tell us in detail about their experiences in South Africa. Some photographs and letters are held at the Australian War Memorial in Canberra.

In the next major conflict between 1914 and 1918 (World War I), a total of 2139 trained nurses served overseas in the Australian Army Nursing Service with the first Australian Imperial Force (Reid et al 1999), the greatest number volunteering from the state of Victoria. The women served in the Middle East, and in the south of Europe, France, England and India. All told, 23 military nurses died on military duty in World War I.

World War II and its aftermath was another period of significance for nurses and nursing. Nurses in the forces were appointed as officers, in senior ranks for the first time, and in charge of men at a time when no comparable positions were open to women in civilian life. These nurses served across North Africa, the Middle East, the south of Europe and parts of Asia in three areas of the Australian military: the Australian Army Nursing Service; the Royal Australian Air Force Nursing Service; and the Royal Australian Naval Nursing Service (Reid et al 1999). Some Australian nurses lost their lives through acts of war, but two well-known events in particular encapsulated the inhumanity of World War II, and drew the attention of the public to the roles of ordinary women who risked their lives in their work as military nurses.

The sinking of the *Vyner Brooke*

Vivian Bullwinkel was 26 years of age when she enlisted in the Australian Army Nursing Service, and served in an army general hospital in Singapore. Just before the fall of Singapore to the Japanese army in February 1942, Bullwinkel and 64 other Australian Army Nursing sisters, including Betty Jeffrey, were evacuated with 265 passengers on a small coastal steamer, the *Vyner Brooke* (Australian War Memorial undated).

The *Vyner Brooke* was one of several vessels attacked by Japanese bombers. Several on board died when the steamer sank, but others managed to swim ashore to Bangka Island and landed as two separate parties. Two days after the sinking, a party of Japanese soldiers discovered one party of survivors from the *Vyner Brooke* and ordered them to march into the sea. Twenty-one Australian nurses were shot and killed; Vivian Bullwinkel was the only survivor of the shooting. After hiding for 12 days in the jungle with a wounded British soldier, Bullwinkel surrendered to the Japanese and spent the next three and a half years as a Japanese prisoner of war with the other party of 31 nurses who had survived the sinking of the *Vyner Brooke* (Morgan 2001, Angell, undated).

The sinking of the *Centaur*

A subsequent shocking act of war occurred close to Australia's shores one year later in May 1943. Not far off the coast of Brisbane, the hospital ship *Centaur* was on its way from Sydney to Papua New Guinea when it was torpedoed by a Japanese submarine. Only one of the 12 nurses on board survived the sinking of the *Centaur* (Commonwealth Department of Veterans Affairs 2000). Sister Eleanor (Ellen) Savage sustained severe injuries to her face and chest, but despite these, Miss Savage managed to assist the 63 injured survivors during the 36 hours that passed until they were rescued (Reid et al 1999).

On the home front

Back home in Australia, wartime was marked by shortages of trained nurses across the nation. Four thousand nurses volunteered out of an estimated workforce of

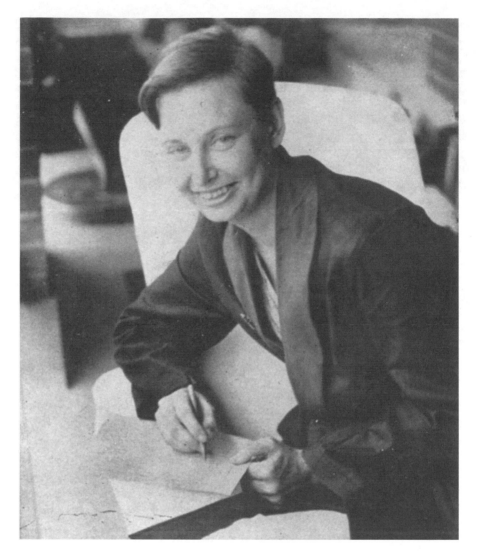

Vivian Bullwinkel.

13,000 (Nelson & Rabach 2002). For the first time 'the nurse of the first part of the twentieth century entered the labour force as part of a mass profession' (Nelson 1997:230). It was difficult to secure staff when armaments factories offered employment opportunities for women that had previously not existed, and women were relocated to jobs previously held by men. Some hospitals attempted to overcome this shortage by extending nursing training from three to four years in some cases. This had an unintended effect of discouraging young women from applying for training. Another strategy to prop up the supply of nurses was to promote the training of 'war emergency nurses' whose training ostensibly consisted of three years in hospitals, and VADs (Voluntary Aid Detachments), who were members of the Australian Red Cross and the Order of St John who usually worked without pay in medical support roles (Reid et al 1999).

Postwar

For the nursing profession at large, there were other important consequences of the war. Nursing was seen in 'manpower' terms from the perspective of national government for the first time. Shortages of staff became so severe that the Directorate of Manpower in 1942 became responsible for the control of the nursing workforce across Australia (Nelson & Rabach 2002). Nurses who wished to work interstate required the permission of this organisation to do so.

After the war, serving nurses were repatriated; adjustment to civilian life must have been difficult for all nurses, but for nurses who had held positions of authority in the military, the lack of positions offering equal status and authority as their officer ranks had done was a problem. In Australian workplaces, women like Miss Annie Sage, Matron-in-Chief of the AANS, were unable to reach the dizzy heights of leadership that military service had offered them. Their aspirations to lift nursing out of the realm of women's work into a more lofty sphere were dashed, as they were unceremoniously devolved of the level of responsibility and authority they had been accustomed to in wartime (Nelson & Rabach 2002).

Members of the VADs who, under the direction of the Army Medical Service, had assumed quite considerable responsibility during the war also had their aspirations crushed. On return to Australia, they were not considered qualified enough to be called 'trained nurses' suitable for registration (Reid et al 1999). Without a career structure and system for postgraduate education and recognition or recompense for experience, the situation for aspirational nurses remained as difficult as it had before the war.

Opportunities for postgraduate study in nursing were limited in the mid-twentieth century. Nurses had recognised that Australian nursing lacked postgraduate education in the tertiary setting, similar to that available to other professions and to nurses overseas. A Royal College of Nursing (RCN) grew out of the Royal Victorian Trained Nurses Association in 1934, but it was a quasi-industrial organisation, which had failed in its attempt to install nursing education at the University of Melbourne. It offered postgraduate courses in teaching, administration and industrial (now occupational health) nursing, and eventually secured funding to lay the foundations for a national college of nursing, but New South Wales declined to participate in this venture (McCoppin & Gardner 1994).

In 1949, New South Wales formed its own college with support from the New South Wales Nurses Association, the Australian Trained Nurses Association and the Institute of Hospital Matrons, and began its own postgraduate courses. The College of Nursing, Australia (RCNA), was established with government support in 1950 with Annie Sage as its inaugural president. The RCNA and College of Nursing have continued to coexist.

The transfer to tertiary education

For undergraduate nurses, the apprentice-style mode of education for nursing and midwifery has predominated since the introduction of pupil nursing in nineteenth century Australia. The education of nurses was managed within institutional and labour force requirements under a 'health' or 'hospitals' government portfolio. Through the 1960s and 1970s, nursing and midwifery education began to be seen as part of a broader education brief, as it was overseas. The New South Wales government was first to redirect nursing education to the education portfolio in 1977 and the then colleges of advanced education assumed responsibility for the education of nurses. Tertiary education for all nurses was formally adopted under a plan announced in August 1984 by the federal government (Russell 2000), and postgraduate education in midwifery transferred into the tertiary sector in the 1990s, and, very recently, midwifery has been offered as a discrete educational path, independent of nursing.

Emerging streams of specialisation

Just as the transfer of education to the tertiary sector signalled a new way of thinking about nurses and their preparation for practice, opportunities for nurses have opened up in tandem with twentieth century developments in the treatment of disease and new ways of understanding health and illness. Whereas in the immediate postwar years, postgraduate nurses could only specialise in teaching or administration, the development of sophisticated new treatments called for nurses with a sound understanding of biomedicine who could work machines and new technologies. Improved anaesthetic methods allowed previously haemodynamically unstable cases to survive with skilled nursing and medical care. This new strand of 'special' care for critically ill people by nurses in the 1970s has been accorded as the beginnings of intensive care nursing units (Fairman & Lynaugh 1988).

The development of adult intensive care in the 1960s and 1970s was followed by intensive care units for preterm and critically ill babies who had previously little chance of survival. These innovations offered nurses other opportunities to expand their skills. Examples of other fields in nursing as specific career paths for specialist practitioners are stomal therapy, diabetes education, mental health, women's health, cancer nursing, tissue transplant nursing and health promotion. The majority of these fields are commonly accepted as specialisations of nursing, but the idea that midwifery is a profession in its own right and not a branch of nursing is a little more contentious. It is the notion of separate histories of nursing and midwifery that we consider next.

SEPARATE HISTORIES OF NURSING AND MIDWIFERY

Since the late nineteenth and early twentieth centuries when the voluntary regulation of nursing was introduced in many parts of the English-speaking world, midwifery has been closely associated with nursing in Australia. The movement for voluntary regulation was primarily driven by those with an interest in nursing, and aimed to differentiate trained practitioners from untrained people as a way of raising nursing's status. The idea that midwifery was separate from nursing arose from the earliest days of voluntary regulation when registration as a midwife, and often as a gynaecology nurse, was recorded quite separately from that for general nurses. Other so-called 'branches' of nursing existed too; mental, tubercular, infectious, and eye and ear nursing came about because the nurses who practised them had trained in hospitals devoted to these specialties. Through voluntary regulation policies of the Australian Trained Nurses Association and the Royal Victorian Trained Nurses Association, the latter four 'branches' were largely absorbed into what became known as 'general' nursing education.

Midwifery, however, remained an anomaly, as did gynaecology nursing, because both of these specialities dealt with women only. To cope with recurring shortages of midwives, especially in rural areas, courses in midwifery known as 'direct entry' midwifery (i.e. without first being a nurse) were available in most states of Australia up to the 1950s. Gynaecology nursing too was deemed inadequate to be called general training and these pupils had to serve time in other hospitals to gain sufficient experience. The practice of midwifery by women who had not completed general nursing education was increasingly frowned upon by professional organisations of doctors and nurses, and direct-entry midwifery was phased out. In its place, all midwifery education was undertaken in Australia only after successfully completing general nursing training. In the meantime, gynaecology nursing was absorbed into general education.

The 'new' midwifery

In recent years, a worldwide movement of consumers and midwives has agitated to cleave midwifery away from nursing. This separation, its supporters say, will reinstate the independence of the profession, and restore the autonomy and professional satisfaction of midwives. It will also reduce medical interference in pregnancy, labour and birth, because the 'new midwifery' is a partnership between women and midwives who approach pregnancy and birth as normal physiological processes and not illness-states (Australian College of Midwives Incorporated (Victorian Branch) 1999).

Following this logic, a background in nursing (which concerns the care of the sick) is argued to be inappropriate preparation for midwifery practice because it brings an unnecessary focus on illness and complications, with the result that midwives whose primary education is in nursing are more likely to support intervention and the medicalisation of birth. Australia is following worldwide trends to institute midwifery education (a Bachelor of Midwifery), which is separate and distinct from nursing, like that established in other countries, including the Netherlands, the United Kingdom, New Zealand and parts of Canada.

Midwifery's past

With this renewed attention on midwifery, there has been increasing interest in recording aspects of midwifery's past in Australia, evidenced by recent biographical narratives of pioneering midwives, and of midwifery heritage (Gaff-Smith 2003, 2004). In thinking about the possible distinctions between nursing and midwifery, we offer two notes of caution. First, it is tempting to imagine the past as a comfortable place where the sagacity of midwives enabled natural birth to happen, and that any medical interference was unwelcome. These kinds of references to the past as 'heritage' reinforce our sense of 'what we value in the past . . . [that is] defined largely in terms of what we value or repudiate in the present' (Davison 2000:121), so it is perhaps unsurprising that nostalgic aspects of occupational history are the ones chosen to reinstate the place of the midwife in history. Critically, these narratives do not extend their vision of the past to incorporate the evidence of malpractice and negligence by midwives, or to recall the plight of women before the application of anaesethesia and caesarean section in maternity care. In ascertaining a more realistic and less romantic separate history of nursing and midwifery, their past(s) have to be considered whatever that past includes (Nelson 1997).

Our second note of caution concerns how we see the past from our present standpoint. If we do this in contemporary terms, we apply the murky vision of 'presentism', described by the historian John Tosh as a view fraught with problems (Tosh 2002). As an example of applying presentism to the notion of profession, consider the contemporary language that we use in health. The meanings we ascribe to 'health', 'healthcare' or 'health services', or 'midwifery', 'nursing', 'practitioner' or 'regulation', are likely to be removed from the meanings of these terms as they were used in the nineteenth century. Similarly, to define a profession in the nineteenth century from a twenty-first century perspective will colour our view considerably. To take a contemporary snapshot of a modern midwife and to attempt to locate this image in the past is present-mindedness (Tosh 2002), an approach that writers of traditional histories of nursing used in the past to promote their ideas about nursing and midwifery because this method suited the promotion of an ideology.

To arrive at separate histories of nursing and midwifery, then, is easier said than done because there are few records in existence that illuminate midwifery and/or nursing practice. This is because, we contend, the work was not considered 'professional' work, as we might imagine it. It was simply ordinary and mundane work for those who adopted it. If we take a definition of midwifery and nursing from the view of contemporary practitioners, we run the risk of not seeing midwifery and nursing, and midwives and nurses, as they were in the past because men and women alike were engaged as attendants in cases of sickness and also at childbirth.

Without archival records through which we might explore this type of work in the Australian community, it is not possible to determine if women as midwives only took midwifery cases, or if women as nurses did only nursing. It is likely that midwives did *midwifery*, but that they *nursed* their midwifery patients, not differentiating between sickness and health in the way that contemporary discussions about midwifery have done. We can speculate that a midwife may have attended maternity cases, but it seems logical that they may also have attended children with measles, mumps, whooping cough, diarrhoea and diphtheria.

What is at issue here is the delineation of the *actual* practice and perhaps accompanying notions of a professional 'identity', but an absence of personal records of the work done at the time means that we cannot say for certain who practised what and how. Neither can we be certain about who may have possessed a professional 'identity' as a midwife in the same way that a contemporary midwife has a professional identity. What we can say with certainty is that midwives did not have exclusive 'rights' to this work and that the field of 'women's health practice' was clearly contested territory. In general terms, midwifery and nursing were jobs done by various people, most of whom had no sense of a professional identity. They were simply occupations until they came to be redefined and shaped by the emergence of the movement for voluntary regulation and its push for professionalisation.

A midwifery 'identity'

There are possible exceptions to any generalisation, and here we consider one example pertaining to midwifery. In a small number of cases, we can speculate that at least in the first half of the nineteenth century some midwives may have held an occupational identity.

An examination of an early Tasmanian newspaper, the *Hobart Town Courier*, reveals that at least three women claimed formal education in midwifery from Dr John Thatcher's Edinburgh Lying-in Hospital: Mrs MacTavish in 1824; Mrs Miller in 1836 (Kelly 1977); and Mrs Sarah Barfoot in 1837 (*Hobart Town Courier*). Sarah Barfoot later worked in Melbourne and at Emerald Hill (now South Melbourne). Mrs Barfoot used a local newspaper, *The Argus*, to place an advertisement as a midwife in July 1848, and was listed as a midwife in a local business directory, the *Sands and*

McDougall directories, between 1862 and 1881. Elsewhere, in local council records, Mrs Barfoot nominated her occupation over a 20-year period as either 'midwife' or 'accoucheur' (*Emerald Hill Rate Books* 1864–81). The *Sands and McDougall directories* provided separate lists for nurses and midwives, but we can only speculate about whether this organisation of title is an indication of professional conscious, identity or scope of practice.

The regulation of midwifery practice was achieved in some of the Australian states well before that for nursing. Contrary to some contemporary views, we argue that this was not effected because parliaments wanted to recognise midwifery as a separate and autonomous profession. Rather, the propensity of midwives to work on their own terms without medical supervision was the central concern of those aiming to regulate midwives' practice. Midwives were known to provide advice to women about ways to avoid pregnancy and to procure abortions when unwanted pregnancies were discovered.

At the turn of the twentieth century, as the new federation of Australia was born, there was concern that Australia was going to experience 'race suicide', a term used by President Roosevelt to describe a similar fall in the number of births in America (Grimshaw 1994). Midwives' contribution to an already depleted population of human potential was a threat to security and future national aspirations. This was the primary reason behind moves to contain midwifery practice through legislation; it was not put in place to endorse midwifery as an occupation independent of nursing.

Midwifery and nursing have been inextricably woven as two occupational strands, which at times were one and the same, and at other times may have been distinct. We know that, broadly speaking, nursing and midwifery of eighteenth, nineteenth and even early twentieth centuries in Australia were not mutually exclusive, and therefore did not constitute independent professions. There was no neat practice division to delineate along occupational lines, which makes claims of separate histories less than convincing. Perhaps more research will illuminate a midwifery history that is more tangible.

CONCLUSION

In this discussion of Australian nursing's past we have broadly surveyed where nursing has come from, the path it has followed, and important influences and milestones throughout its evolution. There are many aspects of nursing history that we have not discussed, but are worthy of examination by researchers in the field. Some areas for future research include: the contribution of women combining nursing with their evangelical missionary work; how the workforce has been shaped by world events and globalisation; the role of Aboriginal women as nurses; and aspects of nursing practice (e.g. doing, organising, planning and implementing the care of others).

A sense of our history helps to explain the shaping of nursing and midwifery as professions, and many more insights into the ways that nursing and midwifery have evolved can be gained when we study aspects of our professional past. A broader understanding of the past in Australian nursing may guide planning and practice in the future, but a central message in studying our past is that nursing and midwifery must accept their pasts 'warts and all' (Nelson 1997:234). Only this pursuit will provide a realistic vision of nursing's and midwifery's history in the Australian context.

REFLECTIVE QUESTIONS

1 How does knowing about nursing's past help us to understand the present and the future?

2 What have been the major historical influences on nursing and midwifery?

3 What new questions could be asked about aspects of Australian nursing history?

RECOMMENDED READINGS

Fairman J, Lynaugh J E 1998 *Critical care nursing: a history*. University of Pennsylvania Press, Pennsylvania.

Nelson S 2001 *Say little, do much: nurses, nuns, and hospitals in the nineteenth century*. University of Pennsylvania Press, Pennsylvania.

Reverby S 1988 *Ordered to care: the dilemma of American nursing, 1885–1945*. Cambridge University Press, Boston.

Rosenberg C E 1987 *The care of strangers: the rise of America's hospital system*. John Hopkins University Press, Baltimore.

Russell R L 1990 *From Nightingale to now: nurse education in Australia*. W B Saunders Balliere Tindall, Sydney.

CHAPTER THREE

The art and science of nursing

Judith M Parker

LEARNING OBJECTIVES

Upon completion of this chapter, the reader should have gained:

▲ an understanding of the development of ideas about nursing as an art and a science within an historical context;

▲ an appreciation of the meaning of the art of nursing within the Florence Nightingale school of thought;

▲ an appreciation of debates about the art and science of nursing in the US context;

▲ an appreciation of emerging ideas about art and science and the relationships between them in the current context of healthcare; and

▲ insight into the implications of these ideas for current nursing education, practice and research.

KEY WORDS

Art, science, nursing, gender, aesthetics, enlightenment, contemporary

NURSING: AN ART AND SCIENCE?

What is nursing? Is nursing an art? Is nursing a science? Is nursing both an art and a science? Is nursing neither an art nor a science? Over the years there has been extensive debate in the nursing literature about the art and science of nursing. Why are questions about the nature of nursing posed in these terms? What is it about how knowledge and practices are understood in our society that invites us to ask these questions about nursing? What are the implications of these perceptions for education, practice and research in nursing?

This chapter seeks to explore some of these questions. It considers some of the history of the development of ideas about modern nursing as an art and a science. More specifically, it examines the division between art and science, and explores the impact that this separation has had upon ideas about nursing.

Two particular developments in the history of nursing ideas are discussed, one stemming from the United Kingdom, and the other from the United States. The first development, often described as the Florence Nightingale school of thought, represents the first expression of nursing as an art in modern times. In this development, nursing as an art is conceived of in relation to the character of the nurse and the importance of character training in nursing education programs. The second is the impact of the development of nursing ideas within the university context of the United States. Of particular note in this discussion are the attempts to construct closed systems of thought through nursing theory development and the production of nursing science. It was in this context that contradictions between nursing as an art and as a science began to be recognised and attempts made to reconcile the two.

The chapter then examines some of the implications of these ideas for nursing in the contemporary context where many of the binary divisions that occurred historically, including those between art and science, are collapsing. It concludes with a discussion of the art and science of nursing within the emerging milieus of healthcare delivery.

WHAT IS AN ART? WHAT IS A SCIENCE?

Many modern ideas about art and science have their origins in the scientific revolution of the seventeenth century and the eighteenth century 'age of reason' that was generated by the philosophical movement known as the French Enlightenment.

The scientific revolution was a quest to understand, control and manipulate nature through rational, empirical means. As Capra pointed out in 1982:

> This development was brought about by revolutionary changes in physics and astronomy, culminating in the achievements of Copernicus, Galileo and Newton. The science of the seventeenth century was based on a new method of inquiry, advocated forcefully by Francis Bacon, which involved the mathematical description of nature and the analytical method of reasoning conceived by the genius of Descartes (Capra 1982:54).

The Enlightenment project had the aim of civilising all, of implementing its ideal of social betterment through the power of reason. It was based on beliefs in the universal superiority of the knowledge and values produced by Western science and culture. Those who believed in the democratic ideals of the Enlightenment sought to perfect humankind through reason and create a better world, a civilised and cultured one aided by the new knowledge produced by science (Parker & Gibbs 1998). Two ways of thinking about art can be linked to the Enlightenment, one concerning the cultural production of knowledge and the other the art of living.

A separation of the arts and the sciences occurred in the educational structures and processes that emerged in the wake of the Enlightenment period and with the rise of modern professions. Knowledge came to be packaged into the two domains of sciences and arts within university faculties, and a division emerged between those who were educated in the sciences and those who were educated in the arts (humanities). Each of these produced different ways of thinking and acting, and different types of knowledge. According to C P Snow (1964), writing of the United Kingdom, scientific training produces 'doers' and training in the arts produces 'thinkers' (intellectuals). He argued that by the 1950s, the science/art professional rift was so deep that the two groups worked completely independently of each other, a trend he saw as potentially dangerous for society.

Another way of thinking about art that emerged out of the Enlightenment concerns the art of living. The search for human perfectibility, which was a major plank of the Enlightenment, became linked to a philosophy of humanism, which, as Nelson (1995:37) points out, '. . . stresses the centrality of the human subject and sets freedom as the subject's destiny'. The human subject, however, was male, and rationality was understood to be a masculine attribute. The art of living for men was linked to the pursuit of freedom through rationality, as 'doers' and 'thinkers'.

Women were seen as neither free nor rational. They were understood '. . . as an essential nature defined by purposeful organic functions' (Berriot-Salvadore 1993:387). Medical discourse defined the feminine ideal in terms of natural determinism as '. . . the mother, the guardian of virtues and eternal values' (p 388). Thus, while men, defined as human subjects, were separated and freed from the constraints of nature via reason and culture, women, defined in relation to nature and the feminine, were not. Nature and culture merged in this understanding of the feminine, and women were defined on natural and moral grounds. Good women exercised their womanly arts and civilised others through the practice of these arts. By and large women were excluded from education into the professions.

ART, SCIENCE AND MODERN NURSING

The constitution of modern secular professional nursing as it has evolved since the days of Florence Nightingale has been influenced by some of these ideas. Of particular importance to this discussion is how the divisions that occurred between art and science were managed in nursing. These will be considered first in relation to the Florence Nightingale school of thought stemming from Britain and then in relation to university-based nursing in the United States.

The Florence Nightingale school of thought

The Florence Nightingale school of thought developed and was sustained within the nurse training schools that sprang up in hospitals, not only in Britain, but also in

Australia, New Zealand and other countries. I argue that within nursing education and practice, nursing as an art was seen to involve the character of the nurse in the exercise of feminine virtues, and the importance of character training in the development of nursing as a female profession/occupation. In this context, science was out of place: the scientific enterprise was a male one and, in the hospital and medical context, belonged to the doctor.

Nursing in nineteenth century industrial England was regarded as an inferior, undesirable occupation practised by morally suspect women. In *Martin Chuzzlewit*, Dickens epitomised the nineteenth century English nurse in the character of Mrs Gamp, writing that '. . . it was difficult to enjoy her company without being conscious of a smell of spirits' (1910:312–13). The contrast of Florence Nightingale's work in the Crimea, and the subsequent publicity, brought about her identification in the public mind as a 'ministering angel' (*The Times*, London, 20 November 1854). This image was instrumental in elevating secular nursing to a female vocation based on Enlightenment ideals of the womanly virtues and the exercise of the womanly arts through the care of the sick. Indeed, Florence Nightingale described nursing as '. . . the finest of the fine arts' (Donahue 1996).

Enormous effort went into the attempts to position nursing as epitomising feminine ideals of the good woman. Nursing transgressed many prevailing ideas about the role of women in society and it was extremely difficult for nursing to gain acceptance as a legitimate and respectable occupation. Mrs Gamp and the 'bad woman' were never far beneath the surface; it is therefore not surprising that Florence Nightingale and her followers placed so much emphasis upon ensuring appropriate character formation among nurses in training (Parker 1990).

The first Florence Nightingale training school began at St Thomas' Hospital in London in 1860 and became the model for many training schools in Britain and its overseas territories in the latter half of the nineteenth century (Trembath & Hellier 1987). Student nurses were judged on their qualities of trustworthiness, neatness, quietness, sobriety, honesty and truthfulness (Smith 1982). Additionally, nurses were trained to ensure they did not wish to usurp any of the doctor's functions. Isabella Rathie, the first trained Matron of the Melbourne Hospital, noted, '. . . we are in a great measure the handmaid of the medical man and our function in this particular is to be obedient in every detail' (Rathie, cited in Trembath & Hellier 1987:19).

Thus, the division between art and science as it was manifest within modern secular professional nursing of the Nightingale school of thought can be described as a gendered division. Nursing as a feminine art was developed through character training that resulted in non-assertiveness, obedience and compliance with medical directives. Specific nursing arts comprised nursing procedures such as bathing, bed-making, positioning patients and comforting techniques. While some science content was included in nursing courses, '[t]here was minimal, if any, application of science content in nursing practice' (Peplau 1987:8). Nor were nurses educated in arts subjects of the university, which produced the thinkers of society, for that was primarily the sphere of men. Rather they were instilled with womanly virtues.

Nursing education was a process of systematically inculcating a task orientation and the moulding of a set of appropriate attitudes within hospital training schools to produce nurses who exemplified the feminine ideal. Science belonged to the rational and objective world of men, of which medicine was one domain. Men were subjects (minds), while women were objects (bodies); nurses were therefore not positioned as rational subjects shaping the Enlightenment project and their own destinies, but rather as passive and compliant objects, subservient to medicine.

Hospital-based nurse training lasted for more than one hundred years in Australia and much longer in Britain. Many changes occurred over that time, including considerable strengthening of the science content, particularly from the 1950s onwards. However, the gendering of nursing as a feminine art, developed in the restrictive environment of the hospital, placed limitations upon the possibilities for nursing to develop as a modern profession. It also limited the possibilities for nurses to develop knowledge, skills and attitudes in ways that would enable them to act as autonomous subjects. Nevertheless, it equipped them powerfully to work as moral agents engaged in socially significant work and to develop in-depth knowledge of the human condition in sickness and in suffering, albeit in an unarticulated, scientifically untested form.

Nursing in the university

In the United States, a 4-year entry-to-practice program had been established within a university by 1919. Within this system, it was possible to ensure the development of knowledge in a systematic and orderly way. By the late 1950s programs for training nurse scientists had developed in a number of major universities, which stimulated interest in theoretical and scientific bases of practice. These developments were supported by a huge federal investment in nursing education during the 1960s and early 1970s (Gortner 1983). In the period from the late 1950s to the early 1980s theories of nursing proliferated as nurse scholars sought to include in the concept of nursing an understanding of biological, behavioural, social and cultural factors in health and illness. Of particular note in this discussion were the attempts made to produce closed systems of thought through nursing theory development and the creation of nursing science.

This scientific orientation in nursing, however, came into conflict with ideas about the art of nursing. These stemmed not only from the Nightingale school of thought, but also from consideration of the art of nursing in relation to humanism and the nature of the human subject, by this time conceived of as including women. It is in this context that most of the debates about the art and science of nursing have occurred.

Nursing as a science

As has already been noted, a significant feature of the modern era has been the rise of professions, each clearly delineated by a separate body of knowledge. In the early modern era, nursing could not be regarded as a profession because it was seen to be subservient to and complicit in the medical tasks of diagnosis and treatment. With the location of nursing education within universities, and with the goal of securing professional status for nurses, a major task was to establish its own scientific base, separate from that of medicine.

One early nursing theorist, Johnson (1961), distinguished medicine from nursing by arguing that while the scientific basis of medical knowledge was biological systems, the scientific basis of nursing was behavioural systems. She proposed a behavioural subsystem model of the person '. . . with behaviour understood as the sum total of physical, biological and social factors/behaviours' (Parker 1995:334). These ideas were further developed by Roy (1980), who conceived of the person as an open, adaptive system, and nursing as the science and practice of promoting adaptation.

Other theorists, however, argued that these approaches did not sufficiently distinguish nursing from medicine. Like medical knowledge, the knowledge produced through study of systems was oversimplistic and mechanistic. Nursing, by contrast, needed to be conceptualised in broader, more encompassing, terms (e.g. Levine 1971). Ideas about nursing as a holistic science were developed by writers such as Rogers (1970) who conceived of the person as an energy field, coextensive with the environment, identified in terms of unified wholeness, openness, pattern, organisation and sentience.

Other writers further differentiated nursing science from medical science by emphasising nursing's caring function in opposition to medicine's curative function. Watson (1985a), for example, pulled together two of the central ideas of the modern era by describing nursing as a humanistic science, with caring the central unifying dimension of nursing (Cohen 1991).

Thus, with the shift of nursing education to universities in the United States, strong schools of nursing thought emerged. Each was developed in opposition to medicine, and understood nursing as a behavioural science, a holistic science or a caring science. These conceptual models for nursing practice were the work of a number of nursing intellectuals who had undertaken higher degree work in a range of disciplines, particularly in social sciences and education. Each model was designed to capture the complex dimensions of nursing, although, naturally enough, each one tended to reflect the disciplinary base of its author.

Following the establishment of the basis for nursing science through these models, there were calls to test the models against practical experience and refine them. However, progress was slow as Flaskerud and Halloran pointed out in 1980, and Fawcett in 1984. There was also concern that the proliferation of models would weaken nursing's claims to be seen as a profession based in a single unique body of knowledge. Fawcett made the point that '[t]he discipline of nursing will advance only through continuous and systematic development and testing of nursing knowledge' (p 84). Nursing authors sought to concentrate on the common ground in nursing conceptual models. Fawcett, for example, proposed a 'metaparadigm' (an explanatory framework) for nursing built on the central concepts of the discipline—person, environment, health and nursing—and attempts were made to further unify nursing knowledge around these concepts.

Many nurses, however, rejected nursing theories altogether as a means of establishing a science base for nursing. Nursing administrators and clinicians were particularly vocal in their rejection following frustrating experiences of trying to implement them in practice. Nursing theories were seen to reinforce the splits between the theory and practice of nursing, between the education students received and the realities of healthcare service provision, and between nursing thinkers (academics in universities) and nursing doers (nursing administrators and clinicians). In their attempts to develop nursing science through the advancement of nursing theory, nursing theorists, not surprisingly, replicated the binary modes of thought and the dividing practices of the general society.

While nursing theory was being developed, attempts were also being made to construct nursing science knowledge in ways that were linked more closely to practice. The nursing diagnosis movement attracted strong support following the 'First national conference on the classification of nursing diagnosis' held in Missouri in 1973. Nursing diagnosis was developed to identify and classify the phenomenon of nursing, to develop a common language for nursing and to facilitate the development and testing of nursing concepts and techniques. However, by 1983 the first broad-scoped critical rejection of nursing diagnosis emerged (Kritek 1985).

This more practice-focused approach to developing nursing science suffered from the same fundamental problem as the theory-based approach. Once again, nursing was attempting to develop its science in opposition to medicine by identifying a discipline-specific scientific knowledge base that would legitimate nursing's claims as a separate profession. In doing this, nursing opened itself to some of the same type of critiques that were made of medicine. The creation of a dedicated nursing language separated nursing not only from medicine but, more importantly, from patients. When viewed through the nursing diagnosis lens, the patients were reduced to objects of nursing diagnoses and treatments, a positioning that was in opposition to nursing's understanding of the patient as a holistic subject.

Two broad approaches to the development of nursing science have been identified: one that focused on defining the domain of nursing theoretically and then testing propositions empirically; and another that focused on the phenomenon of nursing practice and on developing ways of defining and classifying them. Both approaches were consistent with prevailing philosophies of science. Neither appears to have been successful in providing a discipline-specific body of knowledge that would justify nursing's claims to professional autonomy and power.

Nursing as an art

Nursing's power seems to rest more in its moral claims than in its science base. Ideas that stem from the Nightingale school about the nature of nursing art as an expression of the essential goodness of feminine virtues persist in contemporary nursing practice. Peplau (1987), writing about the United States but presenting a view widely held internationally, points out that nursing has been called the conscience of the healthcare system, which '. . . suggests that nurses are major keepers of the morality, goodness, honesty, and ethics of client care' (p 9).

This positioning of nurses on the moral high ground in the battlefield of healthcare provision has been sustained by beliefs that nurses exemplify feminine ideals, and appears to have wide community support. It points to an ongoing belief in the Nightingale legacy that presents nurses as good women. It also suggests that nurses and nursing organisations recognise and exploit the ways in which this characterisation of nursing serves wider political agendas and social functions. Additionally, it supports the idea of nursing as a caring and holistic art that sets itself in opposition to the rationality and reductive practices of scientific medicine and healthcare organisation. As Tanya Buchanan (1999) has noted: the 'Nightingale discourse generates myths about nursing that . . . appear to be eternal truths. We need to see past it' (p 30).

And indeed, ideas that the art of nursing stems from essential female virtues have been challenged within the university setting. The essence of nursing has been claimed to lie in its humanistic philosophy and the artistic practice that flows from this philosophy. In a much-quoted paper, Munhall (1982) argued that nursing has identified itself as a humanistic discipline, adhering to a basic philosophy '. . . that focuses on individuality and the belief that the actions of men [sic] are in some sense free' (p 176).

Munhall focuses attention on the extent to which university-based nursing education in the United States moved away from the Nightingale school of nursing thought based

43

on female character training, and drew more upon a precisely set out philosophy of the discipline to provide the basis for artistic practice. However, this placed nursing philosophy in opposition to prevailing notions of nursing science. As Munhall pointed out, because nursing subscribed to a humanistic philosophy as well as a scientific research orientation, '. . . incongruities, paradoxes, and conflicting ideologies' (1982: 176) resulted between philosophy and research.

Munhall also draws attention to the attempts made within nursing education to accommodate both a scientific and humanistic (arts) orientation. This suggests that professional university-based nursing education in the United States attempted to bridge the divide between the sciences and the arts that had been identified by C P Snow in the British higher education context. Nursing in the university aimed to produce practitioners who were both scientists in orientation and humanists in practice.

However, in educational preparation, the aims and scope of scientific and arts training differ significantly, and the transfer of both scientific and humanistic orientations to the realities of practice is a complex process.

Many writers have noted that the differing orientations of art and science have resulted in problems for nursing practice. Peplau (1987), for example, notes that science and art are both essential for excellence in the performance of nursing's mission, but points out the difficulty for a discipline of accommodating these two forms of professional behaviour:

> Combining both the art and science of nursing, seeing and bringing to bear the distinctive characteristics of each form and of the relation between them, imposes a complexity in professional nursing that virtually defies description (Peplau 1987:9).

Holden (1991), an Australian nurse, argues that the split between the arts and the sciences seriously complicates the notion of nursing. She points out that the caring role in nursing constrains nursing into the domain of the arts, while nursing that embraces high technology pushes into the domain of science. Jennings (1986) suggests that it is not a matter of choosing *either* art *or* science, but rather skilfully blending both for the betterment of nursing.

Peplau (1987) supports Jenning's view, pointing out that both science and art come together in practice, so that:

> There is surely a seamless quality, a graceful and delicately balanced movement, between art and science portrayed by experienced expert nurses that transcends as it uses the differences between these forms (Peplau 1987:14).

She suggests further that this transcending of the differing forms of art and science enables nursing to be practised not only as a helping art, but also as 'an enabling, empowering or transforming art'. People she notes '. . . are touched (literally and figuratively) and sometimes changed at a very personal level by the art nurses practice' (p 9).

The aesthetic dimension—the creative expression—of nursing has received increasing attention over the last two decades. It has built particularly upon the work of Carper who noted in 1978 that the primary emphasis in the professional literature of the time was being placed on the development of the science of nursing. She pointed out:

There is, nonetheless, what might be described as a tacit admission that nursing is, at least in part, an art. Not much effort is made to elaborate or to make explicit this aesthetic pattern of knowing in nursing—other than to vaguely associate the 'art' with the general category of manual and/or technical skills involved in nursing practice (Carper 1978:16).

Chinn and Watson (1994) have been very influential in further developing ideas about aesthetics and nursing, drawing upon notions of nursing as a caring science. Subsequently, Chinn et al (1997) described the development of aesthetic enquiry in nursing and the conceptualisation that has emerged is of nursing as an art form. Further work along these lines was undertaken by Johnson who conducted a philosophical analysis of conceptualisations of nursing art as a means of contributing to debate on the specific abilities required for artistic creation in nursing (1993, 1994, 1996).

Despite these developments, other writers (e.g. Darbyshire 1994a, 1994b, Lafferty 1997) have suggested that science content is still emphasised in nursing curricula at the expense of humanities content, and that, as a result, humanistic aspects of care believed to be essential to the artistic component of nursing are not being addressed sufficiently. Lafferty argues that nursing's dual identity as an art and a science requires a balance and calls for the promotion and acquisition of aesthetic knowledge by nursing students. She suggests that studying literature is a way of fostering this. Darbyshire makes a similar point, arguing that nursing as an art and a science is in danger of becoming a cliché unless attempts are made to reverse the marginalisation of arts and humanities within nursing curricula.

It can be seen that nursing as a contemporary secular profession has developed out of ideas about the essential nature of women, wherein nursing has been regarded as an art practised by virtuous women. This essentialist notion of nursing as a gender-based art may help account for the continuing failure to attract equal numbers of men into nursing. This view has also resulted in nurses sometimes regarding themselves, and being regarded by others, as the conscience of the healthcare system. Nursing as a gendered art is a continuing thread in professional nursing.

However, this notion was challenged significantly by the shift of nursing education into universities in the United States and by the attempts that have been made to discuss nursing as a science and a humanistic art. The literature explored indicates that nursing lies somewhat uneasily in the domains of both science and art, a division that stemmed from dividing practices in the cultural production of knowledge. Nursing developments, too, have replicated many of these dividing practices.

NURSING AND CONTEMPORARY HEALTHCARE

Many of the old divisions of the modern era are collapsing in both contemporary higher education and the health sector. This is certainly true in Australia, with implications for practices that sustained the conceptual, methodological and practical separations between art and science in nursing. The clear division between arts and sciences in higher education that reinforced the arts/sciences divide in knowledge development and the professions is clearly breaking down. It is becoming less possible for professions to define themselves in relation to discrete bodies of discipline-specific knowledge. The continuing knowledge explosion, together with the information technologies now available, are resulting in new fields of scientific enquiry and the proliferation of new professions that draw upon knowledge from a range of sources.

The nexus between professional knowledge and power is being subverted in a number of ways, not least through the processes of mass higher education and the access consumers now have to information that enables them to make their own decisions, independently of professional advice. These changes are taking place in a wider context in which global market influences are strengthening and humanist principles are weakening. This is an era of market contestability, privatisation, accountability and competition. It is an era in which performance is measured and evaluated on the basis of outcomes.

The 'reinvention' of nursing

The healthcare sector is rapidly transforming in response to demands for identifiable, quantifiable indicators of cost-effective quality outcomes. Clinical areas are responding to the changes being wrought in diagnosis and treatment through the use of new investigative and surgical technologies. Nursing, like many other professions, is seeking to 'reinvent' itself to meet emerging challenges (Parker & Rickard 1999).

The reinvention of nursing, I would suggest, is occurring on several fronts, all of which have implications for the art and science of nursing. Measures are being undertaken in nursing education, research and practice to ensure that nurses have the necessary repertoire of knowledge and skills to play a part in the transformations currently underway that are aimed at cost-effective quality outcomes of healthcare (Parker 2001). Efforts are being made to identify the nursing practices that positively influence health outcomes. Nurses are investigating traditional nursing practices to determine both their continuing appropriateness and the skill level necessary for their implementation.

Competencies for general, specialist and advanced practice are being refined to ensure greater accountability in relation to consumers, within the profession, in relation to other health professionals, and with regard to various contexts of practice (ANCI 1998). Nurses, in collaboration with other health professionals, are also contributing to the development, testing, implementation and evaluation of standardised clinical pathways. They are developing evidence-based nursing practices and contributing to developments in evidence-based healthcare (Parker et al 2000, Parker 2002, Pape 2003). They are working with consumers of health services to satisfy their learning needs.

What is becoming clear in this aspect of its reinvention is that nursing is shifting away from attempts to define itself as an autonomous profession with its own discipline-specific body of nursing science knowledge. As it moves into an interdisciplinary, team-based and consumer-oriented approach to practice and research, it is drawing upon current science/technology and information systems, and focusing upon nursing contributions to health outcomes and accountability for practices.

Nurses today need to draw substantially upon scientific knowledge to inform their practice, and scientific training needs to be a significant component of nursing education programs. At the same time nurses can contribute to the development of scientific knowledge in interdisciplinary and nursing-specific research projects. Questions for—and about—nursing emerge out of what nurses ask about their practices and the people and communities that they serve.

But how is the art of nursing manifest in this reinvention of the discipline? In a multitude of ways, I would suggest. We live today in an era of diversity, multiplicity and hybrid practices. Nursing can be practised as a gendered art; as a humanistic, aesthetic endeavour; and it can take fragments from both of these traditions and draw upon others as well. It can take up aspects of traditional art forms such as music, movement and touch, and incorporate them in diverse ways into repertoires of skilful practice.

In all of the multiplicity that is the art of nursing there is, however, a continuing thread, expressed as support of the sense of wholeness and integrity of individuals and communities rendered vulnerable through sickness and suffering.

CONCLUSION

In the current climate many nurses are expressing reservations about the market-driven approach and the economic ethic that underlie contemporary health reforms. They are worried that standardised approaches to care will compromise their ability to meet the demands of particular and unique situations. They are troubled that the increasing rationalisation of health services is causing fragmentation of services, despite the rhetoric of continuity of care. They are concerned that greater reliance upon advanced technologies is resulting in delivery of dehumanised services.

It is important that compliance with current healthcare reforms and resistance to them are not seen to be mutually exclusive endeavours. We can no longer think about the art and science of nursing as mutually exclusive endeavours. We can no longer claim that nursing is a holistic and artistic enterprise with humanistic and expressive concerns developed in opposition to the scientific, technical and instrumental dimensions of care (Parker 1995). The therapeutic tools and technologies of care we use are not separate from us: they are part of us and we are part of them. As they change, so we change. As we change, they change too. They are integral to our self-expression as nurses. The art of nursing, then, involves the perception and understanding of the inseparability of expression and technology.

Working within the framework of a standardised pathway does not prevent a nurse from recognising the individual and unique needs of particular patients. An aesthetic sensibility recognises the extent to which there is congruence between the standard (form) and the individual (content). Aesthetic integrity is responsive nursing in which standard and individual, form and content, become shaped into wholeness. An aesthetic sensibility facilitates expression of the art of nursing as part of the complex, ambiguous and technologically expressive milieus in which nurses work. An aesthetic sensibility is responsive to unified experiences both for recipients and providers of healthcare. It resists fragmented experience and can also '. . . empower people who are . . . sick, weak, vulnerable or disturbed to demand that attention is given to the particularities, complexities and ambiguities of their individual situation' (Parker 1995:2).

Nursing as art and/or science has been addressed somewhat differently at different times and in different contexts. A continuing thread nonetheless exists, which demonstrates the significance that nursing has given as a discipline and a profession to both science and art, and the nature of their relationship in nursing. Modern secular professional nursing since its beginnings last century has been and continues to be a complex set of practices that contains many anomalies and contradictions. The art and science of nursing manifests itself within a broader and changing social, cultural and political agenda. Nursing's social mandate acknowledges the art and science of nursing. The challenge for nurses in the contemporary healthcare context is to exercise that mandate judiciously and creatively.

REFLECTIVE QUESTIONS

1 What do you think are the main reasons nursing has come to be viewed as an art?

2 Why has nursing made consistent attempts to align itself with science?

3 How do you think the art and science of nursing can interrelate in the current contexts of healthcare?

RECOMMENDED READINGS

Carper B 1978 Fundamental patterns of knowing in nursing. *Advances in Nursing Science* 1:13–23.

Chinn P L, Maeve M K, Bostick C 1997 Aesthetic inquiry and the art of nursing. *Scholarly Inquiry for Nursing Practice* 11(2):83–100.

Johnson J L 1996 The perceptual aspect of nursing art: sources of accord and discord. *Scholarly Inquiry for Nursing Practice: An International Journal* 10(4):307–27.

Watson J 1985 *Nursing: human science and human care*. Appleton Century Crofts, Norwalk, Connecticut.

CHAPTER FOUR

Heroines, hookers and harridans: exploring popular images and representations of nurses and nursing

Philip Darbyshire

LEARNING OBJECTIVES

By reflecting on this chapter, readers will be able to:

▲ explain the importance of the question of nursing's image for contemporary nursing;

▲ describe the various prevalent stereotypes of the nurse and nursing and try to explain the persistence of these;

▲ debate the issue of whether nurses *really* wish to abandon the 'overworked angel' image;

▲ explain the difficulties involved in proposing a 'realistic' portrayal of nurses and nursing; and

▲ propose a strategy or small-scale project that could help promote alternative media representations of nurses and nursing.

KEY WORDS
Images, iconography, media, stereotypes, portrayal, mythical, realism

POPULAR IMAGES

Over the last 30 years, there has been a growing interest in the study of popular images of nurses and nursing, and it seems that every conceivable aspect of the image of nurses has been scrutinised. Writers have focused on images of nurses and nursing on television, in cinema, in novels and short stories, in news coverage and elsewhere. Why this fascination with the image of nurses? With the possible exception of doctors, why is there no comparable body of inquiry literature regarding the image of teachers, social workers, physiotherapists, accountants, occupational therapists or other professional groups?

In this chapter I will explore some of the early history and iconography of nurses and nursing in order to clarify the origins of many of the issues and 'images of nursing' which are so hotly contested and debated today. The 'so what?' question is important here. Why, when there are so many other pressing issues and concerns facing nursing and healthcare, should we worry about nursing's image? Delacour argues that:

> Certainly it is important that we analyse the process through which dysfunctional images and discourses are maintained. Moreover, it is useful to regard reading media as a politically situated and critical activity for the nursing profession (Delacour 1991:413).

Developing a critical and questioning view of our historical and contemporary representations is thus important for every nurse's personal and professional development. What we should strive for is to move beyond the 'knee-jerk' response that this or that image is good or bad, and to develop the critical thinking and analytic qualities that help us understand both the production, meaning(s) and possible effects of popular images of the nurse and nursing.

NURSING'S EARLY ICONOGRAPHY

Representations and images of nursing are as old as nursing and healing themselves. By tracing the origins of modern nursing back to antiquity and to the earliest accounts of babies, pregnant women, family and other members of early communities being cared for, usually by women, we can see that, '[t]he nurse as saintly domestic is no modern invention' (Kampen 1988:36). The earliest Greco-Roman depictions were almost entirely of 'baby nurses' and the image of the 'modern' nurse as tender of the sick or wounded was not to appear until the fourteenth century (Kampen 1988:16).

With the emergence of religious orders and associated charitable service came a new iconography of nursing, which showed women extending their care practices from the immediate household and family arena to the care of strangers. This was not always welcomed, however, and the Middle Ages in Europe especially saw the slaughter of millions of 'wise women' who were burnt as witches (Darbyshire 1985). In fifteenth century depictions of 'nurses' working with the sick, Kampen makes the significant observation that:

Several features common to scenes of nursing sisters help to define the nature of their role: they nurse patients who are most often men lying in bed; they work in a distinctive location that does not look like a house; they wear distinctive costumes; their activities are domestic and religious rather than specifically medical; and most important, they are never subordinated to patients and doctors (Kampen 1988:23).

It is salutary to think that with the exception of the last phrase, this description would have fitted any typical Victorian Infirmary almost 500 years later. So powerful is this depiction of nurses as tenders of the prostrate sick, reinforced no doubt by the iconographic imagery of Florence Nightingale wending her ethereal way through the wards of Scutari Hospital during the Crimean War, that nursing has often been seen in the public mind as being exclusively focused on this particular form of acute care nursing. McCoppin and Gardner (1994) noted how this one-dimensional view of nursing and nurses can occlude the view of all other forms and areas of nursing, which can somehow be deemed to be 'less than' or 'other than' 'real nursing', which of course was deemed to be practised exclusively at the bedsides of sick people:

> The stereotypical view of nurses as working only in acute care, high technology areas often portrayed in the media makes it very difficult to provide the alternative view of nurses working within the community which is more difficult to make attention grabbing (McCoppin & Gardner 1994:156).

It is not only the various forms of community nursing which may be seen as less than 'real nursing', but also the myriad other 'nursings', such as working in mental health, health promotion, school nursing, working with people with learning/intellectual disabilities and many others.

This masking of what, even in 1986 was over half of the whole nursing workforce (Dunn 1985–86), is significant as it can help narrow and restrict students' and other nurses' perceptions of what nursing fundamentally 'is'. For example, in Kiger's study of student nurses in Scotland, she found that '[t]he picture of adult medical-surgical nursing as typical of real nursing persisted throughout [the students' concept of] working with people' (Kiger 1993). The 'real nurse as general nurse' is, however, but one of many distortions and misrepresentations that have plagued nursing since its inception. Why nursing should be such a fertile ground for image construction and manipulation is a hugely complex issue and one that has been discussed and argued over many years. One way of beginning to understand the heady brew of images, social constructions, myths and contradictions, and 'realities', which form the image(s) of nurses and nursing, is to look more carefully at the persistence and power of the major stereotypes of nurses that still exist in either blatant or more subtle forms even today.

NURSING'S STEREOTYPES

Perhaps it could be considered something of a backhanded compliment that there are so many stereotypes associated with nursing. At least we are not seen as bland and instantly forgettable! The problem is often, however, that the major stereotypes can be so unrelentingly negative in their connotations and so wholly untenable in their relationship to any notion of a 'reality' of nursing. (This notion of *a single* nursing reality is itself contentious and I shall return to this later.)

The problem with any stereotype is that it can become so pervasive that its effects become more than merely an annoyance. As Delacour observes:

> . . . even stereotypes regarded as dubious may, after a measure of exposure, become internalized and naturalized; they are thereby metamorphosed into categories of the normal, the real, and the healthy and desirable (Delacour 1991:413).

If the sole problem with nursing stereotypes was just that some get-well cards, tabloid newspaper stories or 'X-rated' films portrayed nurses as oversexualised bimbos, then perhaps we could laugh it off, but when the effects of stereotyping are more serious, then there is more at stake than nursing's collective need to 'lighten up'.

The images and perceptions of nursing, both within the profession and in society in general, are important for several reasons. We live in an era where image and the marketing of image has never been more important, and while we can certainly maintain that the 'core business' of nursing is caring for the health and wellbeing of people, we would be foolish to ignore the importance of nursing's image. If we are to attract creative, committed, intelligent and passionate people into nursing, then nursing needs to be seen as every bit as worthwhile and challenging a career as any other in the fields of healthcare or social service. The persistence of hackneyed old stereotypes does nothing to enhance the attractiveness of nursing as a career.

Muff (1982:211) has suggested six 'major nursing stereotypes': angel of mercy, handmaiden to the physician, woman in white, sex symbol/idiot, battleaxe and torturer. Dunn (1985–86:2) credits the average tabloid newspaper with even less imagination, being interested in only three types of nurse: the angel, the battleaxe and the nymphomaniac.

Angels with pretty faces

If nursing iconography has an enduring stereotypic image, it must surely be the nurse as 'angel'. While much of the earliest artwork and imagery of nurses showed nurses ministering to the sick in various quasi-religious ways and settings, nurses in Australia, even in the late 1800s, were 'redefining the image of nurses as motivated primarily by self-sacrifice' (Bashford 1997). However, it was Florence Nightingale's story that captured the public imagination and stimulated a swathe of hagiographic accounts (which critic Leslie Fiedler (1988:103) called 'shameless schlock'), and movies such as *The white angel* and *The lady with the lamp* (Jones 1988b, Kalisch & Kalisch 1983b). So powerful were these images of the angelic presence which lit up the wards of Scutari with her lamp, that Florence Nightingale became easily identified as the soul or spirit of nursing and as the embodiment of selfless, devoted, compassionate care which borders on the saintly.

Despite some of the more recent, critical and balanced scholarship concerning the life and work of Florence Nightingale (e.g. Hektor 1994), the stereotype of the nurse as selfless angel is still prevalent, especially in the public imagination. There are several difficulties here. At first glance it may seem no bad thing to think that society views nurses as 'angels'. Who wouldn't like to be thought of in such a 'positive' light? Which nurse would not like to think that she was capable of such profound caring, which could earn such adoration? Is this not just being held in high regard by society? Don't we feel good when opinion polls put nurses near the top of the list for perceived honesty, trustworthiness and hard work? Jane Salvage perceptively pointed out that nurses often collude in sustaining the selfless angel stereotype while professing to scorn it. As she noted, '[t]he trouble is we are secretly flattered by the myths, especially those emphasising dedication and high-minded self-sacrifice'(Salvage 1983:14).

However, buying into the angel stereotype may be a Faustian bargain, for there is a price to pay for this. 'Angels' may be saintly, but such perfection is impossible for mere mortal nurses to achieve or maintain. Nurses are, after all, only human. Nor do angels seem to require any education or experience, their sanctity being more of a divine gift. For real nurses, however, becoming a skilled and competent nurse is hard work. We may be born with particular dispositions and talents, but we cannot be 'born nurses'. That will take more than an accident of birth. Such shafts of grace as we achieve are often hard won through our sustained engagement in the lives of those people who place their trust in us.

Doctor's handmaidens

If the angel myth is a remnant of nursing's religious order origins, then the unquestioning obedience of the doctor's handmaiden owes much to nursing's military origins. This stereotype touts the image of the nurse as a kind of 'lady in waiting' or the doctor's 'right-hand woman'. This has been a hugely influential media view of nursing for decades, that essentially the nurse is there to provide faithful and obedient service to the doctor and like the angel myth, this view has often been sustained by nurses themselves who were flattered by the idea that 'their' doctors or 'their' consultant says that he or she couldn't manage without them. In her analysis of nurses' image in postwar Britain, Hallam noted also that:

> Within the broadcasting environment, nursing's professional discourse of 'service' was interpreted as service to medicine; nurses themselves did little to challenge the picture (Hallam 1998:37).

In this sense, the handmaiden stereotype may be less mythical than nursing would like to acknowledge. While nationally and internationally, particular nurses and nursing projects/initiatives have led healthcare advances (often in *collaboration* with medical colleagues), there are still many nurses who work with doctors who seem not to recognise nurses' ability and responsibility to make an equal contribution to care and who assume that the nurse's role is to make coffee, not decisions. Despite claims of teamwork and 'multidisciplinary' cooperation, some nurses continue to work in 'teams' where teamwork is lots of people doing what one person says, and that one person is usually a doctor.

The battleaxe or monstrous figure

For images to be powerful and long lasting they must be capable of being both sustained and subverted. The battleaxe figure is in many ways a magnificent subversion of other stereotypes of the nurse, what Hunter calls in a slightly different context, the translocated ideal (Hunter 1988). Where the 'angel' is often portrayed as pretty, feminine, Caucasian, slim, caring, white-clad for purity, fun, deferential and loved by patients, the battleaxe or matron figure was almost the exact opposite—tyrannical, fearsome, asexual, cruel, monstrously large, dark-clad, and set on crushing all fun and individuality.

On a BBC radio program that I compiled several years ago, I listened to a recording of a 1960s radio quiz show where one of the male panelists joked that the tragedy of nurses is that they were one day destined to become matrons. Matrons, like other nurses who refuse to fit the accepted stereotype of the pretty, kind, compliant nurse, are banished to the moral margins of societal acceptance where they become objects of fear or ridicule. Think here of 'bad' nurses like Charles Dickens' Mrs Gamp (Summers 1997), Ken Kesey's 'Big Nurse/Nurse Ratched' from *One flew over the cuckoo's nest* (Darbyshire 1995), Annie Wilkes from Stephen King's *Misery*, and the more comic figures of Hattie Jacques from the *Carry on* film series or Matron Dorothy from Australia's 1990 television series, *Let the blood run free* (Delacour 1991).

The battleaxe stereotype cries out for a feminist analysis that reveals the fate of any nurse who does not comply with the mythical norms of the ideal nurse and who challenges male power (usually patients and doctors). Worse than this, perhaps, is that the battleaxe figure is a powerful woman who is unattracted to them (Darbyshire 1995), thus proving that she cannot be a 'real' nurse, as one of the most prevalent and damaging stereotypes is the nurse as an easily available 'sex bomb'.

Naughty nurses and nymphomaniacs

When I was a lecturer in Scotland, I would discuss the question of nurses' image with the first-year students who had just begun their course. I asked them what a common reaction would be at a party if they happened to mention that they were a nurse. After the laughter and ribaldry had settled, it was clear that a common, if not thankfully universal, reaction from some men was a 'knowing grin' and some suggestion that a night of unbridled sexual abandon may lie ahead. For this reason, many of the students said that they would make up an occupation rather than 'admit' to being a nurse.

Why is the 'naughty nurse' stereotype so prevalent? Why are there no 'naughty lawyer' sexual stereotypes? Why are there no pornographic films made about the adventures of a group of occupational therapy students? Why don't sex shops sell physiotherapist uniforms? What is it about nurses that makes them such a target?

This is a deep and complex issue, but consider the following points in relation to Hunter's notion of a 'translocated ideal' (Hunter 1988). Nursing is utterly implicated in social power relations, between nurses and doctors, nurses and other nurses, nurses and patients, nurses and relatives, and more. When patients enter hospital, the traditional power relations are reversed and they find themselves vulnerable and dependent rather than strong and in control. At a societal level (for not every male patient will see his situation in this way), one way of redressing this balance is to metaphorically (or perhaps even practically) sexualise the encounters between nurses and patients.

We also know that nurses' practices in relation to patients' bodies are part of this process. Nurses are exceptionally privileged in that we are intimate body workers. Nurses have access to people's most private body areas and bodily functions (Lawler 1991). One of the most important practices that a nurse develops is the ability to work with patients' intimate body parts without sexualising the encounter. To transgress this boundary would be both embarrassing and dangerous. In an almost too painful to watch scene in Dennis Potter's television play *The singing detective*, a nurse is having to anoint the 'Philip Marlowe', lead character's genital areas with crème as he has extremely debilitating psoriasis and cannot do this for himself. As the nurse applies his crème he becomes sexually aroused, and, despite trying desperately to divert this thoughts with a litany of the most boring and asexual things he can think of, he develops an erection. The nurse, however, wants to get the procedure done and continues crèming, causing him to ejaculate and suffer an agony of humiliation.

Fagin and Diers are clear on the damaging implications of conflating sexualisation and intimate body work:

> Thanks to the worst of this kind of thinking, nursing is a metaphor for sex. Having seen and touched the bodies of strangers, nurses are perceived as willing and able sexual partners (Fagin & Diers 1983:117).

The naughty nurse stereotype also encourages the subversion of another ideal, that of the saintly purity of the nurse as angel. Beneath the pristine white uniform, tightly bunched and restrained hair and sheepish obedience to authority lies the pornographers win–win scenario. Either the nurse is really a 'sex-bomb' being barely held in check by the rules and regulations of the institution and awaiting the slightest excuse to release all of this pent-up passion, or she really is completely subservient to (male) authority, in which case she will willingly agree to all and every sexual demand.

If you think that these scenarios are far-fetched, consider a feature that ran several years ago in the UK tabloid newspaper *The Sun*, which aroused furious public opposition. The feature had the headline 'Calling all you naughty nurses', and read thus:

> Yes, we know you're out there. Lots and lots of people tell stories about those saucy times when temperatures soared in the wards. Who hasn't heard about the time the young nurse turned a bed bath into a saucy romp? And delighted male patients are always revealing how they got some very special medicine from the attractive sister when the screens were drawn. So come on folks. Let's hear from the naughty night nurses—and their happy patients about the fun times in Britain's hospitals. We're opening our own special phone line between 10 a.m. and 6 p.m. today. Ring the number below and tell us your stories.

Such was the wave of protest from nursing organisations and others that the feature was withdrawn within days.

NURSING'S IMAGE: BLAME 'THE MEDIA'?

For any nurse who wanted to know 'who was to blame' for the worst excesses and misrepresentations of nursing's image, 'the media' in general offer a clear if rather too easy target. Too easy perhaps because we assume that 'the media' is almost automatically the most pervasive form of image transmission. Yet a study of 1155 people in the United States found that less than 10% of the respondents felt that they received their information from the media. Most said that their opinions came from first-hand impressions gained during visits to a hospital (Begany 1994). Delacour makes the important point that, often, it is more than *the ways* in which nursing is portrayed, it is that nursing is 'symbolically annihilated by the mass media' (Delacour 1991:418) and virtually ignored. To test this claim, it would be interesting to keep a local and a national newspaper for a month or two with a view to checking how many health stories included authoritative comments from nurses compared with doctors. Many nurses would say that they could confidently predict the results of such a survey well in advance.

Considerable research has been undertaken into the role of the media in constructing and shaping nursing's image. In the United States in particular, the team of Philip and Beatrice Kalisch in the 1980s produced numerous books and papers on many different aspects of this question (Kalisch & Kalisch 1983a, 1983b, 1984, 1987, Kalisch et al

1982, 1983). This criticism of the media in general continues to this day. Holmes, for example, advises that we should (perhaps) give up watching medical soaps on television, as they are 'anodyne and legitimating rather than transformative and critical' (Holmes 1997:137).

While soaps may well be 'anodyne', there are probably few viewers of television serials such as *All Saints* who bemoan that the show is no longer as 'transformative and critical' as it used to be. Blaming genres for not being what we would wish them to be is surely tilting at windmills. To simply stop watching 'soaps' because we disagree with aspects of their portrayal of nurses and nursing is scarcely a mode of engagement. Nor is it particularly astute to imagine that the media exist to 'accurately' (or should it be positively/flatteringly?) depict nurses and their work. Much as we may dislike the notion, the mass media exist primarily as a profit-making business. It is not nursing's tame public relations machine.

There is also an argument to be made that criticisms of the portrayals of nurses often seem to misunderstand the different genres of representation. For example, criticising a film like *Carry on nurse*, or a series like *Let the blood run free*, for giving a false image of nurses and nursing makes little sense. These are not documentaries and their purpose was never to represent the 'reality' of nursing. They are comedies, and they work by upsetting or translocating our understandings and expectations of nursing. Condemning a *Carry on* film for not being a true-to-life account of nursing is like criticising Thursday for not being the Blue Mountains.

While a 'blame the media' approach has a seductive simplicity, it is unlikely to achieve any significant results. However, working with the media in order to help create more 'realistic' portrayals of nursing's work, as Buresh and Gordon's (2003) exemplary work shows, is a much more productive strategy. In the early days of the filming of *ER*, there was virtually no consultation with nurses or emergency room departments. US emergency room nurses, however, did more than complain or stop watching, they became proactive and contacted the producers regularly with comments, and criticisms, but also with offers of help, storyline ideas, and the names of subspecialty ER nurses who were willing to help the show 'get it right'.

NURSING'S IMAGE: DEPICTING 'REALITY'?

In a news report, the warning of Joanne Rule, former head of the Royal College of Nursing (UK) public relations office was repeated, that 'if nursing were to succeed finally in shaking off the "angel" image it so professes to hate, it might be replaced by an image that it hated even more' (Rule 1995). One of the significant difficulties in challenging potentially damaging images of nursing is that it is very difficult to give an agreed account of what a 'good portrayal' should look like. As Bashford noted in her study of how early Australian nurses challenged their systems:

> . . . resistance was never straightforward. Often, rather than new discourses offering empowering new subject positions, they produced confusion, contradiction and insecurity. Women were asked to think about their work in religious terms in one moment and in one context, in scientific terms in another, and as a type of professionalism in another (Bashford 1997:67).

This historical dilemma will seem blindingly contemporary to today's nurses who are struggling with very similar issues around nurses' 'expanded role' and what this means for nursing's identity/identities. The other difficulty in looking for a 'realistic' image of nurses is that it would be a precious and narcissistic stance for nursing to adopt which stated that the only acceptable (and for acceptable ask: Acceptable to whom? To me personally? To nurses at my hospital? To nursing in general?) portrayals of nurses and nursing were those that were 'positive'. It would be reassuring to think that nursing was a little more secure in its role and purpose than to require to be constantly flattered and puffed up by an unrelenting diet of uncritical media comments and compliments. This quest for the 'positive' portrayal of nursing has been questioned by Hallam who argued that:

> This search for a positive image of nursing identity poses two crucial problems. On the one hand, it tends to presume a professional consensus in terms of what this image is or could be . . . [T]he positive image approach can also be critiqued from the viewpoint of media reception; it conceptualises readers and viewers as uncritical receivers of messages who unquestioningly digest the authority of the image (Hallam 1998:33).

Similarly, Cheek has observed that:

> . . . the task is not to look for *real* and authentic representations of nursing, but rather to look for the speaking and representation that is done about nursing (Cheek 1995:239).

This is not to say, however, that no 'positive' images and accounts of nurses and nursing can be found. For example, in his account of his serious injury and recovery, surgeon and rehabilitation specialist Tony Moore describes the artistic and technical expertise of the intensive care nurses who gave him a blanket bath:

> They worked like a ballet corps in slow motion, softly moving me forwards, to the side, sponging, touching, towelling with clean tenderness, and when one gently washed my genitals I felt nothing but the compassion of her care (Moore 1991:11).

Richard Selzer was another surgeon who found himself a patient in intensive care following legionnaires' disease. He is hugely embarrassed by his dependency and incontinence, but again, his nurses are memorably skilled in what he calls 'the forgiveness of the flesh' (Selzer 1993:56). Unlike the unfortunate 'Philip Marlowe' in *The singing detective*, Selzer's nurses spare him the embarrassment and pain that could so easily become part of his intimate body care. One nurse who makes such a profound difference to Selzer's care and recovery is Patrick, whom Selzer describes as being 'the sort of nurse who can draw the pus out of a carbuncle with his gaze alone, and turn it into a jewel' (Selzer 1993:56). Selzer is quite emphatic that the power of skilled nurse caring is not merely 'nice to get' but that it is actually transformative. He describes his being carried back to bed by Patrick following a tub bath as the moment when his 'molecules rearranged themselves'. 'It is the true moment of cure' (Selzer 1993:93) he says.

Read these authors' accounts of their care and then consider that bathing patients is considered by some to be 'basic' nursing care, where, for 'basic', read 'unimportant and thus able to be undertaken by virtually anyone'. There are many other 'positive' accounts in literature and popular culture of nurses and nursing which are valued, appreciated and which have a markedly beneficial effect on the recipient. However, care is needed not to fall into the trap of 'collecting' these accounts as a kind of trophy for nursing. If we are to cultivate and develop our questioning and critical powers, then the positive accounts also need to be questioned and discussed.

NURSING'S IMAGE: FROM AFFRONT TO ACTION

During the past two decades, there has been a plethora of research and discussion regarding nursing's image and the portrayals of nursing. We are now much more aware of the forces that shape and maintain many of popular culture's images of nurses and nursing. Perhaps the next two decades will see nurses moving from this position of greater awareness to one of more positive action. By this I mean that it is no longer enough to be outraged at the 'negative images' and stereotypes that we will continue to encounter. Indignation or 'refusing to watch' are not strategies for change. Nor will it be enough to merely call for negative images of nurses to be withdrawn or 'banned'.

The most difficult task ahead is for nurses and nursing to *use* the media in a much more 'streetwise' way than we have in the past. If we do not like the images that are being presented, then we have a responsibility to provide alternatives. If we think that media reports and stories about nursing are inaccurate or inadequate, then we need to interest the media in alternatives. If we feel that the media completely ignores a particularly important program, service or aspect of nursing, then why not alert them to this and highlight the importance of what it is that they are missing? No media like to feel that they are missing something interesting or important, especially in their local area.

Delacour lists excellent questions that we should ask about the images and representations of nurses and nursing:

> Who has speaking rights? Who says what? Which position? On behalf of whom? Who is silenced? What are the assumptions? What is privileged in the text? What is ignored, glossed over or marginalised? What is the target audience and how is the reading/viewing position constructed to promote a 'preferred' reading. Which genre and its codes and effects? What type of publication/program and resultant status of discourse? How are power and knowledge articulated? How are gender, sexuality, roles and relationship, race, class, deviance and normality constructed? Which rhetorical devices? Which linguistic features? (Delacour 1991:419)

These are questions that do not naively assume that there is a right or wrong image, but that begin the task of unpacking and exploring this complex yet highly revealing area wherein we can learn so much about ourselves, our society and those for whom we care.

To these questions we should ask some others, which will help us be more active in redressing nursing's image. We should ask questions such as: What images would we want to see in the media? How can we show the positive power of nursing to local and national media? Why would/should the media be interested in this program/ innovation/nursing development? How can we 'sell' this idea or story to the media in such a way that they can't ignore it? Whose expertise and support could we call upon to help us do this? (Clark 1989, Monahan 1996, Strasen 1992).

In short, we now know a great deal about representations of nurses and nursing in the various media and popular culture. Our task now as nurses is not simply to 'adapt' to, or merely observe and comment on future changes, but to get out there and make the changes happen.

REFLECTIVE QUESTIONS

1   Discuss with a group of your peers the reactions that you have encountered, both favourable and unfavourable, when you have told people that you are a nurse/student nurse, and how you feel about such reactions.

2   Use Delacour's questions (listed above) to critique and question some selected images of nurses/nursing (e.g. from a film, documentary, novel or medical 'soap').

3   Plan how you would go about creating your own media story about nurses or nursing. What would you choose as the issue (e.g. a nurse-led clinical initiative, an ethical dilemma, a particularly successful patient outcome, an exciting new approach in nursing education, or a particular nurse who is doing something really special in an area)? How would you go about interesting the media in the story, and how would you present it?

RECOMMENDED READINGS

Donahue M P, Donahue P M 1996 *Nursing: the finest art*. Mosby-Year Book, St Louis.
Jones A 1988 *Images of nurses: perspectives from history, art, and literature*. University of Pennsylvania Press, Pennsylvania.
Salvage J 1985 *The politics of nursing*. Heinemann, London.

CHAPTER FIVE

On philosophy: nursing and the politics of truth

Kim Walker

LEARNING OBJECTIVES

By reflecting on this chapter, readers will be able to:

▲ articulate the relationship between the discipline of philosophy and the discipline of nursing;

▲ identify philosophical positions that have been influential in shaping nursing as a practice and scholarly discipline;

▲ describe the relationship between philosophy and the ways it informs thought and action generally; and

▲ appreciate how nurses might begin to engage philosophy as a way of reflecting on nursing's relation to the truth.

KEY WORDS
Philosophy, essentialism, naturalism, humanism, holism, anti-intellectualism, feminism, gender, postmodernism

Every philosophy conceals another philosophy; every opinion is also a hiding place, every word a mask (Nietzsche, cited in Hayman 1997:38).

What is the value of the will to truth? Why should we not prefer untruth or uncertainty or ignorance? The answer is that we do. Our instinct for self-preservation teaches us to be superficial (Nietzsche, cited in Hayman 1997:36).

WHY PHILOSOPHY?

Why indeed! What interest would nurses have in philosophy, which is, after all, something usually seen as the province of bespectacled professors locked away in their ivory towers? Undoubtedly though, philosophy in many guises has informed nursing from its very beginnings, but sometimes without our consent or complete understanding of the consequences. Therefore, it is for me a fascinating challenge to explore the most significant philosophical positions that have shaped—and continue to inform—our profession in order to better understand why contemporary nurses might think and act the way they do. This is the cut and thrust of my chapter: a journey *into* philosophy *out* of nursing, but simultaneously a journey *into* nursing *out* of philosophy.

My history as a nurse is tightly bound up with a life as someone who has always asked difficult questions of the world and who, consequently, has spent more years than he cares to remember struggling with seemingly countless contradictions and inconsistencies lived out between articulating philosophies of nursing and engaging in it as a practice (Walker 1993). In living through and finding ways to better understand these things, I have journeyed through diverse and often complex philosophical territories—journeys, it could be argued, that have provided me with the credentials to contribute to this text.

Therefore, in this chapter, I want to explore with you the ways many different philosophies—each with their own histories and effects—have variously enabled and disabled what passes for the 'truth' of nursing. And this is why philosophy is perhaps best thought of as 'a way of reflecting not so much on what is true and false but *on our relationship to the truth*' (Foucault, cited in Lotringer 1989:201, emphasis added). Throughout, I attempt to show how certain truths about what it is to be a nurse and 'do' nursing have been decided *for* us, but not necessarily *by* us. These truths have generally made it difficult for nursing to position itself as a serious discipline (in terms of its 'body of knowledge') and authoritative profession (in terms of nurses' capacity to make decisions on their own behalf and be recognised for their contribution to the wellbeing of humankind). But it is our *relationship* to these truths and the effects they create in the minds and actions of ourselves and others that we need most to interrogate. Let me begin this work by putting forward a couple of truths to which I subscribe.

Nursing first and foremost is a practice; it only comes to true (or real) expression in action. Moreover, nursing, as an intractably social and relational activity, is bound up in and manifests itself by way of ceaseless acts of communication and interaction with others. Language is at the core of this activity and is the most significant medium through which we construct and interpret our worlds. Philosophy is primarily a linguistic phenomenon in the sense that it is about words and ideas. There is no other place to start thinking philosophically about nursing than nursing's origins in language. This discussion will lead us nicely towards a more sophisticated analysis of how philosophy might actually be embedded in nurses' everyday talking and moving-about-in-the-world as active agents in that world's creation. With luck, it will encourage you to read more on this fascinating topic, and, if that is the case, then I have achieved more than I could hope for!

WHAT'S IN A NAME?

Absolutely everything. We make sense of the world by differentiating objects and ideas from each other by means of the way in which something means something only because it is not something else. Moreover, the relation between an object or idea and its name is complex and multiple; that a 'nurse' is the creature we have come to know as 'nurse' is unquestionably a function of history (in this case, the history of the origins of words), culture (the interplay of people in societies of shared understandings) and the politics of knowledge (how some ideas and truths come to dominate at the expense of others). Language is the slippery medium burdened with the responsibility for allowing humans to communicate through shared vocabularies—generated by our various formal and informal educations—about our lived experiences and the interpretations we ascribe to them in order to render our lives both accessible and meaningful.

If we reflect on the complexity of the linguistic structures we employ to engage with one another, it becomes easier to appreciate what a miracle effective communication really is. Most *words* have more than one form and one meaning; most *sentences* can be made sense of in a number of ways depending on syntax, grammar and context; all *stories* harbour multiple possibilities for interpretation; and all stories are themselves framed within even more sophisticated *narrative structures* we call myth, metaphor, discourse and ideology, to mention the more common of these.

The sheer complexity of language and its expression renders the communicative act far more dense and opaque than we usually care to acknowledge, and we let language 'have its way with us' much more often than we ought to allow. In other words, we seldom stop to ask questions at a deep level about what is said and why because we normally operate only on the surface of language and its various structures and mechanisms. Not so here, however! Against this brief introduction to the sophistication of language, let's move on with our journey into philosophy by taking a closer than usual look at the word 'nurse'.

If we consult the *Oxford English dictionary* and carefully examine the various entries we discover that 'nurse' is both a noun and a verb. A noun that at the same time enacts its very meaning as a verb limits the potential for confusion: a nurse nurses. Superficially, this congruence between noun and verb seems logical and constructive. At a deeper level, however, it is unhelpful in so far as it leaves no room for alternate understandings of what a nurse might be and/or do. So we are left with two terms that define themselves only in relation to themselves—a kind of linguistic bind or tautology, which, as you will come to discover, is rather bereft of philosophical and practical worth.

As a noun, 'nurse' first appeared in late Medieval England at which time (1450) its primary meaning was: 'A woman employed to suckle, and to take charge of, an infant'. It also meant 'One who takes care of, looks after, or advises another'. A little later (1526), this definition was extended slightly to incorporate: 'A person, usually a woman, who attends or waits upon the sick; now *esp*. one trained for this purpose'. Already it becomes obvious that the nurse is in no way a neutral term; it is highly charged socially, politically and emotionally.

If we examine the word as a verb, again we see the notion of a woman suckling an infant (1535), fostering, tending, cherishing (a thing) (1542), and waiting upon or attending to (a person who is ill) (1736). Finally, in 1861, the verb finally makes explicit the meaning it has today: 'to perform the duties of a sick-nurse'. This last meaning and its appearance in the English language appeared 12 months after the establishment of the first Nightingale schools of nursing in 1860 (see Cuff & Gordon Pugh (1924:3) for more). Such a phenomenon highlights the profoundly incestuous relationship between language and reality: they are mutually constructing of each other. In the preface to her 'Notes on nursing', Nightingale makes the following very telling statement:

> Every woman . . . has, at one time or another of her life, charge of the personal health of somebody, whether child or invalid—in other words, every woman is a nurse (Nightingale 1969:3).

As exemplified in the definitions above, for Nightingale to be a nurse is to be a woman first; this idea reinforces both the necessity and centrality of nursing as a human caring activity that has always fallen to women. But it also seriously disables the potential for nursing to be anything but merely women's work in a world that even today values men's work in every way more than women's. This is a double bind the grip of which will likely never relent in its capacity to constrain the possibilities for nurses to exercise power in any way commensurate with, for example, medicine's capacity to do so.

THE ESSENTIAL NURSE

Embedded within the discussion above are the manifestations of a particular philosophical position (actually an existential philosophical position concerning what it means to be a human being), namely: *essentialism*. This philosophy allows someone to claim the truth that 'a man is a man down to his very thumbs, and a woman is a woman down to her little toes' (Thomson & Thomson 1911:4); or that women are 'longer lived' than men because 'their constitution has staying powers, probably wrapped up with femaleness' (Thomson & Thomson 1911:7). In other words, there is something *inherently* female about women and equally something *inherently* male about men; this is what is called an 'essence' and it is self-evident and needs no further explanation (so you can appreciate how seductive an idea this is to those who want simplicity and certainty to prevail).

Essentialism has its roots in another philosophical viewpoint: *biological determinism* (anatomy and physiology exclusively determine whether we are male or female; boys/men have a penis; girls/women have vaginas; function follows form). Essentialism draws on this determinism very strongly to posit an essence—or a universal, immutable and sex-specific set of qualities and behaviours—of maleness and femaleness, as I suggested above.

But essentialism is also closely related to another significant philosophical stance, both embraced by and reflected in early conceptions of nursing: *naturalism*. Consider the following remarks from the previously cited Thomson and Thomson text, *The position of woman: actual and ideal*:

It seems consistent that men should fight, if there is fighting to be done; and that women should nurse, if there is nursing necessary. Man hunted and explored, women made the home and brought up the children . . . [a] woman is *naturally* a teacher of the young, a domesticator, a gardener, and so on (Thomson & Thomson 1911:15, emphasis in the original).

Furthermore, these authors justify their remarks:

When we say that this or that occupational differentiation is natural to women we do not simply mean it is sanctioned by convention. We mean that it is congruent with *femaleness*, that it occurs in many races and countries, and that it has stood for a long time the test of eliminative selection (Thomson & Thomson 1911:15–16, emphasis added).

In this statement the link between essentialism and naturalism is bald-faced. Naturalism also posits a timeless and universal femaleness and maleness inherited since the origin of the species and it is simply 'God-given' in the great order of beings (reflect, for example, on the concept of 'human nature' and how much of human behaviour we 'explain away' by this concept without giving it another thought). Indeed, naturalism still exerts enormous influence in the ways the world of work is carved into hierarchies of who is 'naturally' better equipped to do certain types of work and who not; consider that it was only in the last couple of decades that women were able to become airline pilots because of the fear that their hormonal fluctuations might render them temporarily unable to be in command of their emotions and therefore endanger the lives of their passengers. The very idea of a woman in charge of an airplane was for a very long time anathema to the airline industry (not to mention the travelling public) and probably still is to many.

If we examine nursing education texts throughout the last century we can see the significance of essentialism, naturalism and biological determinism in the ways nursing has been inextricably linked to the female of the species and how this has shaped the form and content of nursing education and, ultimately, what a nurse is and does (e.g. Watson 1908, Cuff & Gordon Pugh 1924, Burbridge 1935, Nixon & Wakeley 1948, Hansen 1958, Brackman Keane 1969). This reality pretty much fully explains why even in the early twenty-first century only about 10% of the world's nurses are men. And by now you should be better able to appreciate how—as Nietzsche (cited in Hayman 1997:38) put it: 'Every philosophy conceals another philosophy'.

By way of advancing the analysis of how philosophies insert themselves into nursing, I want to draw on the work of a very significant philosopher whose work has deeply influenced my own, namely Michel Foucault (1926–84). Much of Foucault's early intellectual project was to explore how 'knowledge' (and philosophy as a form of knowledge) came to be constructed in so limited and uncompromising a way (Foucault 1970, 1972, 1978). In his work he unpacked the various forces and structures at play in the development of the modern or civilised Western world, and advanced the still quite radical notion that truth and its effects is intimately connected to knowledge production, which in turn is bound up in the exercise of power (Foucault 1978).

These three things—knowledge, truth and power—all interact through language in such a way so as to produce certain disciplines (such as science and the law). These disciplines, in turn, generate an authority for themselves by enabling those subscribing to the discipline to speak of and define the disciplines' territory, address specific audiences and, in so doing, compete for supremacy of position among the various disciplines. In the process, the disciplines' disciples would have us believe that certain truths are more significant than others; indeed, how some are absolute.

This is how science as a discipline has come to dominate our contemporary times as the most revered form of knowledge; indeed, it is *the* truth of things for many communities of professionals. Nursing too has been seduced by the authority of science and has been very concerned to define itself as a science in order to augment its authority and prestige. There is also a chapter in this text dedicated to exploring this notion of nursing as a science (Ch 3), and I will not enter this debate directly (although as you read into this chapter you will discover how certain philosophies closely linked with science have influenced and expedited nursing's development as a science).

(HU)MANKIND AND ITS PHILOSOPHIES OF SELF-DEFINITION AND WORLDLY DEFINITION

Undoubtedly, given the historical epoch in which modern nursing was conceived, much of nursing's theory and philosophical development has been strongly humanist in orientation. *Humanism* is perhaps the most influential philosophy of the last 400 years because of the ways it has shaped government, religion, politics and much else besides. Humanism, in a word, posits that humans are the sovereigns of their kingdom, which is to say, the world as we know it. Humans are able to so claim because they, unlike any other member of the animal kingdom, are possessed of an intelligence, which provides the higher order functions such as language and the capacity for rational thought. Indeed, humanism posits that the human beings *are* the rational authors of their own lives because they possess a stable, coherent and self-same identity, which enables their capacity to act purposefully on the world around them to their own benefit (see McLaren 1988, Rogers 1980, Weedon 1997, Lather 1991b, Johnson 1994).

Humanism is especially attractive to a profession such as nursing, which clearly has humans and their interests, needs and wants as the main focus of, and reason for, its very existence. However, humanism is also a gendered philosophy, which again creates problems for nursing's unproblematic appropriation of it as a defining force in curriculum and practice. Reflect for a moment on the concept of 'mankind': why is it that the term for the collective of men and women, of humanity, is gendered male? Even today after decades of feminist thought and activism, I hear humanity referred to as mankind more often than not. This reality serves to highlight, once again, the deeply political nature of language and the philosophies underpinning it. Everything 'man' does is given greater value than that which woman does, as Irigaray reminds us:

> Man seems to have wanted, directly or indirectly, to give the universe his own gender as he wanted to give his own name to his children, his wife, his possessions. This has significant bearing on the sexes' relationships to the world, to things, to objects. In fact, anything believed to have value belongs to men and is marked by their gender. Apart from possessions in the strict sense that man attributes to himself, he gives

his own gender to God [le Dieu], to the sun [le soleil], and also, in the guise of the neuter, to the laws of the cosmos and of the social or individual order. He doesn't even question the genealogy of his attribution (Irigaray 1993:31–2).

Nursing then, as a deeply female gendered profession, has always to contend with the ever-present reality of patriarchy: a world created by men, for men and to whom women are sometimes equal but, mostly, are not. Humanism is therefore best understood as a philosophy in the service of patriarchy, and to illustrate just how influential humanism has been in nursing let me cite from a couple of the numerous American scholars who led the development of nursing theories from the 1950s through to the late 1980s (a period when humanist thought was especially influential in a number of other disciplines including psychology, education and organisational theory). As you will see, these nurse scholars share a deep commitment to situating the unique, individual human being at the heart of their theories around which invariably wind the core concepts of environment, health and nursing.

For Imogene King (1981, 1987) and her interpersonal/systems interaction model of nursing, humans are 'open systems interacting with environment' (King 1981:10) and are viewed as 'rational, sentient, reacting, social, controlling, purposeful, time-oriented, and action-oriented' beings (King 1987:107). Calista Roy takes a similar line in her work when she asserts that the individual 'shares in creative power; behaves purposefully, not in a sequence of cause and effect; possesses intrinsic holism; and strives to maintain integrity and realise the need for relationships' (Barone & Roy 1996:66). Moreover, the individual in society is best understood in the context of the 'purposefulness of human existence; unity of purpose of humankind; activity and creativity for the common good; and value and meaning of life' (Roy & Andrews 1999:83).

Clearly the autonomous, self-defining human being is accorded primacy in these statements, which exemplify the logic of humanism and its emphasis on the significance of human relationships, sentience and rationality, and the forward-thrust of human life. And as you can see, another important philosophical position is given voice in these theorists' work: *holism* or the idea that the whole is greater than the sum of its parts. The idea of the 'whole' or complete human being is another important facet of the philosophy of humanism, and the philosophy and language of holism currently dominates the rhetoric of healthcare policy and practice. Holism is particularly appealing for a human-centred service because it allows practitioners to imagine they are taking into account every aspect of their clients' needs and wants. Holism defines the human as a bio–psycho–social–spiritual being. You will already have come across this language I'm sure.

Holism is the philosophical opposite of *reductionism*: the idea that every whole can be broken up into its constituent parts. Medicine, for example, is essentially a reductionist science in that the human mind–body complex is reduced to ever-smaller components, as medical knowledge seeks to understand the total or whole organism by breaking it into its various organ systems and structures, examining their tissues and cells, and eventually looking at the cells and their components at the microscopic level. Modern medicine has made reductionism into a highly sophisticated science from which the various medical specialties and subspecialties arise—for example, neurology (the study of the nervous system) or neuroendocrinology (the study of the hormones of the nervous system).

Medicine—as a science—is essentially founded on the philosophy of *empiricism*, or the notion that the only true knowledge is derived from the rigours of experimental method. Empiricism encourages reductionism in the way it insists on increasingly rigorous examination of cause-and-effect relationships at the finest level of detail. Hence, we have the appearance of disciplines such as microbiology (the study of pathological organisms) and microphysics (the study of atomic particles). These disciplines strongly influence the development of nursing as a science and without which it would undoubtedly look more like an art or craft than the highly technologically driven and biomedically oriented profession it is today.

Nursing has become ever-more reductionist throughout the twentieth century, as it too has been obliged to follow medicine down this philosophical and practical path; the trouble is that reductionism inherently devalues the total organism. Reductionism sits very awkwardly with nursing's need to be seen to be caring for a whole human being. So we live with a considerable tension in nursing—preaching one philosophy (holism), while mostly practising its absolute antithesis (reductionism). This paradox has come about largely through the influence of another significant philosophical position: *Cartesianism*.

Rene Descartes was an Enlightenment philosopher (1596–1650) deeply committed to the project of harnessing scientific thought and method in order to better understand and intervene in the world. He coined the now famous phrase: *I think, therefore I am*. This maxim became the founding principle of what it is to be a modern human being and further endorsed humanism as the defining philosophy for society's men and women.

Cartesianism was forged on the anvil of another important philosophical doctrine: *rationalism*, the notion that the only way to truth is through the deliberations of the rational human mind. Descartes' key insight was that the only thing he could not doubt as a rational thinking creature was the fact that his thinking *proved* his existence as a sentient human being. He could be sure of his capacity to reason, but he could not be sure of what his senses (via his body) told him; consequently, he regarded the body 'as a source of interference in, and a danger to, the operation of reason' (Grosz 1994:5). This led him to assert that the 'mind and body are distinct entities. In his view, the mind exists in time only, whereas the body, unlike the mind, is physical and has extension in space' (Benner & Wrubel 1989:33).

This idea that the thinking mind is completely separate from a non-thinking body (Cartesianism) is responsible for the way modern medicine and healthcare still tend to treat problems of the mind with one science (psychology/psychiatry) and problems of the body with another (medicine/surgery). In contemporary healthcare we even go so far as to treat people with problems of the mind in one institution (the psychiatric hospital/clinic) and problems of the body in another (the general hospital).

Descartes' then-radical ideas also spawned a related philosophy: *mechanism*. Descartes thought the world and human beings could be analysed and problems diagnosed by understanding them as something rather like a machine (the clock to be precise). Just as the clock has a variety of interconnected parts, each of which needs to be delicately attuned to the others in order for the clock to function smoothly, so too, the world and human beings could be understood. Therefore, in mechanistic philosophy the human body is explained as if it were simply a very complex machine with interconnecting parts. When something fails or doesn't work properly, it is merely a matter of locating the malfunction and putting it right. Modern surgery certainly makes sense of the human body in this way. So too, it can be argued, does nursing, given that philosophical frameworks for clinical practice are themselves predicated on strongly medical models of health and illness, which are, in turn, reductionist, mechanistic and, ultimately, Cartesian.

For a compelling example of how Cartesianism, reductionism and mechanism influence the everyday practice of nursing, I suggest you read Fassett and Gallagher's (1998) fascinating tale *Just a head: stories in a body*. This text brings to vivid expression the issues discussed above, and is a salutary reminder of the perils these philosophies inflict on real-life human actors and those charged with their care.

By now I expect you are a little perplexed by all these 'isms' and the incredible interconnectedness of them all. Indeed, this is why the study of philosophy is not only strenuous, but also profoundly rewarding (intellectually speaking). As humankind has sought ever-more sophisticated frameworks for making sense of themselves and their worlds, scholars have begun to appreciate how no one truth about those worlds is capable of defining them without the support of many others.

Of course, certain truths (as I hope you are beginning to realise) capture people's imaginations and win their hearts more than others. This depends entirely on how, where and when one is positioned in the world. Living in Enlightenment Europe (from the early sixteenth to the late eighteenth centuries) would have been a very heady experience because this is when much of the philosophical material I have been discussing came into being. It has only been in the last century that serious critiques and challenges to many of the doctrines espoused over these pages—to the 'received truths' they have generated—began to appear. These received truths became influential simply with the passing of time and in the absence of better alternatives.

THE TYRANNY OF 'ISMS': POSTMODERN PHILOSOPHY AS LIBERATOR

I want now to make clear the philosophical ideas that have informed my writing and, in doing so, will return us to the place from which we began. For as must by now be fairly obvious to you, there is a sort of circuitous and mutually reinforcing logic operating between all these different but related philosophical positions. You will recall I mentioned early in the chapter how nursing hasn't always been aware of how philosophy inserts itself into our everyday thinking and behaving, and this is partly the reason why. The philosophies I have been unpacking here are experienced only subliminally by most of us in the sense that we have assimilated them into our ways of thinking to the point where we cannot actually think at all without their influence.

Postmodern philosophy, however, provides us with a rather neat reality check in respect of this problem. I have found it enormously useful as I have grappled with how I have come to be the nurse I am and why. In bringing to a close this admittedly superficial and rather attenuated discussion on nursing and the politics of truth, I would like to suggest a way forward for nursing's relationship to philosophy, which has been rather fraught with a certain ambivalence, if not hostility. I make this seemingly alarmist assertion with good reason. The gender issue that I have belaboured throughout is at the root of my concerns. Let me explain. Elizabeth Grosz, an Australian feminist scholar reminds us:

> As a discipline, philosophy has surreptitiously excluded femininity, and ultimately women, from its practices through its usually implicit coding of femininity with the unreason associated with the body (Grosz 1994:4).

As I have attempted to trace the influence of particular philosophies on nursing, it might have struck you that there is a peculiar logic at play within and/or between them. Either the philosophy is inflexible because its truth claims rest on the basis of their (seeming) self-evidence (essentialism, naturalism, biological determinism) or a philosophy is wedded to a particular thinker's ideas (Cartesianism, mechanism). Conversely, the philosophy may be the product of a whole line of thinkers over an extended period who mutually reinforce the veracity of its propositions over this time and thereby cement its worth in the collective psyche of humanity (empiricism, rationalism, science). Or, differently again, one philosophical viewpoint tends to sit uncomfortably in relation with, and is often all but cancelled out by, its opposites (holism versus reductionism).

Postmodern philosophy is a creature born of these tensions to which I have just given voice. Postmodernism attempts to understand how these tensions arise and what effects they invoke. Postmodernism is not one philosophy, but a hybrid of many, and its value lies in its insistence that Truth (as absolute and unimpeachable) is a necessary figment of the philosophical imagination that is now rather bankrupt in the sense that clearly *multiple* truths abound—not all of which are useful, some of which are plainly dangerous, but also many of which can be decidedly illuminating of the human condition and advance its development.

Postmodernism has received plenty of flak ever since it first appeared on the cultural landscape in the early 1960s. Its antagonists argue that it is philosophically and politically corrupt because it disallows any single claim to the truth in favour of all truths being relative. This *relativism* is said to be exceedingly unhelpful because it does not help people adjudicate between competing claims to the truth and therefore disenfranchises them in many ways. I agree postmodernism in its extreme relativistic forms is problematic for these reasons, but this is not the version I subscribe to. Some truths are more helpful than others and we need to be able to figure out how to differentiate between them and make decisions on the basis of our analyses. This has been the work of this chapter; I have tried to show how certain philosophical positions have produced a set of truths about what nursing is and what it is to be a nurse. Others, too, have been busy this last decade or so exploring nursing from postmodern positions, and shedding light on complex and fascinating issues and concerns hitherto unthought (e.g. Brennan 1998, Latimer 1998, Parker & Gibbs 1998, Whittaker 1998, Anderson, 2004, Pryce 2004, Parker 2004).

Postmodern philosophy, then, is best thought of as a radical questioning of all that has passed in the name of philosophy. Such questioning temporarily decentres the authority of previous philosophies and, in doing so, opens the way for new and hopefully more constructive ways of reflecting on our relationship to the (many) truths that shape our everyday worlds. Why does Grosz voice her concern above in relation to philosophy's exclusion of femininity and women from its development and ongoing construction? Once again the answer lies in the problem of gender.

Postmodern philosophers have uncovered a powerful effect of knowledge production they call 'binary logic' or 'dichotomous thinking'. Once again, as Grosz tells us:

. . . feminists and philosophers seem to share a common view of the human subject as a being made up of two dichotomously opposed characteristics: mind and body, thought and extension, reason and passion, psychology and biology (Grosz 1994:3).

You will now be familiar with how this logic manifests in some of the philosophies we have been discussing on these pages.

As Grosz continues to explain, this

. . . bifurcation of being is not simply a neutral division of an otherwise all-encompassing descriptive field. Dichotomous thinking necessarily hierarchies and ranks the two polarised terms so that one becomes the privileged term and the other its suppressed, subordinated, negative counterpart . . . [b]ody is thus what is not mind, what is distinct from and other than the privileged term (Grosz 1994:3).

It is equally significant that this mind/body opposition is linked to a whole series of related oppositions which, by association, can function in place of the mind/body pairing.

For example, as Grosz puts it:

[T]he mind/body relation is frequently correlated with the distinctions between: Reason and passion, sense and sensibility, inside and outside, self and other, depth and surface, reality and appearance, mechanism and vitalism . . . temporality and spatiality, psychology and physiology, form and matter, and so on (Grosz 1994:3).

What is absolutely pivotal to this hierarchy of opposing terms is that the first term (e.g. mind) is assigned the male gender—and, as Irigaray reminded us earlier (1993), everything of value man has assigned his name to. Consequently, the second, subordinated term in the logic of binaries is relegated the female gender. This is how the great gender divide actually works: not only is it merely a reflection of the inequality of the species in terms of who gets to do what in the world (as my earlier discussion emphasised), it actually produces this inequality because it is deeply reinforced at the level of language. Indeed, language subtly authorises so much of what we do without our ever realising it, and this is why I have insisted on the uncontestable centrality of language as not just reflecting the world so we can give it meaning, but that it actually brings the world into view in highly particular ways.

Thus the female of the species is associated with the human body, whereas the male claims the human mind; similarly, reason is linked with the mind and with men, passion with women and the body. Intellectual work is therefore most properly men's work, whereas caring (which is intimately associated with the body) is consigned to women. And these distinctions are non-negotiable and irreversible. This is why Grosz (1994) can claim that philosophy has largely neglected to include women in its development because it simply never entered men's minds to do so. Women, men have argued, are much less well-suited to engage in this kind of work, but are naturally, essentially and biologically best suited to nurture, suckle, care for and assist others in the care of their bodies. And so we are returned to our definitions of nursing and to Nightingale's injunction that to be a nurse is first to be a woman!

LAST WORDS: TOWARDS A FEMINIST POSTMODERN PHILOSOPHY FOR NURSES

Ironically, nursing and *feminism* have never been happy bedfellows. This is partly because, as 'naturally' women's work, feminists have been rather disinclined towards the study of nursing, seeing little point in making so obviously female gendered an occupation the object of their philosophical gaze (which of course merely reflects and endorses the largely misogynist leanings of masculinist philosophy and its history). Nurses, too, have generally been reluctant to embrace feminism for the very reason that it exposes all the inequities and tensions conjured up in the very idea that nursing is naturally women's work; to be sure, many, if not most, nurses have wanted to believe the truth that nursing is all but exclusively women's work because it has matched their (largely uncritical) version of what it means to be a woman in the first place. That said, I believe feminism and postmodern philosophy can and must be considered as an ally for nurses and nursing. This is because feminism squarely places women on the philosophical and political agenda and lets nothing escape its scrutiny, as it pursues ever-more cogent truths about what it means to be a woman.

Postmodernism, as I hope you now better understand through my attempts here to demonstrate how it works in practice, seeks to unsettle the hard-baked certainties of previous philosophical positions by pointing out the often shaky and untenable foundations on which they rest. Therefore, combining feminism and postmodernism seems a sensible way to proceed if nursing and philosophy are to have a more meaningful relationship and if nurses are to better understand and critique the repressive and less enabling philosophies that have previously kept us in our places (read doctors' 'handmaidens' and patients' 'angels of mercy'). However, this journey to another philosophical home for nursing is not likely to be easy.

Perhaps the most significant obstacle we have to moving forward in this endeavour is the profound anti-intellectualism nursing's history and culture has produced (Walker 1997). This anti-intellectualism is born of the same dichotomous thinking I discussed above. If a nurse's very raison d'être is wound around her (essentially/ naturally/biologically determined) feminine capacity to care for and nurture others, and that caring/nurturing work is closely related to people's bodies while it also requires the fairly heavy investment and cooperation of nurses' own bodies (nursing being generally hard physical labour), then you can appreciate how purely intellectual work (i.e. philosophy) is not likely to receive much attention let alone a high priority in nursing. Without a doubt, it is difficult to know quite how to inspire nurses to even 'think philosophically' let alone engage in the rigours of actually producing philosophical writings. But perhaps this is not what is at issue anyway.

As Silverman (1994:233) tells us, 'philosophy begins in wonder for it has to have something to wonder about'. A place to begin such a project of 'wondering' in nursing is to ask how and why nursing has been cluttered with definitions—not all of them written by nurses—about who or what a nurse is (and can be) and what she or he does (or could do). The work of this chapter has been to start this process of asking questions about our identity and the powerful and largely intangible influences that have come to shape our sense of what it means to be a nurse. As you might now be more aware, in many ways we have not been the rational authors of our life the philosophers such as Descartes would have us believe, because the script was 'always already' written for us by others (who certainly were not nurses).

As nurses and nursing engage with the vicissitudes of life in a new era and with the legacy of our history now more explicit and available to all, perhaps we can begin to imagine a relationship with philosophy that enables us to re-vision and re-fashion ourselves in ways that truly reflect the contribution our knowledge, skills and actions have on those in our care. While I have brushed over the whole issue of 'caring' as a philosophy for nursing (and there is another chapter in this text devoted to this idea (Ch 6)), there can be no doubt in my mind at least that a feminist and postmodern philosophy of caring holds considerable promise for nursing in terms of providing guidance and intellectual succour to the profession. As I said in the closing words to my chapter in the first edition of *Contexts of nursing*, and which are certainly no less relevant now:

> The most appropriate philosophical discourse for nursing is one that is demonstrably feminist in that it places gender firmly on the agenda; [it must also be] overtly critical in that it asks difficult questions about all those concerns with which nursing has been struggling for so long. But it must do this within a context that helps us devise strategies for change at the level of *practice*. Indeed, the relationship between nursing and philosophy must begin with the practice of nursing and end there. Why else, if nursing is 'in the "truth" of things', a practice discipline, would we bother? (Walker 2000:64)

REFLECTIVE QUESTIONS

1 How and why are the times in which nurses find themselves influenced by the history of philosophy?

2 Why is our thinking and acting not always apparent to us and sometimes even in conflict?

3 How can we challenge the received wisdoms through which we live, in order to live differently, if not better, than perhaps we do?

RECOMMENDED READINGS

Cahoone L ed 1996 *From modernism to postmodernism: an anthology*. Blackwell Science, Oxford.

Foucault M 1997 In S Lotringer & L Hochroth (eds) *The politics of truth*. Semiotext(e), New York.

Heidegger M 1982 *On the way to language*. Harper & Row, San Fransisco.

Lentricchia F, McLaughlin T eds 1990 *Critical terms for literary study*. University of Chicago Press, Chicago.

Shotter J 1994 *The cultural politics of everyday life*. Open University Press, Buckingham.

CHAPTER SIX

Nursing care and nurse caring: issues, concerns, debates

Debra Jackson & Sally Borbasi

LEARNING OBJECTIVES

This chapter will:

- ▲ introduce caring as a professional concept that is entwined with understandings about nurses and nursing;

- ▲ explore caring as a theoretical concept;

- ▲ discuss perceptions of nurse caring from the perspective of patients/ clients;

- ▲ provide an overview of issues related to care and cure;

- ▲ critique caring as the basis of the discipline of nursing; and

- ▲ contemplate threats to nurse caring.

KEY WORDS
Caring, clinical nursing, cure, work, patients/clients

NURSING AND CARING

The concept of caring is intertwined with nursing—some literature even states that caring and nursing are synonymous (Wilkin & Slevin 2004)—and has been identified as central to the theory and practice of nurses. Several major theories of nursing recognise caring as one of the foundational elements of nursing (Watson 1985b, Leininger 1986, Boykin & Schoenhofer 2001, Watson et al 2005). Efforts to theorise caring, and understand it as a concept that is able to be compatible with, and integral to, the practice of nursing, has occupied a lot of energy in nursing for a number of years, and is an area that continues to attract the attention of nurse scholars from all over the world. The close relationship of nursing and caring is able to be seen in the many definitions and perspectives of nursing which position caring as inherent and central to the nursing role (e.g. Benner 1984, Leininger 1984, Rawnsley 1990, Swanson 1993, Watson 1988, Bassett 2002, Watson et al 2005).

At first glance, the concept of caring may appear to be simple and uncomplicated. It is a generic word and one that is widely used in the general lexicon—meaning that it is not 'owned' specifically by nursing and nor does it apply only to nurses and nursing. General dictionary definitions of caring define it in simple terms. However, when used in relation to nursing, the concept of care cannot be oversimplified. Terms such as *nursing care* and *nurse caring* carry certain meanings and understandings. In these contexts, care is a complex, multidimensional concept that is positioned as the characteristic that distinguishes nursing, and sets it apart from other health-related activities (Jackson & Borbasi 2000). Although a caring perspective is not unique to nursing, it is widely accepted that nursing has an essential role to care for the health of individuals, families and communities, and many believe the care given by nurses has the potential to restore health (Benner et al 1999, Watson & Foster 2003).

In this chapter we introduce caring as a professional concept, and acquaint you with some of the major arguments and viewpoints associated with caring in general and nurse caring in particular. In writing this chapter we have drawn on a substantial body of international literature that reflects some of the major perspectives of nurse caring that have been published over the past 20 years. In reading it, you will gain an appreciation of the longitudinal and international nature of the debates and discussions around caring. Furthermore, you will see that many of the issues remain unresolved, and that this is one debate that will continue into your own nursing careers.

CARING AS A THEORETICAL CONCEPT

The complexity around such a seemingly uncomplicated and simple concept such as caring can be seen when one considers the plethora of literature devoted to it. Even a cursory database search on caring will generate copious literature on the subject. Try it! Upon examining this literature you will see it reveals a multitude of definitions, and various positions on the ways that caring can be conceptualised. For example, in 1990 Rawnsley noted that caring:

. . . has been proposed to be a philosophy and science, an ethic, an interactive set of client expectations and nursing behaviours, expert nursing practice, the hidden work of nursing and a synonym for nursing itself (Rawnsley 1990:42).

There is general agreement about the difficulties associated with defining and positioning caring (Beck 1999, Paley 2001, Bassett 2002). What is more, it has even been suggested that the task of rescuing the concept of caring from its elusivity is impossible, a situation Paley (2001) attributes to problematic suppositions about the nature of knowledge. Nevertheless, even accounting for the difficulties associated with defining caring, the importance of exploring how nurses have theorised and attempted to understand the elusive nature of a concept so central to their practice cannot be underestimated.

Let's look at more of the literature. Many nurses consider caring as being primarily a relationship between nurse and others (Hoover 2002) in which experiences are shared. Consider Pearson (1991:199), for example; he describes the broad, global human concept of caring as 'investing oneself in the experience of another sufficiently enough to become a participant in that person's experience'. Sullivan and Deane (1994) assert that nurse caring prizes human relationships, and is informed by principles of sharing, sincerity, concern and moderation. Wolf et al (1994:107) propose that nurse caring has several tangible dimensions, including 'respectful deference to others, assurance of human presence, positive connectedness, professional knowledge and skill, and attentiveness to the other's experience'.

In addition, caring is understood to have intellectual as well as emotional aspects (Kapborg & Bertero 2003), and in 1992 Pepin suggested two dimensions of caring: love and labour. Love is said to consist of affective (i.e. pertaining to feelings) concepts such as altruism, compassion, emotion, presence, connectedness, nurturance and comfort, and it is this aspect of caring that has dominated the nursing literature (Pepin 1992). Labour refers to the element of care related to toil and service, and encompasses roles, functions, knowledge and tasks. Though Pepin (1992) suggests that this latter dimension of caring has received much less attention in the nursing literature, a number of these issues are discussed in some depth in nursing discourses on topics such as competency and clinical expertise (e.g. Hardy et al 2002).

If we look at feminist and nurse Falk Rafael's (1996:3–17) work, she suggests caring may be considered either 'ordered caring', 'assimilated caring' or 'empowered caring' (p 4). Ordered caring, she proposes, is problematic for nurses because it is about merely following orders; 'it allows only a severely limited scope of caring, one that is devoid of knowledge, power or ethics' (Falk Rafael 1996:11). To illustrate this point, she draws on the example of the kindness and gentleness shown by nurses towards psychiatric patients as they were led towards the Nazi gas chambers. Assimilated caring is described as a form of caring in which the feminine construct of caring is grounded in (male) scientific discourses. This appropriation of a male construct is proposed as giving legitimacy to the essentially female activity of caring. Falk Rafael positions empowered caring as the most desirable and effective form of caring. This form of caring is grounded within a feminist perspective, and involves the use of power, knowledge and ethics. Falk Rafael (1996) proposes the acronym of CARE (credentials, association, research, expertise) to encapsulate the elements of this empowered caring.

Another theorist you may have found through your literature searching proposed holistic caring as a form of nurse caring (Williams 1997). Williams (1997) regards this as a global concept with four dimensions that she names physical caring, interpretive caring, spiritual caring and sensitive caring. No doubt known to you, holism is a concept crucial to the effective practice of nursing, and is a term used to describe the nurse's belief that a 'patient is a person with social, physical, mental, and spiritual components' (Williams 1997:61–2). Holism is positioned as central to notions of professional caring, and is so intrinsic to this, it is often taken for granted—viewed as a 'given', and therefore often not described or examined in discussions on professional caring. The use of a holistic perspective is said to facilitate an ethos that recognises the uniqueness and value inherent in individuals, and allows for the provision of individualised nursing care.

Several theories of nursing have been developed from the standpoint of defining and describing caring practices. Leininger (1986) believes caring is the essence of nursing but dismisses the idea of nurses' care motivated by a sense of duty. Rather, she considers caring as learned because it is an integral part of cultural life. However, factors within various cultures (e.g. gender) may either curtail or facilitate the use of care knowledge by nurses. Watson (1988), another well-known luminary on the subject, writes of a science (and practice) of caring, and conceptualises caring as the ethical and moral ideal of nursing. More recently, a theory of 'nursing as caring' has been offered by Boykin and Schoenhofer (2001) who consider human beings as a species to be innately caring, and that reaching one's full potential in terms of caring is a lifelong process.

EXPERIENCING NURSE CARING: WHAT DO PATIENTS SAY?

Upholding the theory that caring is a concept central to the practice of nurses is not only important for the profession, but is also highly significant for the recipients of that care. Yet if you explore the literature, what patients want has rarely been discussed in nurses' deliberations about the art of caring (Webb 1996). Notwithstanding, it makes sense that if nurses are to claim they are caring professionals, they are obliged to find out what nurse caring means to patients, and how nurses can demonstrate care for patients (Larsson et al 1998). Somewhat ironically it has been the rise of quality improvement processes over the last few years that has spearheaded the interest in patients' views about the care they receive in healthcare settings, and this movement has not been led by nurses, but economists. Another determinant of mounting interest in patients' satisfaction with care is the fact that patients are no longer ill informed, passive recipients of health services, but increasingly informed and active consumers that expect a certain standard of care and are not afraid to litigate should their expectations not be met.

Reflection

- Have you ever been a recipient of a health service?
- What approach/es do you take if the 'care' you receive falls short of your expectations?

- What are your expectations of 'care'?
- Are you able to articulate them?
- If you *have* experienced being a patient, would you say that your perceptions of what constitutes caring were different from those you hold when you practise as a nurse or nursing student?

If we continue our literature searching, some of the published studies over the last decade that have looked at the notion of care from patient and nurse perspectives articulate some of these expectations for us. If we look, for example, at studies that explore patient experiences of being nursed from a qualitative perspective, we can see that a phenomenological study discovered that patients perceive their care can be delivered either in 'detached' mode or through 'engagement' (Kralik et al 1997). The theme of engagement captured psychosocial qualities such as compassion, kindness, cheerfulness, availability, gentleness and friendliness, while detachment reflected negative characteristics such as feeling depersonalised by nurses and being treated roughly by nurses. Findings of this study are particularly interesting because, although nursing is examined from the perspective of patients, it reflects consistencies between patients' views and ideas about nurse caring held by nurses.

Describing a pilot project aimed at eliciting constructions of behaviours and attitudes that embody caring from the perspectives of registered nurses, Dyson (1996) found that nurses conceptualised caring as essentially an interpersonal construct. She identified attributes such as kindness, friendliness, sensitivity, consideration, giving of self, honesty, sincerity and expertise as evidence of caring attitudes and behaviours. Similarly, Wolf (1986) describes nurse-identified caring behaviours as attentive listening, comforting, honesty and so on. However, a 1998 study of patients and nurses, aimed at exploring perceptions of the importance of caring behaviours, revealed significant differences between the views of patients and nurses, with nurses placing a higher value on the emotional affective aspects of caring (Larssen et al 1998).

Indeed if you delve more deeply into the literature it can be seen that patients' views of professional caring may be very different from those proposed by nurses, with nurses often (but not always) embracing psychosocial models of caring, while studies of patients often (but not always) suggesting that patients value caring that is more technical or task-orientated in nature. For example, one study exploring the caring behaviours of hospital nurses from patients' perspectives found physical caring behaviours such as 'monitoring' were ranked much higher than aspects of caring such as 'trusting relationships', which could be considered to be affective or psychosocial in nature (Greenhalgh et al 1998).

Another nursing theorist, Webb (1996), describes studies in which nurses and patients' perceptions of caring were sought. Again, nurses judged the interpersonal aspects of their work as more caring, and yet the patients valued technical know-how and clinical competence above interpersonal dimensions of caring. From these studies it was concluded, because their physical needs had primacy, patients could not focus on aspects other than physical/technical care, whereas for the nurses, clinical competence was taken for granted. Webb's (1996) review indicated that patients consistently value care that is technically competent and tangible in nature; she cautions nurses against placing too much emphasis on the psychological elements of care, and neglecting physical or technical aspects of care. In light of burgeoning technological intervention this advice appears sound. Yet, the difference in perceptions of caring between nurses and patients warrants consideration.

In Western industrialised societies, technological skills and expertise are viewed as high status, and the domain of 'professionals'. In times of vulnerability, such as when people are ill, they like to be assured they are in the care of competent health professionals, and perhaps view technological proficiency as evidence of such competence and expertise. The interpersonal aspects of caring so highly idealised by nurses may be viewed by patients as 'non-professional' caring—the type of caring available to them within their own social worlds, and not something they necessarily seek within a context of professional caring. It has been argued that the caring that occurs at home differs from that occurring in institutions (such as hospitals) and is mainly affective (Pepin 1992). Similarly, from the perspective of nurses, it has been suggested nurses perceive clinical competence as a given, and thus do not regard it as an indicator of nurse caring (Webb 1996).

More recent literature tends to explore nurse caring from the patient satisfaction angle. For example, a Norwegian study demonstrated a gender-related difference in satisfaction with the quality of nursing care between young female patients when compared to young male patients (Foss 2002). Young female patients perceived nurses to be less committed and caring, to have less time and to be less skilled.

Similarly, a Jordanian study that surveyed patients for their opinions of nursing care discovered that male patients tended to have a more positive experience of nursing care than their female counterparts. The most important predictors for satisfaction with care in this study, however, related to the nurse's ability to meet the patient's information needs, the amount of information provided and the time nurses spent with patients. Demonstrating respect and courtesy towards family and friends was considered another major predictor. Patients appreciated those nurses who 'told them what to expect in the next shift, took interest in them as persons, provided them with privacy and perceived them as friends'. The authors surmise the best aspects of nursing care are a 'happy atmosphere, patients' privacy and individualised care' (Ahmad & Alasad 2004:239).

Reflection

- What are your views on the findings by Ahmad and Alasad (2004)?
- Would you tend to agree/disagree with them?

In Sweden a study was conducted into patient satisfaction with nursing care at night (Oleni et al 2004). A number of nurses and patients were surveyed for their opinions. The study found a significant difference between nurses' and patients' assessments of patient care requirements in terms of nursing intervention. The nurses' assessments of nursing care were more positive than patients' perceptions. Patients scored lower for the concepts information and participation, observation and monitoring, and night rest. Again this study demonstrated the importance patients attach to nurses providing them with appropriate and adequate information in order to better place the patient to influence and take responsibility for the care they receive. Patients were less positive about nursing observation and monitoring, and almost a quarter of them were dissatisfied with their ability to rest at night.

If we look at the findings from a review of predominantly quantitative observational studies related to patient satisfaction with the care provided by nurses, patient satisfaction was revealed as contingent on a number of factors (Johansson et al 2002). These included technological competence, as well as being responsive, kind, attentive, calm and encouraging. Insufficient information was shown to be 'perhaps the most common cause of dissatisfaction' (Johansson et al 2002).

Even as we write this chapter the world of healthcare is changing and the way patient care is organised and delivered is undergoing constant reformation. Because it is a commodity limited in resources yet high in demand, the healthcare arena and all who service it are under duress to do more with less. Nurses everywhere are experiencing heavy workloads, long hours and increasingly complex professional demands. This is not a scenario conducive to the provision of personalised care and considered information giving.

Yet in the world of healthcare today it would appear the pendulum is returning to nursing interventions based on feeling as being more important for patient satisfaction than medical–technical interventions (Johansson et al 2002). Caring behaviour considered paramount to patient and family includes the creation of a natural and constructive relationship between nurse and patient—indeed the capacity to 'feel kinship' with the patient is attributed to the best nurses and the value of physical contact, especially if it has a comforting effect, should never be underestimated (Johansson et al 2002).

In essence, as a recent study of patient experience revealed, it is the ability of nurses being able to show that the patient is an important person and that nurses really *care about* them that epitomises the best nurse caring behaviours (Mok & Pui Chi Chiu 2004:482). And, it is undoubtedly, as Lumby (2001) so aptly puts it, patients who must ultimately judge whether we care (p 144). In a technologised world that values profit over people, it is hard to imagine that a nurse who exhibits caring behaviour could fail to make a difference.

CARE AND CURE

As you are no doubt aware, in a relatively short space of time, rapid developments in medical science, nursing knowledge and related health technologies have acted to dramatically improve patient outcomes and prolong life. We are now told that the human genome project and similar advances in science will lead to predicted increases in human life expectancy by as much as 25 years, and living into our hundreds will become commonplace (BBC online).

In most parts of the world, these same technologies have radically and permanently changed the face of nursing (Pepin 1992, Jackson 1995, Sandelowski 1997a), and this has been the catalyst for a discussion in nursing and health that has become known as the 'care/cure' debate (e.g. Baumann et al 1998, Leftwich 1993, King & Norsen 1994, Johnston & Cooper 1997, Webb 1996). For example, Johnston and Cooper (1997) suggest that the healthcare system in the United States was designed to cure illness and disease, rather than care for people and their health. This is the case for many Western healthcare systems, and provides a challenge for those whose main imperative is to care.

Clearly, caring alone will not meet all the health needs patients have but, as Webb (1996) points out, curing strategies may be insufficient unless accompanied by a caring dimension. Similarly, Morse et al (1990:11) pose the question, 'can a cure be realised without caring?' In recent times a number of nursing scholars have published work on the concept of nursing as a therapeutic activity in its own right and the need for effective therapeutic relationships if the patient is to be 'cured' (Ersser 1997, Johns 2001, Freshwater 2002, Ramjan 2004). Williams (1997) too has suggested caring is, in itself, essential to cure. She proposes that caring nurse behaviours have been demonstrated to have positive effects in terms of patients' wellness and, conversely, non-caring behaviours by nurses have been shown to negatively affect patient wellbeing and recovery.

The concepts of care and cure historically have been constructed as binary and oppositional. Moreover, the difference between the roles of nurse and physician is often centred on ideas of the nurse as caring and the physician as curing. Sullivan and Deane (1994; similarly, Caffrey & Caffrey 1994) suggest caring (as nursing) is viewed as a traditionally feminine activity, and has not been conferred the power and status of male-defined activities, of which the physician/curer may more easily lay claim.

Indeed, if we look back over time, we can see it was Florence Nightingale herself who appeared to reject the idea that nurses can have an essential curing role. In her book *Notes on nursing* (Nightingale 1859–1946:74), she states 'nature alone cures', but goes on to say 'what nursing has to do is to put the patient in the best position for nature to act upon him [sic]' (p 75). More recently, in defining professional caring, several scholars have contended these two concepts are not truly antagonistic (e.g. Leftwich 1993, King & Norsen 1994). Nurses identify elements of both caring and curing, and certain science-based skills and knowledge are highly valued as essential to caring (Carper 1978, Beare & Meyers 1994, Wolf et al 1994). Furthermore, patients themselves expect nurses to have a high level of professional proficiency and technical skill, which are associated with 'cure', and construct these as key aspects of professional caring (Ray 1987, Wolf et al 1994, Borbasi 1996).

King and Norsen (1994) contend that notions of 'care/cure' as solely the domain of either nurse (care) or physician (cure) are not helpful or acceptable, as nurses and physicians have both curing and caring dimensions to their practice areas (see also Leftwich 1993). In a similar vein, Webb (1996) urges nurses to overcome the cure/care dichotomy between medicine and nursing, and argues it is no longer important to distinguish the care given by specific professional groups but to focus instead on establishing clear goals of care. Rather than regarding notions of care and cure as being polarised or at opposite extremes then, it is more accurate to say the notions of care/cure are compatible and complementary. Both are acknowledged and accepted as key aspects of nursing's agenda, and both are reflected in the theories of professional caring constructed by nurses (Beare & Meyers 1994, Wolf et al 1994). Moreover, in today's health service we are seeing an increasing emphasis on multidisciplinary approaches to caring.

Having acknowledged that nursing is a composite of care and cure, it is perhaps ironical to note that the circumstances within which nurses find themselves working today probably mitigate against both. While some patients may be fortunate enough to be cured, technological and pharmacological advances have meant most are merely 'contained' in a state of chronic illness. Often these patients are aged with multiple co-morbidities, which makes caring for them extremely complex and, by the same token, nurses, because they are so occupied with administering medical treatments, overlook the nurse caring behaviours so important to patient satisfaction and wellbeing. Have we perhaps reached a stage where neither cure nor care is winning out?

CARING AS THE BASIS OF THE DISCIPLINE OF NURSING

In addition to being complex and multidimensional, caring is also controversial, for among members of the profession, the debates about the centrality of caring to nursing continue (Dyson 1996, Paley 2001, Cloyes 2002). There are conflicting trains of thought and these challenge the relevance and appropriateness of caring as a foundational aspect of nursing. Stockdale and Warelow (2000) raise concerns about the inconsistencies around care and caring, and the ill-defined nature of caring. They point out the difficulties associated with adopting care as the essence of nursing, when there is not a universal accepted definition from which nursing can continue to develop.

Kitson (1987) argues that if nurses choose to align themselves with care rather than cure, with the nurturing processes rather than with technology and treatment, then they will need to identify how to organise and put into operation those skills they possess. Successful execution of the caring role is, she believes, 'intimately bound up with having the necessary space to practice, sufficient room to manoeuvre and to be able to explore new areas of knowledge and expertise' (Kitson 1987:324).

Dunlop (1986) questions whether a science of caring is possible and resolves that, if it is, it will have to take a hermeneutical form (based on hermeneutics)—a 'form that in many ways does violence to our traditional ideas of science', but one that 'challenges the male hegemony of science' (Dunlop 1986:669). In a philosophical critique, Walker (1995) has also highlighted the problem of nurses' attempts to represent nursing as both a discourse of science and a discourse of caring.

The emergence of differing perspective(s) about the nature of nursing has not been without debate, and there are nurses who believe that an emphasis on alliance to concepts such as caring and holism, with their attendant rejection of the natural sciences, will do more harm than good to nursing's attempts to become a credible academic discipline. Indeed, in some quarters there is strident scepticism. Writing in 2002, Paley positions the ideology of caring as 'a slave morality', and goes on to state that:

> It represents an attack on the 'medical-scientific model', motivated by resentment, and designed to establish nursing's superiority. Its effects have been debilitating, and it has prevented nursing from becoming a 'noble' (that is, properly scientific) discipline (Paley 2002:25).

However, meeting the demands of the caring imperative concerned with cure requires that nurses have considerable specialist knowledge of a range of scientific disciplines such as pharmacology, anatomy, physiology, biochemistry, immunology, microbiology and physics. A sound scientific knowledge base is undeniably essential for nursing, given the need for continued development of the discipline and the need to meet the demands of increasingly technological societies; none would argue that competency in the scientific disciplines is not an essential aspect of nursing knowledge and integral to the caring imperative claimed by nursing.

THREATS TO CARING

From much of what we have said so far, it can be seen that the concept of caring is inherently incompatible with the underlying objectives of many of the organisational structures in which nurses find themselves today. In many parts of the (Western) world, healthcare is not intrinsically altruistic; nor is it based on any real system of equity (Lumby 2001). Rather, healthcare tends to be resourced on a fee-for-service basis, and access to healthcare services is therefore linked very strongly with an individual's ability to pay for such services. Healthcare is increasingly looked at with entrepreneurial, rather than philanthropic eyes. To investors, provision of healthcare services may represent an opportunity for profit, and even 'whilst appropriating the language and images of nursing for business purposes, many entrepreneurs treat professional nursing care as a commodity to be whittled away until it becomes impotent' (Jackson & Raftos 1997:38). Although, to be sure, nurses comprise the largest occupational/professional group within the healthcare system, the system itself is based on a set of values that directly challenges and compromises the very essence of nursing.

In the past it was thought that large, impersonal institutions, by their very nature, may devalue caring by providing little incentive or opportunity for nurses to demonstrate behaviours associated with caring, or failing to provide an environment where caring could be expressed (Morse et al 1990). Align that with today's healthcare system, shaped as it is, by overarching economic influences such as cost containment and profit margins, and we have even less of a platform for caring work. Economic imperatives have been the catalyst for reexamining the whole concept of 'patient care', and attempts have been made to reconceptualise traditional care delivery in order to come up with ways of doing more with less resources (Ray 1989, Caplan & Brown 1997, Johnston & Cooper 1997). These new approaches in provision of care are sometimes presented as strategies to improve patient care but, as Williams (1997) suggests, frequently they are more concerned with institutional cost saving, than on quality patient care (similarly, Duffield & Lumby 1994, Lumby 2001).

This positioning of the wealth of an individual as a major indicator for allocation of (increasingly scarce) health resources is, by its very nature, incompatible with nursing's caring imperative, which places a high value on the individual (Chinn 1989, Morse et al 1990, Williams 1997). Care is most likely viewed by nurses as a resource to be allocated on the basis of need rather than ability to pay. These tensions are inherent in the working life of many nurses, and compromise the ability of nurses to provide care in the way idealised by the profession.

This key philosophical difference between nursing's caring imperative, and the underlying ethos of many (Western) healthcare systems, throws nurses and health administrators into a permanent state of possible conflict, and has the potential to become a source of professional tension for nurses (Jackson & Raftos 1997, Johnston & Cooper 1997, Kralic et al 1997). As a result many nurses leave nursing disillusioned with a 'system' that inhibits nurse caring behaviour. As we have experienced on an international scale, this contributes to critical shortages of nursing staff, which places the system, including patients and remaining staff, under even greater duress.

More than a decade ago Ray (1989) attempted to reconcile the seemingly irreconcilable by proposing a theory of caring compatible with the bureaucratic cultures existing within large organisations. She suggested it is essential the discipline of nursing comes to terms with the corporatisation of healthcare, and that a failure to do this would be disastrous for nursing.

> The transformation of American and other western health care systems to corporate enterprises emphasizing competitive management and economic gain seriously challenges nursing's humanistic philosophies and theories and nursing's administrative and clinical practices. The recent refocusing of nursing as a human science and the art and science of human caring places nursing in a vulnerable position. When pitted against the new goal of corporate advancement in health care delivery, nursing faces a loss of self-identity and an increased risk of alienation and confusion in this competitive arena (Ray 1989:31).

Using a grounded theory approach, Ray generated a 'theory of the dynamic structure of caring in a complex organization' (Ray 1989:31), and proposes this as a means by which nurses can practise within bureaucratic health structures without compromising nursing's caring imperative. This theory proposes several 'structural caring categories', which Ray names as political, economic, legal, technological/physiological, educational, social, spiritual/religious and ethical (Ray 1989). However, Caffrey and Caffrey (1994) suggest that caring will never be accommodated as a core value while profit remains a primary motive of healthcare systems.

The truth of this statement is evident in a paper exploring the experience of whistleblowers—registered nurses who attempted to challenge managerial practices that severely compromised the standard of care provided to residents of a long-term care institution (Jackson & Raftos 1997). These nurses described the struggle to maintain their professional integrity by ensuring adequate levels of care, and how they were thwarted in these attempts by the management. The nurses were prevented from providing adequate care by forces external to nursing—forces driven by an economic (rather than a caring) agenda. This suggests that, certainly in some settings, nurses have not yet achieved the level of autonomy necessary for the provision of acceptable and approved standards of professional care.

Insidiously, over the last few years, further threats to nurse caring have emerged, largely in the form of unregulated healthcare workers and the implementation of education and training programs for new breeds of healthcare practitioners (National Health Service Modernisation Agency 2005). While nurses may have expanded and extended their roles at upper echelons in the health system, they need to be constantly on guard at the rear end: never more so than in a time of cost constraint and massive shortfalls in registered nurse numbers. It may well be that nursing, as we know it today, will shortly be overrun by workers who will not only do the job, but do it without any regard to caring as nurses have conceptualised it.

CONCLUDING THOUGHTS

Caring is proclaimed and understood as the basis of modern nursing, and as you are discovering, nurses have produced vast amounts of literature on aspects of care and caring, and how they may be applied in a nursing context. However, while the concept of professional caring is difficult to articulate, it is recognised as being a complex concept involving the development of a range of knowledge, skills and expertise. Professional caring has similarities with non-professional, or informal, caring and applies knowledge derived from various discipline areas to promote the health and wellbeing of people.

The major perspectives of caring recognise the importance of various types of knowledge and, with few exceptions, all allude to the expressive, artistic and scientific perspectives said to construct nursing. Other common themes that characterise the constructions of caring adopted by nurses are holism, compassion, empathy and communication. Evidence suggests that patients, too, view caring as a perceptible concept, and highly value it as an essential and healing aspect of their professional encounters with nurses. However, in contrast to the ways nurses view caring, reflection on what is known about patients' attitudes to nurse caring suggests that, above all, patients want a nurse who demonstrates caring through clinical and technical competence, as well as through interpersonal skills and, increasingly, a person who keeps them informed along each step of their illness trajectory, including informing family and friends.

Accepting caring as the basis of nursing practice and scholarship is not without problems. Issues of autonomy and power are ill at ease with the concept of caring. Servitude and altruism are intrinsically linked to caring, and these do not sit well with nursing's move to professionalism. To provide adequate care takes time and time costs money. Many nurses work within organisational structures whose primary motivation lies with the cost containment or the accumulation of wealth, rather than a mandate to heal—these economic factors may compromise or even be antithetical to nursing's imperative to care.

The caring imperative, therefore, represents a potential source of stress and occupational conflict for nurses. While it is argued that the need for nursing to place caring as a central concept has never been greater, there are concerns that the caring components of nursing are deemed unsophisticated and hence inferior to the therapeutic interventions of medicine and other allied health service providers. There is the potential for caring to become overlooked, to dissipate.

Despite the many creative theories of nurse caring, the tasks of establishing coherent and clear connections between caring and notions such as professionalism, scholarship and autonomy remain incomplete. Nurses are left with many issues to consider and debate. Even as the healthcare system as we know it today is shaped, reshaped and shaped again, in the years to come the conundrum of caring as the basis of nursing practice and scholarship will no doubt continue to captivate and confound nurses.

REFLECTIVE QUESTIONS

1 Think for a moment about why you chose nursing as a career. Did the desire to care for people have any role in your decision making?

2 Take some time to reflect on your experiences of caring for and being cared for. Based on your experiences to date, how would you define caring?

3 Think about some of the ways you show care to the significant people in your life. Do you think that any of these ways of showing care will be the same or similar to how you will show care to your patients/clients as a nurse?

4 Some people view nursing and caring as being synonymous. Do you think this is good for nursing? Why? Why not?

RECOMMENDED READINGS

Boykin A, Schoenhofer S O 2001 *Nursing as caring: a model for transforming practice*. Jones & Bartlett, Publishers, National League for Nursing Press, Sudsbury, Massachusetts.

Brykczynska G ed 1997 *Caring: the compassion and wisdom of nursing*. Arnold Books, London.

Dunlop M 1986 Is a science of caring possible? *Journal of Advanced Nursing* 11(3):661–70.

Lumby J 2001 *Who cares? The changing health care system*. Allen & Unwin, Sydney.

National Health Service Modernisation Agency 2005 *Changing workforce programme: new ways of working in health care*. Accessed 27 January 2005. Available from: http://www.modernnhs.nhs.uk/scripts/default.asp?site_id=65.

Stockdale M, Warelow P 2000 Is the complexity of care a paradox? *Journal of Advanced Nursing* 31(5):1258–64.

CHAPTER SEVEN

The growth of ideas and theory in nursing

Sarah Winch, Amanda Henderson & Debra K Creedy

LEARNING OBJECTIVES

At the completion of this chapter, the reader will be able to:

▲ define the term theory;

▲ describe the terms modernity and postmodernity;

▲ identify the dominant historical and societal trends within the nursing profession;

▲ explain how these trends influence the practice of nursing and accompanying knowledge development; and

▲ differentiate the contribution of theory to research and research to theory.

KEY WORDS

Theory, modernity, postmodernity, knowledge, practice

INTRODUCING THEORY

This chapter aims to help you critically understand the relevance of theory to inform the ongoing development of nursing knowledge and contribute to the improvement of nursing practice. Clinical practice informed by theory gives nurses the necessary foundation to enlighten and restructure healthcare and improve quality of care at all practice levels. We begin with a brief overview of the philosophies, models and theories that underpin contemporary nursing theories. The next section emphasises nursing practice with a focus on knowledge utilisation, with theory and research as tools of practice.

Broadly, we can state that theory refers to any attempt to explain or represent a phenomenon, and ranges from the highly abstract and large scale, to the specific. Theories act as a lens by which to view the world. If you change the thickness of the lens and its shape, then what is being viewed is seen differently, in more or less detail, or expanded or reduced in size. Theories also act like a kaleidoscope, where turning the end of the instrument creates different patterns forming from the same small elements that are present. Theory and the application of theory to human understanding and social phenomena results in key elements (we shall call them variables and ideas) that underpin our understanding of the person and society being emphasised in different ways. Likewise, key philosophical ideas such as the nature of truth, evil and justice may be viewed differently.

When we focus on the process and practice of nursing, the key aspects that need explanation are the nurse, the nursed and the care setting, including practices, processes and organisation. Nursing theories help us make sense of processes and practices. Nursing theories explain why and when nursing takes place, provide an understanding of how the practice of nursing proceeds and also assist with practice change through critique. In this way nursing theories help us understand the practice of nursing, how we interact with the nursed and how we structure our nursing actions to provide nursing care.

Examples of well-known nursing theorists (Tomey & Alligood 1998)

- Faye Glenn Abdellah: twenty-one nursing problems
- Patricia Benner: stress and coping in illness
- Anne Boykin and Sarvina O Schoenhofer: the theory of nursing as caring
- Joyce J Fitzpatrick: rhythm model
- Dorothy Johnson: behavioral system model
- Imogene King: general system's framework/theory of goal attainment
- Katharine Kolcaba: theory of comfort
- Madeleine Leininger: theory of cultural care, diversity and universality/ transcultural nursing model

---

- Myra Levine: conservation model
- Ramona T Mercer: maternal role attainment
- Betty Neuman: nursing systems model
- Margaret Newman: theory of health as expanding consciousness
- Florence Nightingale: environmental adaptation theory
- Dorothea Orem: self-care framework
- Ida Jean Orlando: theory of the nursing process discipline
- Rosemarie Parse: theory of human becoming
- Josephine Paterson and Loretta Zderad: humanistic nursing theory
- Hildegard Peplau: theory of interpersonal relations
- Martha E Rogers: science of unitary human beings
- Nancy Roper, Winifred W Logan and Alison J Tierney: the elements of nursing: a model of nursing based on a model of living
- Callista Roy: adaptation model
- Jean Watson: theory of human caring
- Ernestine Wiedenbach: the helping art of clinical nursing

NURSING AS SOCIAL PROCESS: THE ROLE OF SOCIAL THEORY IN UNDERSTANDING NURSING

Nursing can be viewed as a social and cultural product of society. That is, nursing is an interactive process that always takes place within a social context. Our common understanding of nursing involves a nurse and the nursed (the patient, consumer or client) interacting within a socially and politically constructed system (healthcare facility or provider) that directs actions and responses.

An understanding of the role of social theory is valuable when we seek to answer the 'how' and 'why' questions about nursing and the social context from which it arises. The field of social theory is comprehensive, as it spans all of the social sciences and the humanities. In the following section we provide an overview of two major ways that social theory contributes to nursing. These are: an analysis of modernity and its contribution to the type of world we live in; and a critique of the social milieu that constructs and defines nursing.

Modernity: how social theory informs the way we think

Modernism, and postmodernism, are terms that hold a number of meanings in different contexts. For example, they may refer to specific styles of literature, art and architecture in the nineteenth and twentieth centuries. Or, as we explore here, they can elicit two different ways of thinking, both of which are fundamental to how we understand nursing.

First, we review modernity and postmodernity as a particular set of philosophical beliefs. These provide a useful philosophical framework that we can use to analyse practice-specific theories by tracing the traditions from which they emerge. Our second understanding relates to how nursing as a social process happens within the different time frames that represent the modern and postmodern eras. This provides a broad social and historical context that explains the nature of nursing and the transformations to nursing practice that are initiated through social change. In a later section, we examine modernism and postmodernism as broad cultural configurations that influence how society is organised.

Modernity and the Enlightenment

For many theorists, modernity encompasses a large historical period that emerged in Europe dating from the Renaissance to the present. Philosophical ideas on the nature of knowledge and modern method (Rene Descartes), science as power (Frances Bacon), the state and the science of human nature (Thomas Hobbes) and modern politics and power (Niccolo Machiavelli) construct the early basis of modernity. Later, in the eighteenth century, many of these ideas had their full intellectual flowering in a time known as 'the Enlightenment'. The goal of the Enlightenment project was to replace the ignorance, tradition and superstition present in the church-dominated societies of the Middle Ages, with knowledge that was based on science and reason. This far-reaching period of intellectual development is still prominent in much of contemporary thinking in nursing and other disciplines.

Ideas on the nature of human life that stem from the Enlightenment period reflect a particular belief about the self and the human condition. The modernist concept of 'the self' is a unified, rational, autonomous and essential entity. This means that 'the self' can be observed and studied. It is free, capable of thought and of independent action. This is a description of human beings as active agents doing things for reasons and shaping the world to their own ends. These core ideas about the nature of the self are central to many nursing theorists who see patients and nurses as autonomous beings who are able to be influenced in their behaviours to promote health and wellbeing or to address deficits caused by illness.

The Enlightenment period crystallised a belief in universal goals and human progress towards an ideal through the application of value-neutral knowledge. Knowledge derived from the empirical or natural sciences can be applied to society to increase human progress and happiness, while knowledge from the human sciences can be used to transform society into a scientific, rational culture. These ideas, which Yeatman (1991) terms 'rational utopianism', underpin modernist emancipatory politics—that is, the search for truth and progress through value-free, objective knowledge.

For researchers working within this framework (and this includes most nurses), it is important to select the correct research method, as this endorses 'truth' and provides theory that is an objective reflection of a securely grounded world (Hollinger 1994:59). Society and history are seen as a whole, able to be grasped through totalising methodologies and explained by grand and comprehensive explanations (meta-narratives). In nursing these would take the form of theories of caring or grand theories of nursing.

Research methods based on modernist assumptions promote the ideas of objectivity, and most importantly value neutrality. In this way a society based on science and universal values can be assumed to be truly rational and emancipatory. As such, theory is an objective representation of social reality. Ideas from the Enlightenment period have led to positivism, scientism and an emphasis on technological reason. For example, although ideas about ageing have been present in the wider literature since ancient times, the Enlightenment constructed the idea of 'old age' through medicine, science and philosophy as an essential part of life. Modernity spawned practices of calculation, division and ranking of the population. It was then possible to separate older age as a distinct developmental stage (Katz 1995:69). As such, all human institutions and practices, including hospitals and nurses, can be analysed by science and improved. This central belief is very much a part of healthcare and service provision today.

Modernity is also about order and rationality (logical thinking underpinned by science). This order and stability are maintained in modern societies through the means of 'grand or master narratives'. These are stories about the practices and beliefs present in a society. A 'grand narrative' in Australian culture may be that the family is a 'haven' and a 'central building block' of society. Generally, if we support families to function well, they will raise the next generation properly and care for their sick and elderly. Contemporary healthcare and social policy reflects this type of grand narrative. For example, aged care policy, such as home and community care, is based on supporting families (often aged spouses) to care for their partners. Likewise, early discharge policy and short stays in acute care hospitals rely on a well-organised, functioning family to provide supportive care.

Postmodernity

The central theme of modernity is a belief in the idea of progress in human life through the application of value-free knowledge gained in an objective way (science). However, as the German philosopher Jurgen Habermas and others have established, the twentieth century experience of the Holocaust and nuclear devastation shattered confidence and faith in scientific progress (Harvey 1989:13). Postmodernism (which in our discussion here includes the related although not identical category of poststructuralism) presents an altogether more pessimistic view of the world in general. It seeks to critique or deconstruct grand narratives to reveal the contradictions and instabilities that are inherent in any social organisation or practice. For example, in Australia, community nurses know that the grand narrative involving the family as a source of comfort and support is not always true. Postmodernism, while rejecting grand narratives, prefers 'mini-narratives', stories that explain small practices and local events, rather than large-scale universal or global concepts. These 'mini-narratives' are always locally based on particular situations and do not claim to be universal or generalisable to other contexts, and have great application in promoting understanding of aspects of nursing practice.

Drawn from a complex mix of ideas from theorists such as Hegel, Nietzsche and Weber, the postmodern position is associated with concepts such as irrationality, play, deconstruction, antithesis and indeterminacy (Gillan 1988:34). In a sense these are the opposite of the science-based rationality that underpins modernism. Critics of the Enlightenment, such as the well-known philosopher Nietzsche, argue that truth, knowledge and rationality are not immutable and science itself may rest on faith (Hollinger 1994:8). Postmodernism, taken to its extreme, refutes all claims to truth and reduces theory to narrative or storytelling. Postmodernism abandons the dualism of facts and values, objectivity and subjectivity, descriptions and interpretations, and gives all methodologies a political emphasis, while contextualising all claims, methods and values. Moreover, postmodernism does not accord 'reason' a central and transcendental status.

From the Enlightenment onwards, the idea of the 'subject' has had a central place in thought about the special nature of humanity. For key Enlightenment thinkers, the autonomous subject was the central tenet of civil society. By stark contrast many postmodern thinkers dispute the concept of the sovereign individual or subject, viewing these ideas about the subject as a form of grand narrative that requires deconstruction itself. For postmodernists, individuals are subjects, constituted through a variety of practices and knowledges or discourses in society in which they are positioned at any one point in time. The modernist, humanist concept of a unified, rational, autonomous and essential self is seen as illusory and results from regular positioning within a common, frequently used discourse (Grosz 1993).

Postmodernity has influenced several thinkers and observers of nursing practice including Winch (2005), who argues that this type of analysis can provide a highly analytical view of nursing practice. This view links the minutiae of nursing work with formation of identity (of the subject), and the monitoring and fashioning of patient conduct within broader historical, social and political processes and institutions.

Characterising modern healthcare institutions

The second way by which we may understand modernism and postmodernism is to view them broadly as historical cultural configurations that influence how society is organised. In two to three centuries modern industrial capitalism altered earlier farming or rural societies and set the scene for the society we know in Australia today. In line with the massive social change from the modern to the postmodern, nursing as a social process or cultural product has also been transformed.

Jameson (1984) outlines three primary phases of capitalism in Western industrialised nations that have produced particular cultural practices associated with modernism and postmodernism. These provide a framework for how we may understand healthcare and nursing. The first predates both modernism and postmodernism and is termed *market capitalism*. This occurred in the eighteenth through to the late nineteenth centuries in Western Europe, England and the United States. This phase is associated with particular technological developments such as the steam-driven engine. It is in this phase that nursing began to emerge as a central form of healthcare responsible for cleanliness and hygiene, with the growth of the clinic and the asylum. The work of the nursing theorist Florence Nightingale is prominent in this period.

The second phase, termed *monopoly capitalism*, occurred from the late nineteenth century until the mid-twentieth century, and is associated with modernism, industrialism, the growth of cities, the nuclear family, democracy and social legislation. It is in this phase that we see the growth of particular institutions such as the modern hospital, the development of the health professions and the rise of medicine as the dominant and most powerful form of healthcare.

The third phase, the one that we currently occupy, is a form of multinational or *consumer capitalism*, a postindustrial or postmodern society. Developing after World War II, the third phase encompasses all of the second phase but emphasises new technologies, marketing, selling and consuming commodities, and the growth of the internet. It is in this era that multinational pharmaceutical companies have grown very powerful, seeking to influence medical care and the consumption of particular drugs, ordered through medical practitioners and marketed in some countries, such as the United States, directly to the consumer. Modern managerialism has also crept into healthcare and influenced nursing work, with a focus on healthcare targets and clinical pathways. Health services are now managed as businesses, with patients as consumers.

Our consideration of the modern and postmodern has ranged over a wide number of issues, of which there is no clear agreement among social theorists, philosophers or nursing thinkers. Some argue that we live in truly postmodern times, and we must abandon the quest for truth and justice through the application of science. Others still believe that society is evolving to become a more logical and rational place, despite the odd setback. Nursing over this period of time has ebbed and flowed with the dominant social and cultural practices of the time. What is clear is that the work that nurses do is essential in a civil society. What is less clear in a postmodern, postindustrial time is how that work may be fragmented or reorganised and what nursing may look like in the future.

IMPLICATIONS FOR THE DEVELOPMENT OF A BODY OF KNOWLEDGE

Social theory has influenced how nurses inquire into their profession. This inquiry has explored ways to study human beings, what counts as 'evidence', reflection on practice and analysing the profession itself. Prevailing ideas and theories have been instrumental in how nurses approach and conduct their practice and accordingly the development of professional knowledge. This section provides a brief overview of some of the more dominant ideas and theories that have influenced the discipline of nursing. These influences are significant determinants of how nursing is presently understood and practised.

The contribution of scientific inquiry

From the Enlightenment period onwards, science and reason were perceived to be methods to obtain value-free knowledge in a neutral manner. Prior to the Enlightenment, nursing work had been undertaken by untrained religious people and local women with experience of caring for family members or having babies (Ehrenreich & English 1973). A structured logical analysis of human behaviour began with John Locke (1690) in *An essay concerning human understanding*. Locke espoused the belief that all ideas originate in experience. The inherent premise was that a newborn infant must acquire his or her ideas of this world by observing what goes on around him or her. The limits of understanding are therefore set by the limits of sense and reason. This argument was readily adopted as the dominant philosophy on all aspects of intellectual life during the eighteenth century (Miller 1985). This argument was termed *empiricism*. It referred to the idea that what was known was only possible through sensory experience. Knowledge could therefore be validated (Mitchell 1987).

Florence Nightingale (1820–1910) gave shape and form to what was to become the discipline of nursing by using the scientific methods proposed from the Enlightenment period. Tutored in mathematics as a child, Nightingale systematically collected data and analysed this statistically (Cohen 1984). Nightingale's explanation of the phenomena of concern to nursing marks the beginning of systematic inquiry and the development of a knowledge base (Newman 1983). She applied 'scientific inquiry' to illness generally to derive specific nursing interventions. Nightingale is best known for her carefully collected information in relation to the environment, namely the concepts of ventilation, warmth, light, diet, cleanliness and noise (Tomey & Alligood 1998). Through careful observation, keen documentation and subsequent analysis of these factors, she sought insights into causal relationships on which nursing could make a difference.

Nightingale also needed to persuade influential politicians who championed her cause. She used the dominant method of the day to progress this, namely observation, to collect objective data and logic/reasoning instead of religion and superstition (Ehrenreich & English 1973). Since Nightingale, nurses have approached their practice in a structured and systematic manner. As a discipline, nursing has sought theory in an attempt to describe, explain, predict and control. Nurses have borrowed theory from a range of other disciplines to assist in understanding the core phenomena inherent in nursing. In many situations nurses have modified and adopted theory from these disciplines in an attempt to develop a nursing-specific theory.

The dominance of empiricism in the practice of nursing

Physiological theories based in scientific methods of inquiry were well advanced by the second half of the nineteenth century and provided information about how the body worked (Miller 1985). The biomedical model, the basis of contemporary acute medical practice, arose from this form of investigation. This model views people as biological beings, made of cells, tissues and organs that achieve homeostasis, an internal mechanism that keeps physical and chemical parameters of the body relatively constant. Consistent with the notions of reason and causality that accompanied modernity, how the body functioned could be likened to a machine (Benner & Wrubel 1989, Pearson et al 2005).

The biomedical model has continued to dominate healthcare during the twentieth century (Aronowitz 1998), and has become the dominant paradigm in many areas of practice, not only the medical profession but also for nurses (Pearson et al 2005). For example, during the initial establishment of intensive care areas, nurses frequently learnt with doctors about how the physiological body responded in situations of illness (Fairman 1992). Nurses, who had become responsible for the physical body, were learning more about the physiological responses that accompanied health problems. Potentially this knowledge was instrumental in assisting health restoration, as nurses could act quickly on this information and interventions based on biomedical knowledge could be appropriately administered.

Increasing knowledge of the physiological processes that affect the body has resulted in a plethora of methods and tools to diagnose and prescribe treatment. These methods have largely been controlled by the medical profession, creating a hierarchy based on science in which nursing knowledge has been coerced (Henderson 1994). This situation has arisen primarily because healthcare is directed by the medical profession and provision of care by nurses is largely organised to support interventions directed by the medical profession.

The extensive use of the biomedical model has similarly led to an emphasis on technical-related aspects of the nursing role. This can be partially explained by the observation that during clinical interactions the body is essentially objectified. In the physical interaction the patient experiences his or her body as a scientific object beneath the dispassionate gaze consistent with scientific investigation (Leder 1984). This has inadvertently led to a devaluing of assisting the individual through the experience of their illness (Pearson et al 2005). When disease is conceptualised as the aberrant dysfunction at the tissue, cellular or organ level, the biomedical model is an efficient theoretical framework to explore this function (Benner and Wrubel 1989).

This perspective has been contested by many contemporary nursing theorists working from a postmodern perspective. These theorists (e.g. Rosemarie Parse, Martha Rogers, Jean Watson and Patricia Benner) are interested in the non-technical, or more caring, relational aspects of the nursing role, which examine the minutiae of the daily practice of nursing work and the patient's experience of illness from their own perspective. They argue that this is more akin to the reality of nursing as it is actually practised. Nurses can make an important contribution in such dimensions of patient care. They have a capacity to recognise and explore individuals' spirituality, feelings, situated meaning and ethical concerns that accompany their (the individual's) journey through the illness trajectory, which are lost in a purely biomedical or scientific approach. The work of these postmodern scholars has resulted in a growing appreciation of the experience of illness and also recognition of tacit nursing knowledge (Benner & Wrubel 1989).

THE META-PARADIGM OF NURSING: IDENTIFYING A DISTINCT BODY OF KNOWLEDGE

In line with the emergence of organised society and the modern-day hospital (Bullough & Bullough 1972), during the phase we have identified as *monopoly capitalism*, nursing knowledge grew through a complex mix of practice, science, social and behavioural theories and tradition. This resulted in a body of healthcare knowledge that is respected independently of medicine, although not necessarily seen as equal or as valuable. During the push to obtain professional status, nurses recognised the need to identify core proponents that would assist in the continuous debate and refinement of a unique body of knowledge. To assist with this, a meta-paradigm was sought by which to organise and direct the knowledge that would become nursing's unique focus.

A meta-paradigm of any discipline is a statement or group of statements identifying the relevant phenomena to the discipline (Fawcett 1984). It originates from the term paradigm, used to describe accepted practices and techniques through which a discipline accumulates and refines its knowledge base. According to Kuhn (1970:24), a paradigm assists in the articulation and refinement of the phenomena being explored. Exploration of the scholarly arguments, as they pertain to nursing, identifies four central recurring themes that can arguably be described as constituting a meta-paradigm for nursing. The components of the paradigm are identified as: nursing (as an action); client (human being); environment (of the client and nurse–client); and health. The nurse interacts with the client and the environment for the purpose of facilitating the health of the client (Fawcett 1984, Newman 1983).

These four components facilitate the description and explication of theories in nursing. For example, the model proposed by Roper et al (1990), which addresses clients' activities of daily living, is a development on earlier notions of understanding health. This model recognises the integral part of psychosocial wellbeing on health, and appropriately ensures consideration of environmental factors including communication and capacity to develop relationships. These components of the meta-paradigm are essential because what is meant by nursing is largely influenced by the meanings and the importance attributed to it (Newman 1983). Insights into potential meaning may be derived through an understanding of the shifts and developments in how two of these components are understood, the client and the environment.

Understanding the client

The nomenclature referring to the person receiving the nursing care has changed in line with some of the broad cultural configurations that we mentioned previously. Historically, nursing language uses the term 'patient' to refer to the nursed. In modern times (i.e. the postindustrial age), we have exchanged this term for 'client' and, in some cases, 'consumer'. This interesting change of language is meant to confer an attitude of active participation of the person receiving care.

These changes in nomenclature about the person being nursed are, in part, related to how the individual being nursed is actually viewed—that is, how they are understood as a human being and a person. How the individual is approached and how nursing care is attended to has largely been influenced by how the human body has been conceptualised, which has in turn influenced what practices are perceived to constitute nursing.

According to the biomedical model, health was the maintenance of the body's biological functioning. However, with increasing knowledge about the human body, the conceptualisation of the individual, and accordingly health, has broadened. Methods of scientific inquiry have not only been used to describe the internal operation of the biological body, but also human behaviour. Consistent with empirical research, initially human behaviour was likened to a stimulus–response model—for example, if a person was hungry they sought food. Subsequent to these initial observations and experiments, it was recognised that there was a cognitive component to human behaviour. Individuals could think, plan and make decisions on remembered information.

Acceptance of the cognitive component of the individual has been very influential in broadening the scope of nursing work. The impact of psychological wellbeing on overall health status meant that nurses could have a sphere of influence apart from the technical interventions accompanying tests, procedures and other intrusions into the body.

Aspects of the human condition relating to stress and anxiety are core concepts repeatedly studied in nursing. These concepts frequently accompany deviations of health when experienced by clients, and they are an area in which nurses are readily able to make a difference (Devine & Cook 1986). Many nursing theories have been developed in response to the potential of psychological issues that affect individuals with deviations in their health condition. Theorists using this approach include Peplau and Travelbee (Tomey & Alligood 1998).

Peplau and the theory of interpersonal relations in nursing

In the theory of interpersonal relations in nursing, Peplau (1952) emphasises the importance of the nurse–client relationship. The relationship develops through interlocking and overlapping phases. These are: the orientation phase; the working phase (subdivided into identification and exploitation); and the resolution phase. It 'is educative and therapeutic when nurses and patient can come to know and respect each other as persons who are alike, and yet different, as persons who share in the solution of problems' (Peplau 1952:9).

However, during the early part of the twentieth century, the limitations of experimental research in explaining the human condition were exposed by Sigmund Freud. The work of Freud is powerful in challenging the notion of accepted empiricism. Freud, through recognition of the subconscious of individuals, exposed another form of knowledge that was not acquired through empirical studies (Miller 1985). Freud's work demonstrated the importance of the unconscious and instinctual forces in human conduct (Miller 1985:267). The recognition of this knowledge is influential in postmodernity—there is now acknowledgment that we can learn more about ourselves and how we function within the world apart from rigorous empiric methods. Meanings are understood as specific to the individual or a small group of individuals as 'mini-narratives'.

Understanding the environment

From the inception of this chapter we have argued that the social and cultural environment produces nursing and structures nursing action. Nursing does not occur in a vacuum. Despite this fundamental premise, the various conceptualisations of the environment remain the most ill defined of all the central concepts of the espoused meta-paradigm (Brodie 1984). Kleffel (1991) similarly reviews the perspective of the environment, and concludes that the concept of the environment is important as a domain of nursing knowledge, as it is the nature of the environment as it is conceived in global terms that impacts on nursing.

We have seen how the nature of nursing and transformation of nursing practice can be initiated through shifts in social thoughts and ideas that emerge from the global environment, such as the growth of science as an explanation (from the Enlightenment) or the different ways that nursing work has been produced across the broad epochs of monopoly and postindustrial capitalism. Let us now take a specific example that affects nursing practice and that has become prominent in the postindustrial era—that is, growth of the business model of healthcare.

Among the competing discourses involved in the complex production of healthcare in Western industrial nations, the strength of the business-model-driven health-care system is paramount. The roots of modern managerialism with its stress upon healthcare targets, admissions, discharges and care pathways can be traced to the industrial revolution. This factory-style production of nursing work is a form of Taylorism (Lundy 1996). Taylorism involves taking a professional skill set and breaking it up into component parts, which can then be further classified according to a particular skill level. Workers with less training can participate in what is hitherto a complete professional activity. This provides definite economic benefits, as less of the more highly trained professionals are required. For the nurses working on the factory line, producing regimented segments of nursing care according to prescribed pathways, the scope of what we would term professional nursing practice, is stymied. In a climate that Hofstadter (1963) has termed *unreflective instrumentalism*, there has been a loss of the complexity of nursing and the ability for the high level of analysis and reflection necessary for a practice-based profession to provide the highest level of care.

In this type of business-driven healthcare environment, Ackroyd and Bolton (1999:372) argue that while nurses do retain autonomy from managers, the context of nursing is controlled via the supply of patients. By increasing the number of patients, managers control the time that nurses have to treat. This means that nurses have to work harder if they want to give what they feel is an appropriate level of care. In this way, key parameters of nursing activity are gradually lost to the profession that may wish to control the quality of its work. Thus we can see that awareness of the environment in which nurses practise is revealing—as the environment prescribes the conditions not only in which development of knowledge occurs, but also how that knowledge can be applied.

Concomitantly, it is argued that the nursing profession is starting to mature and that professional nurses have started to examine their behaviours, examine influences on their behaviour and manage their situation to better suit the profession. Nurses are beginning to acknowledge the complexity of the knowledge operating within the profession (Street 1992) and are learning how to best draw on this knowledge. Street (1992) advocates for critical inquiry—that is, the capacity for self-reflection and collaborative analysis to effect rational change. For nurses to enact this, she advocates nurses draw on the work of Habermas (1971), who argues that individuals should act from raised awareness, rather than coercion or habit, as previously recognised in nursing behaviour.

IMPLICATIONS FOR CONTEMPORARY NURSING PRACTICE: THEORETICAL PLURALISM

Nursing has been informed and influenced by many different ideas and trends within modern society. These are evident in the education, practice and research of nursing. The involvement of nurses in understanding their professional practice is imperative so that the foundations upon which they base their practice are not hidden beliefs, but are made overt so that their effects can be considered and further developed to better meet the health needs of the broader community.

The difficulty with the development of theory in nursing is the notion that 'one size fits all'—that is, one theory should account for all the 'truths' in nursing (Emden & Young 1987). Theoretical pluralism as described by Dickoff and James (1984), however, permits the nurse to select and apply the theoretical model appropriate to the particular practice setting and client situation. This approach also allows and acknowledges that the selection and application of a variety of nursing theories and models depends on the depth and breadth of knowledge of the individual nurse. For example, the conceptual and theoretical framework adopted by nurses in a community health clinic may be different from the framework adopted by nurses working in an acute care hospital.

How theory informs the development of the discipline of nursing is somewhat ambiguous—it is essentially an interactive process with research. Arguably, theory and research occur along a continuum, in that research can test the validity of theoretical concepts (Chinn & Jacobs 1987). Alternatively, there is a growing emphasis on research formulating theory (Emden & Young 1987). Data derived from practice are conceptualised; theories are then formulated and inform the intellectual structure organising practice (Benner 1984). Ideally, theory development and research are interactive processes.

Many nursing theories have been largely informed through dominant societal trends rather than emerging from limitations experienced within the practice of nursing. It is therefore not surprising that nurses have not embraced theory in their practice. Similarly, it is recognised that much of nursing research does not attempt to substantiate nursing theory (Donaldson & Crowley 1978). The challenge for nursing is for practitioners to have a comprehensive understanding of ideas, how they have contributed to their practice and how nurses can derive the best outcomes from a systematic organisation of these ideas into theories that inform their own spheres—namely, research, knowledge and practice.

CONCLUDING THOUGHTS

The way you think about people and about nursing has a direct impact on how you approach people, what questions you ask, how that information is processed, and what nursing activities are included in the care offered. The utilisation and application of nursing theory (in the form of philosophies, models and theories) help you think critically for professional practice. Theory and research together lead to systematic inquiry, which informs practice.

REFLECTIVE QUESTIONS

1 To what extent is theory development crucial to nursing and nursing practice?

2 How does the Western industrial healthcare environment affect nursing work in the twenty-first century?

3 How does the conceptual shift of postmodernity affect the development of nursing knowledge in practice?

4 What local situations and conditions operate in your sphere of practice that influence the nursing care you provide?

RECOMMENDED READINGS

Alligood M, Marriner-Tomey A ed 2002 *Nursing theory: utilization and application*, 2nd edn. Mosby, St Louis.
Hollinger R 1994 *Postmodernism and the social sciences: a thematic approach*, pp 169–77. Sage, London.
Pearson A, Vaughan B, FitzGerald M 2005 *Nursing models for practice*, 3rd edn. Butterworth Heinemann, London.

CHAPTER EIGHT

Reflective practice: what, why and how

Kim Usher & Colin Holmes

LEARNING OBJECTIVES

After reading this chapter, students should have gained:

▲ an understanding of the importance and benefits of reflection to a practice-based discipline such as nursing;

▲ insight into the nature of reflection and the ideas of its leading theorists;

▲ an appreciation of the link between self-awareness and professional self-monitoring;

▲ an understanding of the strategies that assist with reflection—for example, reflective writing, journalling, critical incident analysis, clinical supervision, and forms of creative expression; and

▲ insight into the legal and ethical issues surrounding the keeping of professional journals.

KEY WORDS
Reflection, reflective practice, journalling, critical incident analysis, self-awareness

INTRODUCTION

The context in which nursing occurs has changed markedly in the last two decades. As a result of advances in nursing and medical knowledge, and reduced government spending (which has led to a reduction in hospital beds, shorter hospital stays, and more rapid patient turnovers), workers in healthcare institutions are spending much more of their time dealing with acutely ill patients who require specialised care (Usher et al 2001). The role of the nurse is also influenced by cultural, social, economic, historical and political constraints that all affect the ways in which nurses approach and react to certain situations (Taylor 2000).

As a consequence, today's nursing graduates must not only be clinically competent practitioners, but also need to be adept at *critical thinking* in order to understand the complexities of the world and the rapidly changing practice arena (Usher et al 1999). Critical thinking, or the practice of questioning, is necessary so that practitioners integrate relevant information from various sources, examine assumptions, and identify relationships and patterns (Parker & Clare 2000). *Reflective practice* and critical thinking are often used interchangeably, but, while not identical, there is a reflexive relationship. After all, as Lumby (2000:338) explains, '. . . to adopt a critical approach to the world, it is necessary to reflect on the world and one's experiences in it'.

We begin this chapter by introducing you to the *why* of reflection, and explaining why *reflection* is a useful strategy for undergraduate nursing students, as well as registered nurses. We will also provide an overview of the related legislation that requires the use of reflective thinking in practice by registered nurses and makes it a requirement for all students exiting undergraduate university degrees. The next section of the chapter addresses the *why* and *what* of reflective practice, including an overview of the definitions of reflection.

WHY BE REFLECTIVE?

Every workplace presents a complex environment to the new recruit. It is often difficult to understand and appears to abound with multiple decisions, each coupled to a host of different ways in which the desired outcomes could be achieved. Nursing is no different. When you first enter a nursing context, perhaps during your first clinical placement, you will be confronted by discrepancies, such as those between 'ideal' and 'real' practice, and you will experience or witness difficult interpersonal relationships. It is important that these situations do not distract you from your nursing goals. Reflection can help you during these times, as it will assist you to recognise and set aside the emotional content and enable you to learn from otherwise negative experiences. It will help you identify alternative ways you could react in the future, hopefully resulting in more positive outcomes.

Johns (1998) explains how reflection offers a way to bring to the surface the contradictions between what you intend to achieve in a situation and how you actually practise. In other words, being faced with contradiction opens the possibility for change and offers the practitioner the opportunity to achieve desired practice.

One of the outcomes of reflection is thus a process of continuous monitoring and improvement of practice.

Regulatory authorities in Australia have embraced the need for practitioners who are reflective, and require that all nurses engage in some form of reflective activity. This is indicated by their adoption of the Australian Nursing and Midwifery Council (ANMC) competency standards for registered nurses (2000). These are a set of competencies representing the minimum core standards for registration as a nurse in Australia. There are 14 core competency standards that all registered nurses must be able to meet, and reflection is included under 'Competency 5: professional development of self and others'. These competencies have been extended to apply to enrolled nurses and also specialty groups, such as critical care nurses.

The Nursing Council of New Zealand has also incorporated reflection as a key competency for registered nurses. Reflection in the New Zealand competencies comes under communication, professional judgment, management and quality improvement (Nursing Council of New Zealand 2004). The development of midwifery competencies is currently under way in Australia.

Further information about these competencies is available from the following websites:

▲ Australian Nursing and Midwifery Council competencies for registered nurses: http://www.anmc.org.au/

▲ Competencies for the registered nurses' scope of practice in New Zealand: www.nursingcouncil.org.nz/standardsrn.pdf

Encouragement for reflection is also echoed in the education sector, in the *Review of higher education financing and policy (final report): learning for life*, or the 'West Report' as it is commonly known (Department of Employment, Education, Training and Youth Affairs 1998), where reflection is listed as an expected attribute of graduates from all undergraduate university degrees in Australia. In other words, it is a requirement of your undergraduate education that you exit the program of study with the ability to reflect. As a result, all undergraduate degree coordinators are now charged with the responsibility of ensuring their graduates have been provided with the opportunity to develop the skill of reflection.

WHAT IS REFLECTION OR REFLECTIVE PRACTICE?

Reflection comes from the verb *reflectere*, which means to bend or turn backwards (Hancock 1999). This infers that reflection is a process of going back over something after it has already occurred. This might include recalling thoughts and memories, in cognitive acts such as thinking or contemplation, as a way of making sense of the situation so that necessary changes may be identified or made (Taylor 2000). We all reflect on what goes on around us to some extent. If you think about it, we do not generally just walk around in the world without noticing things or thinking about what has happened and how it has impacted on us. Similarly, we all reflect at some level on our practice, but it may only involve thinking about what happened rather than theorising about what happened and looking for ways to improve it in the future.

Thus the type of reflection to be discussed in this chapter is actually a much more purposeful activity that leads to action that is better informed than that which occurred before the reflection took place (Francis 1995). Rolfe et al (2001) argue that not all knowledge for practice comes from textbooks, research journals and lectures, or other classroom activities. Rather, they claim that, in addition to what they call scientific knowledge, practitioners actually 'pick up' practical knowledge from their everyday experience, and reflection is the process of *theorising* about that knowledge. As a result, they claim that reflection provides the practitioner with access to the processes by which he or she makes clinical judgments, which can then be used to justify actions to others or pass on expertise to less experienced colleagues.

Taylor (2000) sees it as necessary to alert clinicians to the intricacies of nursing practice and the knowledge embedded in it. However, Johns (1988) claims that being a reflective practitioner is more than just noticing things by chance in a situation. He suggests that it involves a deep sensitivity to what is happening around us, or '. . . a constant monitoring of self within the situation that ripples along the surface of conscious thought' (Johns 1988:14). It is also important not to assume that improved skill in reflective thinking equals learning, which equals improved nursing practice. A study of reflective thinking in nursing by Teekman (2000) demonstrated that learning from reflection is not something that happens automatically. He identified the importance of coaching by a mentor, and a supportive environment, as ways to reduce the uncritical reinforcement of existing patterns of practice.

Much of the contemporary emphasis on reflective practice in nursing can be attributed to the work of the American educationalist Donald Schön (1983, 1987). Even though he was not the first to write about it, he actually coined the term 'reflective practice' (Teekman 2000), and has been very influential in the way nursing has embraced the notion. Schön (1983) argued that reflection is a strategy whereby professionals become aware of their implicit knowledge base. While he did not attempt to define reflection or reflective practice, he advocated two distinct types of reflection: *reflection-on-action* and *reflection-in-action*. The former, reflection-*on*-action, occurs after the event or action where details are recalled and analysed in some way with the aim of reviewing practice. It has been referred to as a type of cognitive 'postmortem' or an act of looking back at practice (Burton 2000).

Reflection-*in*-action occurs simultaneously or at the same time as practice. That is, reflection-*in*-action is said to occur when the practitioner engages in practice and makes adjustments as a result of relevant feedback. Rolfe (2001) claims that reflection-*in*-action is a more advanced form of reflection and leads to more advanced practice. He describes it as a process whereby the nurse is constantly testing theories and hypotheses in a cyclical process while simultaneously engaged in practice—what he termed 'nursing praxis' in an earlier paper (Rolfe 1993).

Boud et al (1985), however, noted an additional step in the reflective process, that of *pre-reflection*. In other words, they recognised the importance of reflection in anticipation of events. Greenwood (1998:1049) explains how preparing for experience involves the learner becoming aware of what they bring to the event and what they want from it (the personal), the constraints and opportunities the event provides (the context) and how they may acquire what they need from the event (the learning strategies).

THE ROOTS OF REFLECTIVE PRACTICE

The ancient Greek philosopher Plato declared that the unreflective life was a life not worth living. Plato was drawing attention to the view that reflection is a distinctively human activity and without it we would be no more than unthinking automatons, our lives governed by our biological instincts, and forever subject to those forces, human and natural, exerting power over us. Plato saw reflection, in other words, as vital to our identity as a human being, and to our having a mind of our own, and thus to our personal freedom. We are free only to the extent that we are a reflective being.

This idea resurfaced and drove the huge change of thinking that occurred in seventeenth and eighteenth century Europe, which became known as the Enlightenment. Enlightenment philosophers such as John Locke in England, and Jean-Jacques Rousseau in France, argued that human beings are free to think and decide for themselves rather than simply accept the prevailing norms, largely imposed by those in power, and notably by the Christian churches. Today we just accept this as natural, and probably do not think twice about it, but in those days it was a radical and rather dangerous claim.

This history reminds us of several important principles concerning reflection. First, reflection is not an artificial technique that is being imposed by regulatory authorities or universities; rather, it is the refinement of a natural process that is part of being human, and which needs to be nurtured and encouraged. Second, we should always reflect upon, and if necessary challenge, prevailing ways of thinking and acting, even if it occasionally means being unpopular or thought foolish. When it involves 'big issues', this may be hard to do, but reflection and action working together (i.e. 'praxis') is the impetus for change, and ultimately for improvement. This applies in all arenas of human activity, including your local healthcare setting.

Although there are many ways of conceiving reflective processes, even within the same discipline, reflection as we refer to it here is not simply thinking, but rather thinking deeply, systematically, logically and deliberately. Political theorists have emphasised the role of reflection in challenging the status quo, and it plays an important part in the teachings of some political radicals and revolutionaries. Educationalists, such as the American John Dewey, have emphasised the role of reflection in learning and problem solving and have explored how reflection is related to experience. Dewey observed that 'we learn by doing and realising what came of what we did'; this 'realising' is the result of reflection.

Reflection also played an important part in the development of psychology as a discipline during the nineteenth century, in the form of 'introspection'—that is, reflection focused upon oneself. Until the rise of scientific psychology in the 1880s, introspection was the primary source of data for the elucidation of human psychology. An especially important figure, who brings the political and educational aspects together, is the Brazilian Marxist, Paulo Friere. His work is widely cited as the basis for the development of reflective processes in nursing, although nurses have mostly shied away from acknowledging the political revolutionary aspects of his work. Friere's concept of reflection was developed as part of a strategy for educating and politicising the impoverished and largely illiterate peasants of Brazil, and has an explicit emancipatory intent. The key idea, which makes it 'emancipatory', is that reflection and action should work together (as praxis), in order to generate new, enlightened and empowering ways of thinking and behaving.

This is an important way for you to think about reflection because, as a nurse, you will work in complex systems where you may feel powerless and unable to express your concerns and opinions; in this sense, you too may feel 'illiterate'. In order to create a sense of control and of having a worthwhile part to play, you can begin by engaging in reflective processes, and out of these should arise constructive courses of action, which constitute 'praxis', an idea discussed further by Holmes and Warelow (2000).

Nursing's descriptions and adaptations of reflective processes have been clearly explored in a series of chapters in the classic Australian text edited by Gray and Pratt (1991), and you should read these as part of your continuing education as a nurse (Emden 1991, Gray & Forsstrom 1991, Cox et al 1991, Crane 1991, Lumby 1991). The authors explain how reflective processes bring theory and practice together, what forms they can take, and how they can be used by nurses in clinical, educational and research contexts.

The opening remark in Carolyn Emden's brilliant contribution nicely captures the spirit behind these chapters: 'Reflective practice is of pre-eminent interest to nurses', she says, and '[t]o be a *reflective practitioner* suggests professional maturity and a strong commitment to improving practice—a reasonable aspiration for every Registered Nurse' (Emden 1991:335). The work of Boud and his colleagues (1985), which was mentioned earlier, plays an important role here. Emden (1991) explains how his three phases of reflective learning—preparatory, experiential and processing— can be undertaken by you, in your workplace, and provides actual examples of nurses' 'field notes', or written reflections. For Emden (1991), as for most nurse authors, reflective processes are inextricably tied to the 'critical social science paradigm'—that is, the politically informed approach we have noted above, which is interested in identifying and changing irrational, oppressive or counterproductive beliefs and practices (Kemmis 1985).

Perhaps the most important exemplars of this approach in Australian nursing were the School of Nursing at Deakin University, where reflective processes and critical social theory were used as the basis for the undergraduate nursing curriculum from 1988, and subsequently formed part of the Master of Nursing Studies degree, at the Flinders University of South Australia, where they formed part of the Master of Nursing degree from 1991. Most Australian nurse scholars who have written about these topics are in some way linked to these two schools.

Emden (1991) summarises the ways in which reflective processes have the effect of 'educating the emotions'. Reflective processes should be mutually encouraged, and there is an educative element, as you help others by recognising and responding to their needs and sensitivities, as well as your own; reflective processes also help you come to terms with the uncertainty of clinical practice and with its inevitable injustices and inadequacies. Clinical practice is never perfect; it is always constrained by resource shortages and by the failings of the system and those who work in it. It is part of the human condition that we cannot do everything right all the time, and that things sometimes go wrong. Reflective processes enable us to face up to this reality, but at the same time challenge us to overcome the obstacles and aspire to the best possible standards of practice. They contribute to our development as thinkers, practitioners and as people; that is why Emden (1991) referred at the outset to them being the hallmark of the mature professional.

THE BENEFITS OF REFLECTION

We have referred already to some of the benefits that derive from reflective processes, but let us now discuss these in more detail. Friere (1972) insisted that action and reflection must work together, and we can agree with Emden when she describes action as a 'key outcome' of reflection. 'Action' can take many forms. For example, when you reflect upon your practice world and become sensitive to its inadequacies and injustices, you are most likely to want to do something about them, especially as you consider them in relation to individuals' rights. In contrast, action might involve improving your own clinical skills; your reflections having alerted you to shortcomings in your attitudes or skills, and you take action to bring them to a higher standard.

Another benefit of reflection is that it can help you elucidate the theory–practice relationship. Critical social theory insists that this relationship is 'reflexive'; in other words, theory feeds into your practice, and practice informs your theory. This supports the suggestion by nurse theorists Walker and Avant (1983) that reflective processes can be used to help develop clinical practice by helping you to recognise, evaluate and refine your personal nursing theories (i.e. your beliefs about nursing and clinical practice). Indeed, much of Emden's (1991) chapter is about how to use reflection to help elucidate and develop your own theory of nursing. Since critical social theory is closely tied to these conceptions of reflection, it is widely argued that any theory of nursing developed in this way should be consistent with critical social theory, and many nursing scholars have attempted to show how this can work (good places to begin exploring this topic are Holter (1988) and Crane (1991)). This link has become more difficult to sustain, however, as critical social theory has been the subject of criticism in light of alternative ways of thinking about social structures and processes, including 'post-structuralism' and 'postmodernism' (Holmes 1995).

Another positive outcome of reflection, which follows on from its role in the 'education of the emotions' noted above, is that it sensitises us to the plight of the less fortunate and marginalised people in society. We become more sensitive to the suffering, courage and determination of people who are faced with serious illness, and to the problems faced by those who are oppressed, such as mentally disordered and intellectually disabled people, and people who belong to ethnic and religious minorities. This increased sensitivity impels you towards greater engagement with such people, and a willingness to become involved in their problems. Not only are you aiming to improve your clinical performance with all your patients, but also to act as their support and advocate. You are not only motivated to question inadequate practices, but also to generate possible strategies for improvement. Even though it may be challenging, you will find that you cannot do otherwise, and you will enjoy increased levels of job satisfaction because this heightened level of engagement is intrinsically rewarding.

Once again, it is Carolyn Emden who sums up this aspect so accurately. She says:

> The outcomes of reflection are so profound, and so personally enlightening, that you are unable to let them go, or to return to former unquestioning ways. Increasingly, you are likely to recognise, and challenge, those political, social, and historical forces which are unjust, irrational, and oppressive in your professional life: together with colleagues and clients, you will wish to create and implement strategies of empowerment that lead to informed choice and fulfilling forms of action (Emden 1991:352).

We might add that these benefits accrue not just in the context of your work, but also in your life generally. The big claim being made here is that reflection, because it educates your emotions and impels you to action, helps make you a better person and not just a better nurse. Let us now turn to consider the 'how' of reflection.

STRATEGIES FOR REFLECTION

Many strategies can be used for reflection, including writing (e.g. journalling and critical incident anlaysis), and photography, drawing and other forms of creative expression.

Writing

Reflective writing has been advocated as a technique to aid reflection (Usher et al 1999, Rolfe et al 2001). It involves the use of writing as a strategy to assist us to learn from experiences and involves engaging in the reflective process using writing as an instrument. It differs from other forms of writing in that it is undertaken primarily for the purpose of learning and to assist us to develop a deeper understanding of the subject of our reflection (Rolfe et al 2001). Van Manen (1990) says that writing is a reflective activity where we come to know and understand the way in which we know what we know. This can be achieved by writing and rewriting, so that we come to understand something in greater depth, in ways not previously open to us, and in new or more intimate ways. Further, the '. . . act of writing forces a coherence and anchors thinking in a way that permits revisiting and reworking' (Usher et al 1999).

Journalling and *critical incident analysis* are two well-known types of reflective writing, but clinical supervision, poetry, letter, story and group writing activities are also examples of reflective writing.

Journalling

Journal writing has been advocated as a strategy for the development of reflective practice (e.g. Holly 1984, Boud et al 1985, Cox et al 1991, Heath 1998, Usher et al 1999). By the term journal we mean what is commonly referred to as a diary or log. Writing a journal involves the writing of accounts of practice experiences after they occur and allows the writer to take ownership of the content—for example, using the first person and writing about themselves.

However, journal writing offers the practitioner more than the opportunity to recount an experience; it provides an opportunity to return to the experience in its written form and then theorise about the experience from which conclusions are drawn. This type of reflective writing provides for many returns for analysis (Owens et al 1997), and the writer can add, delete or change entries as often as they wish. As a result, it becomes an ongoing critique of the practitioner's thoughts about an experience. Journals have also been described as cathartic because they offer an opportunity to 'work through' problems or difficult situations (Davies & Sharp 2000). The box below lists some journalling techniques, which are taken from Owens et al (1997).

Journalling techniques

- Write a short biography to begin.
- Select a quiet environment where you will not be interrupted.
- Write vividly and as close to the event as possible.

> - Include your initial thoughts, but leave space where you can add comments at a later time.
> - Where possible, make use of diagrams, illustrations, photographs and drawings to aid your memory.
> - Make use of a book and use one side for writing and leave the other for later reflections.

Some students find starting a reflective journal a difficult task, but you should remember that there is no right or wrong way to do it. Cox et al (1991:380–1) identify three challenges that face the newcomer to journalling:

1   valuing journalling so that time and effort are allocated appropriately;

2   removing the 'censor' that inhibits us from writing honestly and accurately; and

3   reviewing the journal critically in order to identify areas of strength and weakness, and new ways of thinking and acting.

The use of a framework or model as a prompt for reflection has been advocated (Heath 1998, Johns 1998, Rolfe et al 2001) and you may find this useful. Have a look at the model proposed by Rolfe et al (2001) in Figure 8.1, and think about how you might use it to aid your reflection.

Taylor (2000:67–8) offers a number of hints that may also be helpful: be spontaneous; express yourself freely; remain open to ideas; choose a time to suit you; be prepared personally; and choose a reflective method. It is also important to avoid the use of abbreviations, and resist the temptation to censor your writing, as this is more likely to assist with the exposure of the 'isms' we hold as an individual.

A further strategy that may also be helpful is the notion of a *critical friend*. Sharing with others opens reflective journal entries to a different perspective. The other person may offer alternative actions that could have been taken or might challenge you to think more deeply about a particular issue (Heath 1998). It is important that the critical friend is someone you trust, as they will be reading your entries and discussing them with you. The role of a critical friend is to support and guide you in your reflection, while posing questions and offering alternatives in a non-judgmental way (Taylor 2000). Duke describes how critical friends have:

> ... acted as a sounding board for my ideas and thoughts, sometimes they have given me an 'expert' view of an area of knowledge new to me, and sometimes they have stimulated a thought that I have then gone on to explore (Duke 2000:152).

Ethical and legal issues related to journalling

One aspect of journalling that became a problem in the early 1990s, when reflective processes were still considered strange and dangerous by those in authority in health services, concerns their ethical and legal status. In short, these concerns were:

- whether journalling required the consent of institutions and individuals to whom they refer;

Descriptive level of reflection	Theory- and knowledge-building level of reflection	Action-oriented (reflexive) level of reflection
What . . . 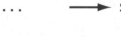	**So what . . .**	**Now what . . .**
. . . is the problem/difficulty/reason for being stuck/reason for feeling bad/reason we don't get on?	. . . does this tell me/teach me/imply/ mean about me/my patient/others/our relationship/my patient's care/the model of care I am using/my attitudes/my patient's attitudes?	. . . do I need to do in order to make things better/stop being stuck/improve my patient's care/resolve the situation/feel better/get on better?
. . . was my role in the situation?		. . . broader issues need to be considered if this action is to be successful?
. . . was I trying to achieve?	. . . was going through my mind as I acted?	. . . might be the consequences of this action?
. . . actions did I take?	. . . did I base my actions on?	
. . . was the response of others?	. . . other knowledge can I bring to the situation?	
. . . were the consequences • for the patient? • for myself? • for others?	• experiential? • personal? • scientific?	
. . . feelings did it evoke • in the patient? • in myself? • in others?	. . . could/should I have done to make it better?	
. . . was good/bad about the experience?	. . . is my new understanding of the situation?	
	. . . broader issues arise from the situation?	

Figure 8.1 Framework for reflection
Source: G Rolfe, D Freshwater & M Jasper 2001 *Critical reflection for nursing and the helping professions: a user's guide,* p 35. Palgrave, New York.

▲ whether journalling was appropriately conducted in work time or in the clinician's own time;

▲ who owned the journals, and who had a right of access to them; and

▲ what status the journals had in law; whether they could, for example, be used as evidence in the court room.

With the formal recognition that clinicians generally, and registered nurses in particular, are required to be 'reflective practitioners', it is now widely accepted that they should be journalling, and that this is part of their clinical work. Intellectual property is a vexed issue in law, and there does not appear to be any precedent set in Australian law as to the obligations of clinicians in relation to journals, but there does appear to be general acceptance that they belong to their authors, and that employers therefore normally have no right of access. You should, however, be able to reassure managers that your reflective journal conforms to the usual ethical standards that apply in healthcare situations—namely, that they are securely stored and accessible only to authorised individuals (such as your supervisors or educators), that you use pseudonyms when referring to particular patients or colleagues, and that they are strictly for your private professional use.

Like all documents, journals may be ordered to be submitted as evidence in courts of law. Although this is extremely unlikely, and most of what appears in a journal may only have the status of 'hearsay evidence', it is wise to bear this possibility in mind. Another principle you should adopt, therefore, is that your journal should always refer to your colleagues and patients in a professional and respectful manner, even though it may express criticism. Your journal is, after all, not a vehicle for catharsis—that is, unrestricted emotional expression—rather, it is the professional documentation of your deeply and carefully considered thoughts.

Critical incident analysis

A critical incident is usually an event that is remembered as important to an individual or one that is provided to a learner for the purpose of reflection. The notion of a critical incident is discussed by Rolfe et al (2001) who outline how the term is negative because it brings to mind something unfortunate or life threatening, something we certainly found in a study that utilised critical incident analysis with nursing students (Usher et al 1999).

Critical incidents, however, should be thought of as events that are meaningful or significant in some way; they need not necessarily be large or major occurrences (Rolfe et al 2001), and they can be negative or positive experiences (Davies & Sharp 2000). Critical incident analysis is thought to lead to:

> . . . a deeper and more profound level of reflection because it goes beyond detailed description of an event that attracted attention, to analysis of and reflection on the meaning of the event (Griffin 2003:208).

A study by Usher et al (1999) found that writing critical incident analyses offered undergraduate nursing students an opportunity to distance themselves from an event and, as a result, come to understand it in new ways.

The box below provides a framework for a critical incident analysis, which has been taken from Davies and Sharp (2000:67–8).

Framework for critical incident analysis

1 Give a concise description of the incident (which relates to the learning outcomes).

---

2 Outline the rationale for choice of incident and its significance and relevance to you.

3 Identify pertinent issues related to the incident.

4 Reflect on and analyse the key issues focusing on: your own involvement; feelings and decision making; the involvement and role of others; identification of any dilemmas or ethical elements; and the rationale for action, drawing on relevant theory evaluation of the situation and the implications for practice and personal learning.

5 Conclusion.

Photography, drawing and other forms of creative expression

Taylor (2000) describes how reflection can be facilitated by creative expression. She explains that it is unclear whether the awareness of the creative expression precedes or follows the reflection, but that it occurs sufficiently to include it as a way of reflective thinking. Some have been inspired to draw or write poetically as a result of events they have experienced, while others have used art forms, such as photography, drawing, painting or music in an attempt to express their reactions. Rolfe et al (2001) explain that these techniques are described as creative because they involve using the imagination to transform experience away from the more accepted ways of analysis to the use of metaphor as a way of creating insight and facilitating learning.

SELF-AWARENESS AND CLINICAL SUPERVISION

In essence, self-awareness is the foundation skill upon which reflective practice is based. It offers individuals the opportunity to see themselves in certain situations and to observe how they affected the situation and the situation affected them (Atkins 2000). In fact, this is what differentiates reflection from other types of mental activity such as logical thinking or problem solving (Boud et al 1985). Reflection is also a very personal experience, as it opens the self up to scrutiny (Johns 1998). As a result, reflection can be disconcerting to the individual, as taken for granted competence and ways of coping are exposed as inadequate.

Self-awareness is also an essential skill for professional monitoring. As a professional you are required to be aware of yourself, and the influence you have on patients and the healthcare context. Consequently, constant and vigilant self-monitoring is an important skill that every nurse needs to develop. Registered nurses need to come to an understanding of their racist, sexist and ageist attitudes, for example, and identify how these impact on their practice. An awareness of your own frailties and susceptibilities is crucial to maintaining high standards of practice.

Many nurses do not care adequately for their own psychological and physical wellbeing, and yet are under pressure from their work and their domestic lives. It is important to consider whether you are going to work tired and distracted; whether you are overanxious, depressed or angry; whether you are going to work with a hangover and suffering the effects of too much alcohol. Many nurses find that the stress of their lives leads them to overuse medications, smoke heavily, or resort to illicit drugs. The reflective practitioner is aware of these tendencies and will take remedial action, seeking appropriate advice and support.

A similar argument applies to any tendency that may ultimately lead to professional misconduct, including inappropriate sexual thoughts, feelings of aggression, and racist, sexist, ageist or other prejudiced attitudes. A reflective practitioner becomes aware of these possibilities, takes action, and thus maintains high standards of practice. This self-monitoring role leads us almost seamlessly into the issue of clinical supervision.

Reflective processes have been linked by many authors to the process of clinical supervision. Marrow et al (1997), for example, outlined ways in which supervision could help develop reflective nursing practice among both supervisors and supervisees, through group supervision sessions, diary writing and so on. More recently, Severinsson (2001) has described how clinical supervision in nursing can be based on a 'reflective practitioner model', citing the work of Schön and Johns, both authors we have mentioned in this chapter. She sees reflective processes as integral to the analysis and understanding of the theory–practice relationship, which is one of the goals of the supervisee, and the consequent development of 'know-how'. She also sees reflection as essential to self-awareness, emotional education, and the development of 'know-what'. Supervision should be 'centred on enhancing the practitioner's ability to "reflect-in-action"' (Severinsson 2001:40)—that is, on the care being provided. She explains that:

> Clinical supervision demands reflection on what care is being provided. Reflection can result in a better understanding of oneself. There is a difference between concentrating on the dissatisfaction within oneself and striving not to repeat what caused it (e.g. feelings of guilt). It is important to find answers to questions such as: Why did I make this mistake? Why did I fail to observe factors of relevance in caring for this patient? A deeper insight into patient needs may thereby be developed (Severinsson 2001:43).

When you think about Severinsson's statement, it is not difficult to see how reflection could become a powerful tool in the supervisory process, and lead to real improvements in patient care.

PROBLEMS, CRITICISMS AND RESPONSES

Despite their endorsement by regulatory authorities and encouragement by educators, the use of reflective processes in nursing is not without critics. Some have argued that the evidence for their effectiveness, in increasing critical thinking, promoting learning and improving practice, remains weak (e.g. Burton 2000). However, there are several counterarguments:

▲ although little research has been conducted on its value to nursing, the concept of reflective practice is supported by empirical research conducted and elaborated over many years, notably in education, and the accumulated evidence as to its value in a variety of disciplines (e.g. science, social work, medicine, law, education) cannot be ignored;

▲ the research results, although limited, are favourable, and there is no evidence that clinicians taking time to engage in critical reflection has any detrimental effects;

▲ there are strong *a priori* (logical) arguments in its favour, such as the argument that a problem is unlikely to be acted upon unless it is recognised as a problem, and that learning entails reflection, and not merely experience or the absorption of facts;

▲ reflective processes acknowledge the value of the experiences and beliefs of all members of a discipline in contributing to its knowledge base and practice development; the alternative is that the views of a privileged group are allowed to dominate; and

▲ reflective processes happen naturally, and one cannot simply stop them without denying an integral part of one's personal identity; the alternative is to be robotic.

Oncology nurses reported reflective practice to be an important aspect of their work and of their support structures (Loftus & McDowell 2000), while the study by Johns (2001) showed that reflective practice serves to reveal the ways in which nurses care.

Finally, for the sake of balance, we should add that there are also a number of theoretical arguments that can be levelled at reflective processes in nursing. Cotton (2001) has brought attention to some of these, notably:

▲ despite its championship by many nursing authorities, reflection remains ill-defined and elusive; she notes Johns' (1998:2) observation that 'it seems an academic pastime to try and define exactly what it [reflective practice] is';

▲ reflection is a strategy for scrutinising private thoughts, a form of policing or surveillance by oneself on behalf of others; this complaint derives from the work of the French philosopher Michel Foucault (1972);

▲ reflection only masquerades as radical; in reality it is aimed at imposing a standardised way of thinking and acting; and

▲ not enough attention is paid to the negative effects of reflection and the problems that arise in trying to be a reflective practitioner.

We believe these are important issues that need to be considered by those who champion reflection, but we do not regard any as fatal to that cause. Our response to these criticisms is, in short, that:

▲ the meaning of words is a matter of convention, and agreement takes time to emerge;

▲ self-scrutiny is a positive feature of professional life; indeed 'profession' is often characterised by such self-regulation;

▲ the aim is to open up the practitioner's mind to possibilities, not to impose rules, and reflective practitioners are therefore more likely to be creative, to challenge the status quo, and to be independent thinkers; and

▲ the problems of reflective practice may have been underestimated, but they are increasingly acknowledged; in any case, this means only that we need to be better at reflective processes, not that they should be abandoned.

You should consider carefully, and reflect upon, the claims we have made in this chapter, and come to a reasoned and practical personal arrangement for your own development as a reflective practitioner. To help you do this, consider the following questions, and undertake some further reading on the subject.

REFLECTIVE QUESTIONS

1 How would you use pre-reflection to prepare yourself for the challenge of clinical practice?

2 Write a paragraph about how you will use reflective processes during your clinical practice. In the paragraph address the following:
    (a) the technique you think would be best suited to you and why;
    (b) whether a framework would help you; and
    (c) the benefits you might receive.

3 How will you use reflective processes to enhance your self-awareness and ensure you practise at the highest possible standard?

4 Why is it important for you as a reflective practitioner to understand the theoretical background of reflection?

RECOMMENDED READINGS

Emden C 1991 Becoming a reflective practitioner. In G Gray & R Pratt (eds) *Towards a discipline of nursing*, pp 335–54. Churchill Livingstone, Melbourne.

Heath H 1998 Keeping a reflective practice diary: a practical guide. *Nurse Education Today* 18:592–8.

Johns C, Freshwater D eds 1998 *Transforming nursing through reflective practice*. Blackwell Science, London.

Rolfe G, Freshwater D, Jasper M 2001 *Critical reflection for nursing and the helping professions: a user's guide*. Palgrave, New York.

Taylor B J 2000 *Reflective practice: a guide for nurses and midwives*. Allen & Unwin, Sydney.

CHAPTER NINE

Research in nursing: concepts and processes

John Daly, Doug Elliott & Esther Chang

LEARNING OBJECTIVES

Upon completion of this chapter, readers should have gained:

▲ an understanding of the role of research in the development of contemporary nursing;

▲ an appreciation of the need for a range of approaches to research in nursing;

▲ basic knowledge and understanding of research processes in nursing;

▲ an appreciation of the contribution of research to the development of knowledge and clinical practice standards in nursing; and

▲ an understanding of research critique and research dissemination processes in nursing.

KEY WORDS

Processes, research traditions, quantitative research, qualitative research, dissemination, critique, evidence

RESEARCH IN NURSING

This chapter introduces the reader to basic concepts and processes of research in nursing. Research has assumed a position of significance in Australian nursing, and there continues to be advances in knowledge development and the sophistication of research approaches.

The concept of research in nursing is not new in the Western world (D'Antonio 1997, Mulhall 1995). In Britain, Florence Nightingale was active in research in nursing in the nineteenth century, though it was not until 1940 that further progress occurred and it was 1963 before the first government-funded post to facilitate research in nursing was established in the Ministry of Health (Mulhall 1995). Nursing research and educational centres were established in some universities in the 1970s. In the United States, government support for research in nursing was initiated in the 1950s (D'Antonio 1997). By that time many universities had nursing degree courses at undergraduate and postgraduate level, as well as a significant number of nurse researchers with doctorates who were able to provide research leadership for the profession.

In Australia and New Zealand it was in the late 1980s when nursing was established as an academic discipline with a significant presence in universities. There continues to be growth in appropriately prepared nurse researchers who can provide research leadership, disciplinary scholarship and contribute to the ongoing professionalisation of nursing throughout Australasia. The nursing discipline, through various professional bodies, has highlighted the important role of research in the continued development of nursing as a practice discipline with a research-based body of knowledge (e.g. Royal College of Nursing Australia 2003). The Australian Nursing and Midwifery Council (2000:3) highlights that a key competency of a registered nurse is the value of research in contributing to developments in nursing and improved standards of care by:

▲ acknowledging the importance of research in improving nursing outcomes;

▲ incorporating research findings into nursing practice; and

▲ contributing to the process of nursing research.

WHAT IS RESEARCH?

Research is a rigorous process of inquiry designed to provide answers to questions about phenomena of concern within an academic discipline or profession. It is defined as 'the systematic study of materials and sources to establish facts and reach new conclusions' (*Compact Oxford English dictionary* 2004:1). Research is a complex subject and field comprised of a number of well-established but diverse traditions. In a chapter such as this, it is possible to present only broad brushstrokes to familiarise the reader with key underpinnings about research processes in nursing. To develop in-depth knowledge and understanding of any one or a range of research traditions, processes and/or methods, further study and reading from a variety of sources will be necessary.

115

Research traditions can be investigated in relation to their philosophical underpinnings, and in the course of your reading of research you will encounter a number of essentially different paradigms. A research paradigm is an overarching framework that is based on values, beliefs and assumptions (Parse 1987). This framework contains theory about the nature of reality and guidelines for the methods to be used in carrying out research using (or within) the paradigm (Parse 2001). In addition, the ideas within the paradigm have implications for the type of knowledge being sought in a research study, the way in which the study will be carried out and the way in which outcomes from the work will be used.

As nursing is a complex field, researchers access a range of approaches, including positivist, feminist and interpretive paradigms. Quality research is labour, skill and resource intensive; therefore, a number of important decisions need to be made before embarking upon a research project. Not least, all research must be ethical, requiring adherence to strict guidelines (National Health and Medical Research Council 1997) and obtaining the necessary approval from institutional human research ethics committees.

Research has the potential to serve a number of purposes in a practice-based discipline such as nursing. Research is necessary to:

▲ test commonly held knowledge or assumptions;

▲ widen understanding of a subject;

▲ stimulate self-action/study;

▲ develop best practice (i.e. research-based practice);

▲ explain behaviours;

▲ allow predictions; and

▲ assist in the formation of a body of nursing knowledge.

The use of research knowledge in practice is the most common contact professional and student nurses have with research. This contact will be through reading, reviewing and critiquing research studies published in the literature. Constructing a review of the relevant literature is often called 'secondary research', while developing and conducting an original study is called 'primary research'. Levels of research use and understanding can be described by the '4 As of research' (Elliott 2003b:7). These are:

1 *Awareness* of and access to the research literature;

2 *Appreciation* or the ability to understand and critique the language of research;

3 *Application* of research findings to local practice settings; and

4 *Ability* to conduct original (primary) research independently or in a team.

The aim of the first three As of research is not to produce research workers, but to cultivate and nurture nurses to:

▲ accept research as a normal and integral aspect of nursing practice;

▲ read and understand research reports;

▲ apply research findings to clinical practice (i.e. evidence-based practice);

- ▲ influence colleagues on the use of research data; and

- ▲ accept responsibility for their own professional development (Crookes & Davies 1998:xii).

That is, not all nurses need to undertake research, but *all nurses* should *use research* in their practice. Some nurses will also undertake original research (the fourth 'A').

WHERE DO WE FIND RESEARCH?

Literally hundreds of research journals, dissertations, reports and books are published each year. One of the most important steps in the research process is conducting a thorough literature review. Students are often faced with the dilemma of how extensive a review is necessary. There is no formula to determine that 20 or 120 articles will provide the necessary background for the study. The number of references will depend on how familiar you are with the area under investigation, and the scope of the review will depend on how much research is available for that topic. Checking the reference list at the end of recent articles can often assist in the process. Experienced researchers know that maintaining an up-to-date review of the literature is an ongoing process throughout any research activity.

To begin with, it is important to differentiate between primary and secondary sources (this is equivalent to primary and secondary research approaches). A primary source is a report written by the study author/s themselves. A primary source includes information on the rationale of the study, its participants, design, methods of collecting data, procedure, results, outcomes, limitations, recommendations and references. Most research articles published in professional journals are primary sources. A secondary source is one that summarises information from primary sources presented by other authors. When an author cites a previous study in the review of literature section, that is a secondary source.

Both primary and secondary sources are important in different circumstances. Secondary sources such as systematic reviews (SRs) are becoming increasingly common as the best available evidence when reviewing clinical practice issues. However, secondary sources should be limited when undertaking your own secondary research (i.e. a literature review), while every effort to obtain relevant primary sources should be an aim of the activity.

Indexes, abstracts and databases

Most libraries now provide reference sources via computer databases to assist students in locating references on a specific topic and to undertake their own computer searches. A computer search will generate complete bibliographic citations, often including abstracts of many articles published in a particular area of interest. A variety of indexes and databases are available, providing bibliographic listings of articles, abstracts, conference proceedings and books. All indexes provide bibliography citations, giving the authors' names, publication date, article title, journal volume and issue number, and pages. Each academic discipline has an index to its collection of journals.

A valuable index and database in the health science literature is the Cumulative Index to Nursing and Allied Health Literature (CINAHL), which has journals from nursing and allied health disciplines listed. Another important index and database is Medline, a bibliography of medical studies (Elliott 2003b). The related database, Pubmed, provides free public access to Medline studies (http://www.ncbi.nlm.nih. gov/entrez). Other important abstract indexes that may be relevant to your topic are: Education Resources Information Centre (ERIC), Psychology Abstracts, Sociological Abstracts, Cancer Therapy Abstracts (CANCERLIT) and Dissertation Abstracts International.

Most indexes and databases use key words or medical subject (MeSH) headings. When a topic is not found in the subject headings, you can search key words that have been adopted by most of the journal publishers. Many journals also publish key words with an article. Most university libraries hold extensive collections of refereed journals across a range of disciplines. Many databases now provide full-text papers online, although this function may be restricted to journal subscribers (check with your professional library for access rights to journals).

Peer-reviewed journals

Peer-reviewed journals serve many important functions, including facilitation of expert review of manuscripts, reporting the findings of research studies or theoretical papers, dissemination of papers that have been approved for publication following peer review, and serving as a resource for scholars and researchers involved in compiling and/or developing knowledge in an area of nursing research or practice. Criteria that must be met before a paper is approved for publication in a refereed journal vary, but all editors will be concerned with maintaining a standard of excellence in regard to scientific merit and the literary standard of the work, and the relevance of the paper in terms of its potential to contribute to knowledge development in the topic area.

There are many peer-reviewed journals in nursing internationally. Each has its own aims, purposes and requirements, which must be followed by nurses wishing to submit their work for peer review with a view to being published in the journal. Most journals have a related website that provides further details for readers and authors.

HOW NURSES CAN USE RESEARCH

Nursing and other health professionals are concerned with improving the quality of patient care and establishing standards for best clinical practice, by examining the current knowledge base of the discipline. Findings from research studies are disseminated at conferences and in professional journals. Some studies are designed to inform practice development by describing a clinical practice, or comparing two (or more) different ways of performing a practice. Other types of studies may shed light on patients' experiences of phenomena that are poorly understood, such as hope or suffering.

The ability to critique studies is therefore a fundamental skill for undergraduate nurses to master in preparation for professional practice as registered nurses. Current registered nurses also need these skills in terms of continuing professional development. However, the skill is not easily attained, and does not magically appear at the end of a single university research course. Rather, the ability is additive and experiential, as it is related to experience, practice and reflection over time. In fact, it is an ability that relates to 'lifelong learning' where we can always learn and improve our skills.

Evidence-based practice

The critique of an individual research paper can be extended to multiple papers on the same topic, resulting in a literature review. This is a common assessment item for university nursing students. There are various tools available to assist readers in critiquing research papers (e.g. Schneider 2003), but the most important factor is exposure and experience in reading research publications.

An adaptation of the narrative literature review is a systematic review (SR), which addresses a well-defined question, provides specific information on the process undertaken to minimise bias in the review process, and uses a systematic approach to assess the quality of each study (Droogan & Cullum 1998). The question for an SR has a specific clinical focus with four components forming the acronym PICO:

P Problem (patient-related or a health issue)
I   Intervention
C Comparison of interventions and/or control practice
O Outcome (that is measurable) (Leslie & Finn 2003:95)

When conducting an SR, the search strategy describes the databases (e.g. CINAHL, Medline) used and any journals searched by hand. Selection of articles is by key words in the article title or abstract, as well as any other filters (e.g. English language, study design). A preliminary review of the abstract enables identification of the papers for inclusion in the SR. The excluded paper may also be noted, including the reasons for exclusion. Included studies are then assessed according to a structured and explicit criteria. An SR may also include the pooling and analysis of data from the studies investigated; this process is called a meta-analysis.

A number of organisations are now developing repositories of SRs to appropriately guide clinical practice (Cochrane 1972). The Cochrane Collaboration was one of the first to develop as an international multidisciplinary collaborative group to systematically review clinical research, and is now represented in many countries including Australia (see http://www.cochranc.org.au). The Cochrane Collaboration aims to develop, maintain and disseminate SRs of healthcare interventions, and includes a database of completed and in-progress reviews, a bibliography of SR abstracts and methodological articles.

The majority of the current SRs are related to medicine. This is not surprising, given the number of studies and journals devoted to topics in the various medical subspecialities. The most powerful and rigorous design (the 'gold standard') for examining cause-and-effect questions in clinical practice is the randomised controlled trial (RCT). Thus, the classification developed for rating the levels of evidence (National Health and Medical Research Council 1999) regard the RCT as providing the best evidence to answer these types of clinical practice questions:

Level I:	a systematic review of all relevant randomised controlled trials (RCTs)
Level II:	at least one properly designed RCT
Level III—1:	well-designed controlled trials without randomisation
Level III—2:	well-designed comparative studies with concurrent controls (e.g. cohort, case-control)
Level III—3:	well-designed time-series studies with historial controls (before–after)
Level IV:	post-test, pretest/post-test

If there is no rigorous scientific evidence available, then the opinions of respected authorities, clinical experience, descriptive studies, or reports of expert committees, can be used to support clinical practice (National Health and Medical Research Council 2000).

The Joanna Briggs Institute for Evidence-Based Nursing and Midwifery (see http://www.joannabriggs.edu.au) and the Centre for Evidence-Based Nursing in the UK (http://www.york.ac.uk/healthsciences/centres/evidence/cebn.htm) conduct SRs of specific clinical practices which are of importance to nurses.

It should be noted, however, that nursing uses a variety of research paradigms and methods to answer questions that cannot be appropriately investigated by RCTs. We therefore need to consider how to evaluate non-RCT observational studies of nursing practice so that these findings can also guide nursing care. Further, how do we incorporate findings from qualitative studies, which have no generalisability to the patient group in question, but which may provide valuable insights of patient experiences in guiding quality nursing practice? One approach has included explicit assessment of the study description, methodological rigour (including documentation, procedure, confirmability of data collection and analysis), analytical preciseness, and theoretical connectedness (Cesario et al 2002).

The development of these necessary frameworks continues to evolve, but are not yet formed or developed to an adequate level nationally or internationally. The goal remains to foster SRs of relevant studies on clinical nursing so that quality nursing practice will be informed by the best available evidence, regardless of the research design.

Developing research questions

Research ideas come from many sources. Some ideas are derived from theoretical considerations, while others arise from the need to solve practical problems or to improve the quality of care. Having a good idea is often not enough—you need to translate that idea into research questions. This section briefly discusses how to develop research questions based on the amount of knowledge and/or theory about the topic, and describes the importance of a thorough review of the literature to identify relevant theory and research.

A research question needs to be clearly stated as an 'explicit query about a problem or issue that can be challenged, examined, and analysed and that will yield useful new information' (Brink & Wood 1993:2). Although there are no specific rules and procedures for asking research questions, the way research questions are worded can have an effect on the research design and methods that follow.

When formulating a research question it is important that you discuss your topic and question with your colleagues or experts in the field, as this will assist you with the development and refinement of the question. Often the initial research question is structured too broadly to provide a feasible project in terms of timeframe and resources. Consider the following example: Do undergraduate students taught in a supportive environment increase their learning capabilities as graduates? Before this can be answered, a number of issues have to be clarified. What exactly is a supportive environment? What does it mean to increase their learning capabilities? How do we measure learning capabilities? How do we determine learning capabilities in graduates? Until you can define the terms and determine how to measure the variables they represent, you cannot answer the original question. Frequently, researchers have to narrow the topic area or, in some cases, the types and number of settings or the number of participants they include in the study. This process of narrowing the topic ultimately must also be consistent with the research design and methods of the study.

Research questions can be classified based on the amount of knowledge and/or theory about the topic area. Questions may be exploratory and descriptive, through to testing or confirmatory. The style of question directs the research approach. Exploratory studies are used when there is little or no literature on either the topic or the population to be researched. Questions at this level are designed to explore the topic or a single population—for example, 'What is . . .?' or 'What are . . .?' the phenomena or concepts of interest. Studies that build on exploratory studies have some existing knowledge and theory about the topic and population. Questions at this level often examine relationships between phenomena or measurable variables— for example, 'What is the relationship . . .?' between two or more concepts. These questions lead to correlation designs, where statistical analysis is used to determine the significance of the relationship between the variables. Questions at a testing or confirmatory level require considerable knowledge about the topic. Research at this level begins at knowing the relationships between variables; therefore questions at level III are designed to examine why this relationship exists, with a rationale and with an explanation. These questions lead to experimental designs.

Reviewing the literature

Whether you begin with a vague idea of a study or a well-developed research plan, every project needs to be considered an extension of previous knowledge. An appropriate review of the literature is therefore a common beginning stage of a study. First, your research question may have been addressed and answered, or a review can be the initial source of ideas for a research question. By being familiar with and understanding what has already been done with existing research and theory in an area, you can devise your research study to explore any newly identified questions. A review will also assist you to establish a theoretical context and rationale for your study. From a practical (methodological) perspective, the review can also reveal appropriate research strategies, measuring instruments, techniques and analysis. The review allows you to learn from the strengths and limitations of other researchers' work in regard to successful outcomes and assumptions, and keeps you current with the research work being undertaken in your area of interest.

NURSING RESEARCH PROCESSES

Research can be either quantitative or qualitative.

Quantitative research

The term 'quantitative research' refers to studies that seek to measure some concept or phenomenon of interest—for example, blood pressure, pain, or student attitudes to learning about research. The quantitative research paradigm is also called positivist, reductionist or empirical. Quantitative reasoning is termed deductive, which means the thinking leads from a known principle to an unknown, and is used to test a particular research hypothesis.

Quantitative research encompasses a range of research designs and associated methods; the most common designs used in healthcare research are listed in Table 9.1.

Table 9.1: Common quantitative research designs

Design	Purpose
Descriptive	Examines characteristics of a single sample; clarifies concepts; generates questions about potential relationships between variables (e.g. case study, cross-sectional analysis)
Correlation	Examines (describes, predicts or tests) relationships between two or more variables, but does not infer a cause-and-effect relationship
Quasi-experiment	Tests a cause-and-effect relationship, but without control or randomisation (e.g. case control, intervention-only)
Experiment	Tests a cause-and-effect relationship using randomisation, manipulation of an intervention and control of other variables (e.g. randomised controlled trial (RCT), laboratory experiment)

Selection of an appropriate design relates to the research question being posed (Sackett & Wennberg 1997). The topic of interest may be framed as a question, objective or research hypothesis. Each design incorporates a number of variations; readers are directed to any number of nursing research texts for amplification of these designs (e.g. Burns & Grove 2005, Crookes & Davies 2004, Roberts & Taylor 1998, Schneider et al 2003).

Quantitative studies rely on sampling a smaller group of individuals who have similar (representative) characteristics to the overall population of interest. Inclusion and/or exclusion criteria (defined in Table 9.2) are developed, which guide the selection of participants. In experimental studies, the explanatory (independent) variable (an intervention) is manipulated by randomly assigning subjects to a treatment or control group, while the outcome (dependent) variable of interest is measured and other related variables are controlled (e.g. RCT).

Measurement of the concepts of interest is conducted using single or multiple 'measuring instruments' (also called tools); these can be physiological (e.g. heart rate monitor, blood glucometer) or psychological/psychometric (e.g. anxiety scales, functional status, quality of life). Ideally, an instrument should exhibit characteristics that are valid, reliable and responsive. Development of new instruments is time-consuming and resource-intensive, as the validity, reliability and responsiveness must be tested, and modification of items (questions) may be required to improve the performance of the instrument. Established instruments generally have had their validity and reliability rigorously tested over time, and have been accepted as useful research tools.

Instrument (measurement) validity refers to whether the instrument actually measures what it is intended to measure. The aim is for an instrument to have appropriate construct validity—that is, the extent that an instrument accurately measures a theoretical construct or trait that is established over time, following repeated use and testing of the instrument in various studies. With any instrument there is the possibility of measurement error. The aim of a good study or instrument is to minimise the chance of that error. There are numerous subforms of construct validity that have been used to describe increasing rigour for testing an instrument's performance (Elliott 2003a). For example:

Table 9.2: Glossary of common quantitative research terms

Term	Meaning
Construct validity	The extent to which a measuring instrument measures a theoretical construct or characteristic
Descriptive statistics	Description of characteristics (e.g. frequency, percentages), but no inference of relationships between variables
Exclusion criteria	A list of characteristics that exclude an individual from being in a study (e.g. less than 24 hours admission in hospital; presence of other illnesses that may influence patient outcomes)
Explanatory variable	Independent variable; the intervention being manipulated to exhibit a change in the outcome variable
Inclusion criteria	A list of the characteristics required for a subject to be included in a study (e.g. patients admitted for cardiac surgery; 16 years or older; English language skills (reading and writing) sufficient to complete the study questionnaires)
Inferential statistics	Statistical procedures used to test an hypothesis about the relationships between two or more variables (e.g. t-tests, analysis of variance, regression modelling) and the application of study findings to the population being studied (generalisability)
Measuring instrument	The tool used to measure the concept of interest (e.g. questionnaire; biochemical test)
Normal distribution	Distribution of scores for a particular variable follow a bell-shape pattern around the mean score for the sample; required to use inferential statistics
Outcome variable	Dependent variable; measurement of the concept being studied
Primary research	Original research conducted with participants (e.g. patients, health professionals, students)
Reliability	The consistency or stability of a measure or instrument on repeated uses
Responsiveness	The ability of a measuring instrument to detect small but important differences of a dynamic characteristic
Sample	A selected group of participants who have similar characteristics to the population from which they were drawn (i.e. representative); allows for generalisation of results from the study sample to the wider population
Secondary research	A process where data from previous primary research studies are reinvestigated (e.g. literature review, systematic review)

▲ content (appears to include all major elements of the concept; often assessed by an expert panel of relevant professionals; includes face validity—on the face of it, the instrument appears to measure the concept);

▲ relationship to other variables of measures (e.g. criterion-related—examines the instrument against another or the 'gold-standard' criteria); and

▲ hypothesis-testing (uses theory to test relationships between concepts).

Reliability relates to the accuracy with which the instrument measures the concept being investigated, and which can be tested in terms of stability (test–retest: similar scores on repeated testing for a stable trait), homogeneity (internal consistency: all parts of the instrument measure the same characteristics), and equivalence (interrater reliability: consistency between observers using the same instrument with the same study participants). There are a number of statistical tests for reliability, which are commonly expressed as a correlation coefficient, ranging from 0.0 to 1.0. A reliability of 0.80 is considered the minimal acceptable coefficient for a developed instrument.

Responsiveness is the ability of an instrument to detect clinically important changes in the variable of interest with a participant (Elliott 2003a:345). This is the opposite characteristic to stability, and relates to the precision of measurement for the instrument. Unfortunately, assessment of this performance characteristic has been minimal when compared to reliability and validity testing.

In addition to the Glossary at the end of this book, Table 9.2 explains some common quantitative research terms used in this chapter. More detailed glossaries are available in specific nursing research texts (e.g. Burns & Grove 2005, Crookes & Davies 1998, Roberts & Taylor 1998, Schneider et al 2003).

Quantitative studies collect numerical data to answer the questions or objectives posed. All information is therefore transformed to numbers prior to data management and analysis. Data analysis procedures can be descriptive or inferential, depending on the design and the levels of measurement for each variable (i.e. nominal, ordinal, interval, ratio). The categories must be mutually exclusive and collectively exhaustive:

▲ *Nominal*: Assigns values to classify characteristics into non-ordered categories (e.g. sex, religion, diagnosis). The assigned numbers do not convey any relative order or weight between the values (e.g. 1 = male, 2 = female; in this instance there is no implication that '1' is ordered higher than '2', or that '2' is twice the score of '1').

▲ *Ordinal*: Values are ordered in a logical way in providing a relative ranking (e.g. pain, levels of mobility, self-care, use of Likert scales—'strongly agree', 'agree', 'undecided', 'disagree', 'strongly disagree').

▲ *Interval*: Values exhibit a rank ordering with equal distance between values (e.g. temperature, scores on a linear analogue scale (from 1 to 10)).

▲ *Ratio*: Values have the above characteristics plus a meaningful baseline or absolute zero (e.g. weight, height, heart rate).

Data management and analysis are commonly undertaken using software packages (e.g. MS Excel spreadsheet software can undertake certain statistical analysis procedures or Statistical Package for the Social Sciences (SPSS) is a comprehensive analysis package). Study designs and methods that provide findings using inferential statistics allow the researcher to 'infer' that the results from a sample of participants (e.g. patients) can be applied to the wider population being investigated. Inferential statistics are further categorised into parametric or non-parametric procedures. Parametric tests are used when the following assumptions are met: the sample was drawn from a normal distribution; random sampling was used; and data were measured at least at interval level.

As beginning research consumers, students must consider the objectives of the study and the related purposes for the statistical tests performed. Table 9.3 can be used to critique papers for consistency between the purpose, the level of measurement, and actual tests that are appropriate to answer those questions. More in-depth information regarding the actual statistical tests is beyond the scope of this chapter, but can be found in comprehensive research texts.

Qualitative research

The term 'qualitative research' spans a range of research designs and approaches. This field of research has its origins in the humanities disciplines such as philosophy, anthropology, history and sociology (Denzin & Lincoln 2000). Qualitative research focuses on human experiences, including accounts of subjective realities, and is conducted in naturalistic settings involving close, often sustained contact between

Table 9.3: Statistical purposes and related parametric and non-parametric tests

Statistical purpose	Parametric test	Non-parametric test
Compares *mean scores* for two independent samples	Two sample (unpaired) *t*-test (*interval/ratio data*)	Mann-Whitney U test (*ordinal data*)
Compares *mean scores* for two sets of observations from the same sample	Paired *t*-test (*interval/ratio data*)	Wilcoxon matched pairs test (*ordinal data*)
Compares *mean scores* for three or more sets of observations	One-way analysis of variance (ANOVA)	Kruskall-Wallis ANOVA by ranks
Compares *proportions* from two samples	Chi-square (χ^2) test	Fisher's exact test
Compares *proportions* from a paired sample	No equivalent	McNemar's test
Assesses strength of straight line *association* between two variables	Product moment correlation coefficient (Pearson's *r*)	Spearman's rank correlation coefficient (r^S)
Describes *relationship* between two variables, allowing one to be *predicted* from the other	Simple linear regression	Non-parametric regression
Describes *relationship* between a dependent variable and several predictor variables	Multiple regression	Non-parametric regression

Source: Adapted from N Burns & S K Grove 2005 *The practice of nursing research: conduct, critique and utilization,* 5th edn, Elsevier/Saunders, St Louis; T Greenhalgh 1997 *How to read a paper: the basics of evidence based medicine,* BMJ Publishing, London; and Z Schneider, D Elliott, G LoBiondo-Wood & J Haber (eds) 2003 *Nursing research: methods, critical appraisal and utilisation,* 2nd edn, Mosby, Sydney.

the researcher and research participants (Denzin & Lincoln 2000, Sarantakos 2005). Naturalistic research is often referred to as field research (Polit et al 2001), because it is conducted in the 'field'. This label may be applied to a range of contexts—for example, a community health centre, an intensive care unit or a participant's home.

The qualitative researcher approaches a study with a particular set of values and beliefs, which is different from the purely quantitative researcher. These differences relate to the world view (ontology) of the researcher, notions about epistemology (ways of knowing) and research methodology (Parse 2001, Sarantakos 2005). For example, in the qualitative or interpretive paradigm, value is placed on individual subjectivity, multiple truths are accommodated and individuals who participate in the study are regarded as active participants and partners in the research (Sarantakos 2005). In the positivist paradigm, the opposite applies and concepts such as control, precision, objectivity, testing, one truth, prediction and cause–effect are valued, while individual perceptions are not considered or trusted.

Qualitative research methods are richly descriptive in nature (Sarantakos 2005) and allow exploration of a range of human experiences, which are of interest in a discipline such as nursing—for example, the experience of suffering for people living with terminal cancer, the characteristics of cultural groups, including their health beliefs, or the question 'What is comfort for recipients of nursing?' It may be possible to study these phenomena using a quantitative approach, but this could be very limiting. Human interaction and intrapersonal and interpersonal communication processes may influence the experience of comfort for recipients of care. Qualitative research approaches would therefore produce richer, more in-depth accounts of this phenomenon.

Sampling approaches in qualitative research deliberately seek people who have lived the experience under investigation. Reasoning in qualitative research is inductive but may involve a process of induction–deduction. The advantage of using a qualitative approach is that the phenomenon may be studied more holistically, taking account of individual and group perspectives (Nieswiadomy 2002), with a focus on the human experience; this is sometimes referred to as 'lived experience' (Parse 2001). In qualitative studies, the researcher's aim is development of a thick description of the experience under investigation—that is, 'a rich and thorough description of the research context' (Polit et al 2001:472).

Qualitative studies are commonly carried out with small numbers of research participants and involve in-depth inquiry into the phenomenon of concern. The data in qualitative research are presented in the form of words rather than numbers. The researcher may interview participants and audio-tape the conversation, which is later transcribed for data analysis. In this way narrative text is often assembled by the researcher in working with the research participants. The text of the interview can be analysed and developed into themes to reflect core ideas or recurring features in the data (Miles & Huberman 1994). This process involves intensive reflection on the part of the researcher. The qualitative paradigm is often referred to as interpretive because as:

> . . . social interaction is a process of interpretation; social reality is constructed through interpretation of the actors; social relations are the result of a process of interaction based on interpretation; and theory building is a process of interpretation (Sarantakos 1993:50).

A range of research approaches are available, depending on the aims or purposes of the study. Each approach incorporates a way of structuring the study, selecting the research participants, collecting and analysing the data. Some examples are provided below. Readers are also directed to nursing and social science research texts for amplification of the approaches to qualitative research described below (Denzin & Lincoln 2000, Munhall & Oiler Boyd 1993, Parse 2001, Sarantakos 2005, Schneider et al 2003).

Phenomenology is a philosophy and a descriptive research method designed to uncover the essence and meaning of lived experiences—for example, suffering or grieving (Parse 2001). 'The phenomenologist investigates subjective phenomena in the belief that critical truths about reality are grounded in people's lived experiences'(Polit et al 2001:214).

Ethnography is a qualitative, theory-building, holistic research approach that is applied to study of the culture of a group (Nieswiadomy 2002, Polit et al 2001).

> In ethnographic research, the researcher frequently lives with the people [being studied] and becomes a part of their culture. The researcher explores with the people their rituals and customs. An entire cultural group may be studied or a subgroup in the culture. The term *culture* may be used in a broad sense to mean an entire tribe of Indians, for example, or in the more narrow sense to mean one nursing care unit (Nieswiadomy 2002:153).

The ethnographer sets out to uncover insiders' (emic) view of the culture under study as opposed to the outsiders' (etic) view (Polit et al 2001).

Grounded theory is a research process designed to lead to generation of theory through study of a particular human context. In grounded theory research studies, 'data are collected and analyzed and then a theory is developed that is "grounded" in the data' (Nieswiadomy 2002:360).

CONCLUSION

An understanding of basic concepts and processes in research is central to professional nursing practice. Ideally, quality nursing care is based on the outcomes of quality research processes. It is envisaged that, in time, one of the hallmarks of the profession of nursing will be the utilisation of research evidence to inform the best, safest and most appropriate care for patients and their families. All nurses engaged in nursing practice require research utilisation skills in order to make judgments about how relevant and applicable research findings are to practice. Nursing is a complex, practice-based discipline in which researchable questions will always require answers in order to extend knowledge. A range of research paradigms and approaches are available to appropriately answer these questions.

In the course of your reading and learning about research processes in nursing you will discover that in some instances researchers use 'triangulation' of both quantitative and qualitative research processes to study a particular area of interest. The evaluative criteria for establishing the scientific validity of qualitative research are the subject of continuing development and debate (e.g. Cesario et al 2002). As the content of this chapter is introductory, you can also expect to learn of other research traditions, paradigms and methods during your undergraduate education.

REFLECTIVE QUESTIONS

1 What processes could be followed in formulating a research problem in nursing?

2 What advantages, if any, might qualitative research designs have over quantitative research designs in clinical nursing research?

3 What are the critical features of a comprehensive review of the literature?

RECOMMENDED READINGS

Borbasi S, Jackson D, Langford R 2004 *Negotiating the maze of nursing research: an interactive learning adventure.* Mosby, Melbourne.
Burns N, Grove S K 2005 *The practice of nursing research: conduct, critique and utilization,* 5th edn. Elsevier/Saunders, St Louis.
Carper B 1978 Fundamental patterns of knowing in nursing. *Advances in Nursing Science* 1(1):13–23.
Crookes P A, Davies S eds 2004 *Research into practice: essential skills for reading and applying research in nursing and health care.* Bailliere Tindall, Edinburgh.
Schneider Z, Elliott D, LoBiondo-Wood G, Haber J eds 2003 *Nursing research: methods, critical appraisal and utilisation,* 2nd edn. Mosby, Sydney.

CHAPTER TEN

Ethics in nursing

Megan-Jane Johnstone

This chapter will:

- ▲ define nursing ethics;

- ▲ outline the development of mainstream bioethics;

- ▲ discuss the relationship between nursing ethics and mainstream bioethics;

- ▲ explore a range of 'everyday' ethical issues that nurses might face in the course of providing nursing care to clients/patients; and

- ▲ discuss five areas in which a re-examination of the ethical issues faced by the nursing profession is warranted.

KEY WORDS
Moral, ethics, nursing ethics, bioethics, social justice

NURSING AND ETHICS

Nurses at all levels and in all areas of practice are confronted every day with having to make morally relevant choices and to take action on the basis of these choices during the course of their work. This 'everyday' occurrence should not be taken to mean, however, that deciding and acting morally in nursing care contexts is simply a matter of habit or 'daily routine', and therefore as something trivial requiring little knowledge, skill or attention. It is to the contrary. As can be readily demonstrated, dealing with everyday ethical problems requires of decision makers an exquisite moral sensibility, 'moral knowing', moral imagination, life experience, virtue (e.g. compassion, empathy, integrity, care, 'decency'), general 'informedness' (e.g. about law, social and cultural processes, human nature, politics), and a deep personal commitment to 'doing what is right'. In some instances 'being moral' also requires political savvy and an ability (personal and otherwise) to overcome the many obstacles that may obstruct or prevent a morally just outcome.

Although it should be otherwise, there are times when deciding to act morally can require enormous courage and even 'moral heroism' on the part of those choosing to take an ethical course of action. This is especially so in the case of nurses who, despite an apparent increase in professional status over the past several decades, continue to lack authority in their own realm of practice, continue to be burdened with enormous responsibilities without the lawful authority to fulfil them, and continue to be forced into silence when what they have to say on important ethical issues threatens the powerful vested interests of others (Johnstone 1994, 2004a, 2004c).

All aspects of nursing (e.g. education, practice, management, leadership and research) have a profound ethical dimension. This dimension of nursing is distinguished from others such as the legal and clinical dimensions by the inherent moral demands to:

▲ promote human wellbeing and welfare;

▲ balance the needs and significant moral interests of different people;

▲ make reliable judgments on what constitutes morally 'right' and 'wrong' conduct; and

▲ provide sound justifications for the decisions and actions taken on the basis of these judgments.

Members of the nursing profession cannot escape these demands or the stringent responsibilities they impose. One reason for this is that no nursing decision or action (however small or trivial) occurs in a moral vacuum, or is free of moral risk or consequence—even the most 'ordinary' of nursing actions can affect significantly the wellbeing, welfare and moral interests of others. This is so whether in a nursing education, practice, management, leadership or research setting.

Nursing codes of ethics around the world make clear that nurses have a stringent moral responsibility to promote and safeguard the wellbeing, welfare and moral interests of people needing and/or receiving nursing care. These codes also variously recognise the responsibility of nurses to balance equally the needs and interests of different people in healthcare contexts. What is often not stated, however, is *how* nurses ought to fulfil their moral responsibilities to deal effectively with the many ethical issues they encounter on a day-to-day basis. 'Dealing effectively' with ethical issues in this instance includes being able to:

▲ identify correctly the most pertinent ethical issues facing nurses (locally and globally) at any given time;

▲ recognise both the short-term and long-term implications of these issues for the nursing profession generally; and

▲ develop strategies for responding effectively to these issues, once identified.

Dealing effectively with ethical issues in nursing also requires at least a rudimentary understanding of:

▲ what nursing ethics are; and

▲ the relationship between nursing ethics and mainstream bioethics.

Let us now consider these two points.

WHAT ARE NURSING ETHICS?

In advancing this discussion, it is important to first provide a brief definition of the notion 'nursing ethics'. Nursing ethics can be defined broadly as the examination of all kinds of ethical (and bioethical) issues from the perspective of nursing theory and practice. In turn, these issues rest on the agreed core concepts of nursing: person, culture, care, health, healing, environment, and nursing itself (i.e. its end and good or *telos*) (Johnstone 2004a:14). In this regard then, and contrary to popular belief, nursing ethics are not synonymous with (and indeed are much greater than) an ethic of care, although an ethic of care has an important place in the overall moral scheme of nursing and nursing ethics.

Unlike other approaches to ethics, nursing ethics recognise the 'distinctive voices' that are nurses', and emphasise the importance of collecting and recording nursing narratives and 'stories from the field' (Benner 1991, 1994, Bishop & Scudder 1990, Parker 1990, Hodge 1993). Collecting and collating stories from the field are regarded as important, since issues invariably emerge from these stories that extend far beyond the 'paramount' issues otherwise espoused by mainstream bioethics (to be identified shortly). Analyses of these stories tend to reveal not only a range of issues that are nurses' 'own', as it were, but a whole different configuration of language, concepts and metaphors for expressing them (Johnstone 2004a:14). As well, these stories often reveal issues otherwise overlooked or marginalised by mainstream bioethics discourse.

Given this, nursing ethics can also be described as 'methodologically and substantively, inquiry from the point of view of nurses' experiences', with nurses' experiences being taken as a more reliable starting point than other mainstream ethics discourses (texts, practices and processes) from which to advance meaningful discussions on nursing ethics and the development of helpful processes for addressing ethical issues in nursing and related healthcare contexts (Johnstone 2004a:14–15).

NURSING ETHICS AND THEIR RELATIONSHIP WITH MAINSTREAM BIOETHICS

Contemporary nursing ethics have been profoundly influenced by the Western mainstream bioethics movement. Whether this influence has been advantageous to the development of nursing ethics, however, remains an open question and one that has yet to be fully explored by the nursing profession (see also Johnstone 2004a).

The term 'bioethics' first found its way into public usage in 1970–71 in the United States (Reich 1994). Although originally only cautiously accepted by a few influential North American academics, the new term quickly 'symbolized and influenced the rise and shaping of the field itself' (Reich 1994:320). Significantly, within three years of its emergence, the new term was accepted and used widely at a public level (Reich 1994:328). Today, both in lay and professional circles, bioethics (and all the issues associated with it as a movement) have become the subject of major interest and debate.

Initially, the term 'bioethics' was used in two different ways. The first (and later marginalised) sense had an 'environmental and evolutionary significance' (Reich 1994:320). The other, competing sense in which the word 'bioethics' was used referred more narrowly to the ethics of medicine and biomedical research. Significantly, it was this latter sense which 'came to dominate the emerging field of bioethics in academic circles and in the mind of the public', and which remains dominant today (Reich 1994:320).

The primary focus of contemporary bioethical debate tends to be on 'exotic' issues such as abortion, euthanasia and assisted suicide (and the associated issue of advanced directives), organ transplantation (and the associated issue of brain death criteria) and reproductive technology (e.g. in vitro fertilisation (IVF), surrogacy, genetic engineering). The debate also focuses on ethics committees, informed consent, confidentiality, the economic rationalisation of healthcare, and research ethics (particularly in regard to randomised clinical trials and experimental surgery). Not only have mainstream bioethics come to refer to and represent the above and other related issues but, controversially, they have given legitimacy to them—through the power of naming—as *the* most pressing (or 'paramount') bioethical concerns of contemporary healthcare in the Western world.

The nursing profession, like other healthcare professions, has responded vigorously to the modern bioethics movement. Since the late 1970s, there has been a plethora of texts and journal articles published specifically on the topic of 'nursing ethics', in which a full range of the popular mainstream bioethical issues have been raised and explored; undoubtedly, these works have made an important contribution to knowledge of the field, and have assisted many nurses in their quest to competently and confidently fulfil the many moral responsibilities associated with their professional practice. Nevertheless, the apparent and possibly obvious practical importance of bioethics to nurses, while recognised, is not without controversy.

One reason for this controversy is that the dominance of the more exotic ethical issues in the nursing literature has sometimes been at the expense of other areas that could be judged as being more relevant to the profession and practice of nursing (Johnstone et al 2004). For example, while much has been written on the ethics of euthanasia and medically assisted suicide (both regarded as 'paramount' issues in the bioethics literature), comparatively little has been written on the unethical economic rationalisation (read 'decline') of expert nursing care services for people at the end stages of their lives.

Similarly, while literature abounds on the subject of promoting patients' rights (abstract entitlements) in healthcare contexts (e.g. the right to confidentiality, the right to give an informed consent to treatment, the right to die), comparatively little has been written on the promotion of patients' genuine wellbeing and welfare (tangible realities), which are sometimes compromised, paradoxically, in the interests of upholding a patient's supposed 'rights' (Johnstone 2004a:179–80). To further complicate the issue, there is much discussion on patients' rights to refuse medical treatment, but virtually nothing is said on patients' entitlements to request that 'everything possible be done', including (and perhaps especially) the provision of quality nursing care from qualified and skilled nurses.

And, to cite one more example, while much has been written on nurses' duties in regard to upholding patients' rights and employer interests, comparatively little has been written on nurses' rights and interests—despite the fact that, compared with other health workers, nurses are at disproportionate risk of being exploited, scapegoated, abused, injured, maimed and even killed during the course of their work (Alspach 1993, Hadfield 1991, Johnstone 1994, 2002, Kinkle 1993). On this point, it is significant that, although nurses are morally entitled to be protected from these abuses, and are not obligated to 'act beyond the call of duty' in situations where their lives and genuine wellbeing are at risk, the issue of nurse exploitation, scapegoating, abuse and violence has rarely been addressed as an ethical issue per se, either in the nursing ethics or mainstream bioethics literature (Johnstone 2002).

IDENTIFYING AND RESPONDING EFFECTIVELY TO ETHICAL ISSUES IN NURSING

It is important to understand that ethical issues in healthcare contexts do not only involve the so-called 'big' or 'exotic' issues (e.g. when to disconnect a 'brain dead' patient from a life-support machine or whether to abort a severely disabled fetus), they also involve fundamental questions about the nature and quality of professional–client relationships. It is also about examining the more fundamental day-to-day practical ethical concerns relating to the precise impact that nurses' decisions and actions (or non-actions) have on the lives and welfare of other human beings and to 'our capacity to do harm to others while claiming scientific and professional legitimacy' (adapted from Lifton 1990:xiii).

While the so-called 'paramount' ethical issues (e.g. abortion, euthanasia) are widely discussed in the mainstream bioethics literature, healthcare professional literature and the lay media, it would be a mistake to conclude that these issues are the only, or indeed the most important, problems facing nurses and healthcare professionals (Johnstone et al 2004). Indeed, there are many other issues which, though less 'exotic', are of equal importance and which are equally deserving of attention. However, because these matters tend to be specific to the different healthcare contexts in which people work, or tend to be 'too political', or both, they do not always get the attention they deserve. The ethical issues faced by nurses working in a variety of healthcare contexts is an example of this.

The kinds of ethical issues faced by nurses are as complex as they are varied. While until recently attention has tended to be focused on the better known bioethical issues already identified, there has been a significant shift in the kinds of ethical issues faced by nurses, and it is becoming increasingly difficult to ignore a range of other issues of relevance to the profession and practice of nursing. These issues include:

▲ 'everyday' practical ethical issues faced by nurses;

▲ a genuine *nursing* perspective on common mainstream bioethical issues; and

▲ (the otherwise neglected) broader social justice issues associated with promoting the wellbeing and significant moral interests of stigmatised and marginalised groups of people.

'Everyday' ethical issues faced by nurses

As stated earlier, nurses have to deal with ethical issues everyday. The nursing ethics literature does not, however, always represent or reflect the reality of these 'everyday' problems for nurses. Instead, this literature has borrowed heavily from mainstream bioethics to shape nursing ethics discourse, and that has sometimes been at the expense of nurses' own experiential wisdom.

There is considerable reason to suggest that the actual lived experiences of nurses would (and do) provide a far more reliable methodological starting point to nursing ethics inquiry than do the 'top down' theories of Western moral philosophy and the field of bioethics that derives from it (Johnstone 2004a:14–15). An examination of nurses' lived experiences would yield important insights into such areas as:

▲ *moral boundaries of nursing* (e.g. nurses as carers being 'in relationship' with others, as opposed to being what the North American philosopher John Rawls (1971) describes famously as, 'detached observers choosing from behind a veil of ignorance');

▲ *catalysts to moral action* (e.g. 'experiential triggers' such as 'the look of suffering in a patient's eyes', as opposed to abstract moral rules and principles);

▲ *operating moral values* (e.g. sympathy, empathy, compassion, human understanding, and a desire 'to do the best we can', rather than an obsession to 'do one's duty');

▲ *ethical decision-making processes* (which tend to be collaborative, communicative, communal and contextualised, rather than independent, private, individual, solo and decontextualised);

▲ *barriers to ethical practice* (which tend to be structural rather than knowledge-based—for example, the power and authority of doctors to determine patient care, organisational norms forcing compliance with the status quo, and negative attitudes and a lack of support from co-workers and managers); and

▲ *need for cathartic moral talking* (e.g. 'talking through' moral concerns in a safe and supportive environment to help relieve the distress that so often arises as a result of trying to be moral in a world that appears to be growing increasingly amoral)—(for a helpful discussion on moral stress/distress/perplexity and moral incident stress debriefing, see Johnstone (1998:83–8)).

What talking with nurses so often reveals is that it is not the so-called paramount ('exotic') bioethical issues that trouble them, but the more fundamental issues of:

▲ how to help a patient in distress in the 'here and now';

▲ how to stop 'things going bad for a patient';

▲ how to best support a relative or chosen carer during times of distress and when the 'system' appears to be against them;

▲ how to make things 'less traumatic' for someone who is suffering;

▲ how to reduce the anxiety and vulnerability of the people being cared for;

▲ where nurses can get help for their own moral distress; and

▲ how to make a difference in contexts where indifference to the moral interests of others is manifest.

The above and other related concerns are all issues worthy of attention and consideration within and outside of the nursing profession. They are also issues that deserve to be recognised as being an integral part of a substantial moral framework and approach that might be appropriately described as nursing ethics.

A nursing perspective on mainstream bioethics

Mainstream bioethics has had as the principal concern the ethics of medicine and biomedical research, and this has been at the expense of the ethical concerns of other healthcare professions, including nursing (Reich 1995b). One major consequence of this has been that the viewpoints of nurses on the ethics of certain medical and healthcare practices have been either invalidated, marginalised, trivialised or ignored altogether (Johnstone 2004a). In some instances, nurses have had their job security threatened and have even lost their jobs for speaking out against, or for exposing, unethical practices in healthcare contexts.

Some examples are the 'unfortunate experiment' case in New Zealand (discussed in Johnstone 1999:22–7), the Pink case in the United Kingdom (Turner 1990, 1992), the noted North American legal cases of *Free versus Holy Cross Hospital* (505 NE 2d 118 (Ill App 1 Dist 1987)) and *Warthen versus Toms River Community Memorial Hospital* (488 A 2d 229 (NJ Super AD 1985)), which are both discussed in Johnstone (1994, 2004a), and more recently the high profile Australian whistleblowing case involving the Campbelltown and Camden hospitals in New South Wales (Johnstone 2004c).

The historical neglect and marginalisation of nurses' concerns and experiences has been seriously problematic for mainstream bioethics. Not only has such oversight rendered mainstream bioethics 'less than complete', but, paradoxically 'unethical', because of its discrimination against a nursing point of view. In failing to give due attention to the concerns and experiences of nurses, mainstream bioethics contributed to the subjugation of the moral voice of nurses and, in so doing, contributed to the subjugation of the moral interests and genuine wellbeing of patients (Johnstone 1999).

Over recent years, however, this situation has changed. As can be readily demonstrated, since the mid-1990s, the 'special' ethical issues faced by nurses have received—and continue to receive—increasing attention in mainstream bioethics discourse. An important example of the changes that have occurred can be found in the 1995 revised edition of the internationally acclaimed *Encyclopedia of bioethics* (discussed at length in Johnstone 1999:31–6), and other works (too numerous to list here), which are now much more inclusive of a nursing point of view than has previously been the case.

It is also evident by the plethora of nursing literature on the topic of ethical issues in nursing that, for all its past neglect of the ethical issues faced by nurses, since its inception in the early 1970s, bioethics has made an enormous contribution to the development of nursing ethics and will continue to do so. Indeed, as nurses have frequently commented informally over the years, the study of bioethics has enabled them to make sense of their moral experiences and has helped them to feel more confident in dealing with ethical issues in their practice—especially those involving the rights and interests of patients.

Broader social justice issues

Earlier, it was explained that the word 'bioethics' has come to refer narrowly to the ethics of medicine and biomedical research. This has not only resulted in the marginalisation of the ethics of other professions (e.g. nursing) (Reich 1995b), but in the marginalisation of other important issues which do not 'fit' with the mainstream ethical concerns of medicine and biomedical research. For example, a cursory glance at the bioethics literature will reveal a scandalous neglect of the ethical issues associated with providing healthcare to highly stigmatised populations—people with mental health problems, the poor, the homeless, the unemployed, the disabled, survivors of child abuse, partner abuse and elder abuse, people from different cultural backgrounds, Aboriginal peoples, refugees, and gay, lesbian and transgendered persons. Significantly, the nursing ethics literature has also been relatively silent in this area.

As long as nurses interact with and care for people from these stigmatised and highly vulnerable groups, they will be faced with having to make morally relevant choices associated with their care. Given this, it is morally imperative that the many special and complex ethical issues inherent in caring for people within these populations are identified and addressed as a matter of priority, and that nurses working in the field are educationally prepared to respond effectively to these special problems when they arise.

ISSUES AND RECOMMENDATIONS

It is timely to raise important questions about the nature and future directions of contemporary nursing ethics. I do not suggest that the better known issues of abortion, euthanasia, organ transplantation, reproductive technology, patients' rights to informed consent, confidentiality, and so forth are not important. Clearly, they are important, and will continue to be as long as people are confronted with having to make morally relevant choices related to these issues. There is room to suggest, however, that these more 'mainstream' issues *might not have the same priority in different healthcare contexts, nor necessarily be the most important ethical issues* that nurses, and indeed other health professionals and the community at large, need to be grappling with at this present time.

A re-examination of the kinds of ethical issues faced by nurses today is warranted, as is the need to make visible the experiences of nurses in trying to be moral in contexts which can be—and for the most part are—extremely demanding at both a personal and a professional level. While it has not been possible to identify or do justice to all the 'new' ethical issues that nurses face, perhaps the brief discussion given here will provide a catalyst for further discussion and reflection on the nursing profession's global task of making visible and, through this, giving legitimacy to what might be appropriately described as the distinctive field of 'nursing ethics'.

In particular, attention needs to be given to identifying, considering and responding effectively (at local, national and global levels) to issues relevant to the following key areas:

- ▲ *nursing education*: for example, the ethics of ethics education for nurses (what to teach, how to teach, when to teach, whether teaching ethics is possible, cross-cultural considerations); designing curricula to prepare nurses in 'preventive ethics'; devising and teaching an 'ethics of personality' (e.g. What does it mean to be a virtuous or 'decent' human being? Are nurses as 'decent' as they could be? Is virtue enough to fulfil the task of ethics? Can virtue/decency be taught?); preparing nurses to take a stand (e.g. against unscrupulous practices, conscientious objection, action lobbying on local policy issues, broader social justice issues, professional ethical issues, law reforms relevant to nursing ethics); global ethics (e.g. environmental, cultural and political concerns); and ethical issues in nursing education itself;

- ▲ *nursing practice*: for example, the ingredients of and the processes which facilitate the ethical practice of nursing; 'everyday' issues versus large philosophical issues; the nature and implications of the moral boundaries of nursing and nursing relationships; catalysts to moral action; guiding moral values; ethical decision-making processes; barriers to ethical practice; moral distress; institutional/management support of nurses dealing with moral quandaries; formulation of position statements by professional nursing organisations; the unacceptable moral consequences of the economic rationalisation of nursing care provided by qualified and skilled nurses; and the increasing use by healthcare agencies of lower paid, unqualified carers;

- ▲ *nursing management*: for example, how best to prepare nurse managers not just to manage ethically (e.g. treat employees fairly), but to manage ethical problems effectively in the workplace (e.g. using their positions to develop an ethical culture within the workplace, supporting staff, providing a 'safe place' for cathartic moral talking, institutional/unit policy development, resource mobilisation);

- ▲ *nursing leadership*: for example, advancing inquiry into the relatively new field of leadership ethics and how best to prepare nurse leaders to *lead ethically* (see also Johnstone 2004b); and

- ▲ *nursing research*: for example, improving recognition of philosophic inquiry (of which ethics inquiry is a form) as a legitimate and important form of research within nursing; developing an ethics research agenda (involving all research approaches); facilitation of research into ethical issues in nursing; keeping visible the nursing profession's experience of ethical issues; developing nursing ethics theory; and ethical issues in nursing research itself.

CONCLUSION

Nurses in all areas and levels of practice are confronted with ethical issues on a daily basis. In order to deal effectively with these issues, nurses must be able to identify correctly the ethical issues facing them, recognise the short-term and long-term implication of these issues for the broader nursing profession, and develop strategies for ensuring moral outcomes to the ethical issues encountered in work-related contexts. Achieving these outcomes, however, requires a constant reappraisal of nursing ethics education, ethical nursing practice, ethical nursing management, nursing leadership ethics, and nursing ethics research. By undertaking such a reappraisal, members of the nursing profession will be able to ensure that they are well situated to meet the complex challenges and responsibilities of ethical nursing practice that inevitably lie ahead.

REFLECTIVE QUESTIONS

1 Nurses are faced with ethical issues every day. In your view, what are the most pertinent and pressing ethical issues facing nurses today? What are some of the professional implications of these ethical issues for the nursing profession generally, and how might nurses best deal with these issues both locally and globally?

2 How, if at all, might the study of nursing ethics assist nurses to practise nursing in an ethically just, caring and responsible manner?

3 What is the future of nursing ethics, and what influence, if any, do you envisage it will have on the broader field of healthcare ethics generally?

RECOMMENDED READINGS

Berglund C 2004 *Ethics for health care*, 2nd edn. Oxford University Press, Melbourne.

Fry S, Johnstone M 2002 *Ethics in nursing practice: a guide to ethical decision making*, 2nd revised edn. Blackwell Science/International Council of Nurses, London UK/Geneva.

Johnstone M 2004 *Bioethics: a nursing perspective*, 4th edn. Churchill Livingstone/ Elsevier, Sydney.

Storch J, Rodney P, Starzomski R 2004 *Toward a moral horizon: nursing ethics for leadership and practice*. Pearson/Prentice-Hall, Toronto.

CHAPTER ELEVEN

An introduction to legal aspects of nursing practice

Judith Mair

LEARNING OBJECTIVES

Upon completion of this chapter, the reader will have gained insights into:

▲ the basics of the Australian legal system;

▲ basic principles of law applicable to nursing practice;

▲ the legal rights of patients;

▲ the role of the criminal law in nursing practice; and

▲ legal rules governing the registration and discipline of nursing.

KEY WORDS
Litigation, common law, precedents, legislation, assault, safety, negligence, duty of care, consent

INTRODUCTION

Today, more than ever, nurses have to consider the legal implications of their practice. Litigation against healthcare professionals has increased as healthcare consumers become more aware of their legal rights and, as the law develops, to recognise more factual circumstances that can give rise to a legal action. Operating alongside these changes is a higher patient expectation of a good outcome from the delivery of healthcare services.

This chapter serves as an introduction to law relevant to nursing practice. This introduction is necessarily brief, and does not cover all aspects of the law that affect nursing practice. Nurses should develop a deeper understanding of the legal system in which they practice, and the laws that govern clinical practice, through lectures and further reading.

THE COMMON LAW BASIS

The common law developed in England from the fourteenth century and became the basis of the legal systems of countries that were colonised by England. Thus the English common law forms the basis of the legal systems of, among others, Australia, New Zealand, Canada and the United States. It is within these jurisdictions, as well as in England, that law relevant to nursing practice has developed.

The primary source of law in common law countries is a combination of common law and legislation. Common law consists of the application of legal principles developed in past cases to determine the outcome of present cases. Common law is based upon the doctrine of precedent (i.e. by looking at how cases have been decided in the past). Cases that have an important impact on the common law are reported in law reports relevant to particular courts. Less important cases are unreported but can still be accessed.

Precedents are either binding or authoritative. *Binding precedents* are those laid down by a high court in a hierarchy of courts, which a lower court must follow. In the absence of a binding local precedent, a court may apply *authoritative precedents*, which are binding principles developed in courts of other jurisdictions, and which appear to be good law applicable to the local jurisdiction.

The common law remains the major source of law covering clinical practice. For example, the law relating to assault, false imprisonment, negligence and negligent advice is found within cases in which relevant principles of law recognising the right of persons to individual autonomy and bodily integrity have been developed.

The second type of law is *legislation*, or statutory law, which is law developed by parliamentarians through the parliamentary process. An individual piece of legislation is referred to as a statute or an Act of parliament. Legislation is important in that legislative provisions prevail where there is any inconsistency with the common law. Thus parliamentary law can be used to change the law where it is considered that the common law is deficient.

Legislation can create new law that is not known at common law. An example of this is the statutory definition of brain death, which has enabled the removal of organs from a person whose brain has ceased to function but whose heart and lung activity is being sustained artificially.

Nurses practising in Australia need to be aware that, under the Australian system of Federation, the law can and often does differ from state to state or territory. As well as state-by-state and territory differences, the federal government has power, by virtue of the Constitution, to make laws that are binding on all states and territories (i.e. the *Commonwealth of Australia Constitution Act*). In some cases, this law-making power is exclusive to the federal government (e.g. the defence power). In other cases, the states and territories have a concurrent power to make law (e.g. taxation). However, in the latter case, a federal law will override a state/territory law where the federal law is intended to cover the field or there is an inconsistency between a valid federal law and a state/territory law (section 109 of the Constitution). Where the federal government has no power to make law, the states and territories have residual power. Most health law, such as the regulation of hospitals and nursing practice, falls within state/territory law.

Differences in law from state to state and territory are less obvious in common law cases. In the absence of any binding judgment from the High Court of Australia, judges in the superior courts of each state and territory are free to interpret and apply the common law as cases come before them for adjudication. However, judges generally adhere to the principles developed in previous common law cases heard locally, or from other respected common law courts.

It is within parliamentary law that significant differences can arise. Legislation in one jurisdiction (state/territory) does not bind people in another jurisdiction unless the legislation has valid extraterritorial application. Even in this latter case, there must be some connection with the state/territory promulgating (proclaiming) the law. Thus a criminal offence which is found in one state/territory statute cannot serve to convict a person where the offence occurs in a state/territory which does not have such an offence embodied within its legislation. Individual states/territories may enact parliamentary law to govern particular matters, while other states/territories may leave such matters to be covered by common law. For example, not all states/territories have legislated to control the reproductive technologies.

Law is divided into civil and criminal. *Civil law* involves legal actions taken by complainants against another or others seeking a civil remedy for a legally recognised wrong—for example, a complainant (the plaintiff) seeking compensation for pain and suffering as a result of a nurse giving an injection incorrectly. The negligent practitioner is normally referred to as the defendant in the case. The task (onus) of proving the case rests with the plaintiff on the balance of probabilities.

The *criminal law* consists of prosecutions brought on behalf of the state/territory to punish breaches of criminal offences, and a guilty verdict results in a fine and/or custodial sentence. The onus of proving a criminal offence lies with the prosecution, which must prove its case beyond a reasonable doubt. The criminal law of murder and manslaughter, criminal assault and criminal negligence are some of the major criminal offences that can apply to nursing practice.

Legislation in all jurisdictions provides for limitation periods to apply for civil claims in the courts (e.g. *Limitation Act 1969* (NSW)). An aggrieved party must commence an action within the specified limitation period; otherwise the claim will become statute barred. Limitation periods vary from jurisdiction to jurisdiction, but most are around three to seven years after the cause of action arises, or, in some cases, when the plaintiff first becomes aware that a cause of action exists. Notwithstanding that a limitation period has lapsed, it is usually possible to apply to a court to extend a limitation period in prescribed circumstances (e.g. a person who contracts HIV through a blood transfusion may not be aware that they have contracted the disease until some time after the expiration of a limitation period).

Whatever limitation period applies, most jurisdictions suspend the limitation period while an injured party is a minor. Therefore, a child who suffers an injury as a result of alleged negligence is not affected by a limitation period until reaching majority. A person acting as 'tutor' for the child may take action on behalf of the child in the child's name prior to majority. If this is done, the evidence necessary to prove the case is more easily available soon after the event than later.

Unless specifically stated, no limitation periods apply to most criminal offences. Thus a nurse who causes the death of a patient intentionally or recklessly could be charged with murder or manslaughter many years after the event should evidence to support such a charge arise.

CIVIL LAW

As noted above, civil law involves legal actions taken by complainants against another, or others, seeking a civil remedy for a legally recognised wrong. Nurses need to work within the context of civil law, as it relates to: patient safety; negligent advice; patient consent; patient freedom of movement; and patients' property.

Patient safety

By the very nature of their practice, nurses are engaged in close physical contact with patients. Some of the procedures performed by nursing staff pose risks to patients should the procedures be performed without due care and skill. If a patient suffers harm as a result of a nurse's failure to perform nursing duties at the standard to be expected of the nurse in the circumstances, then the patient has a right to sue in negligence to recover compensation.

Negligence is a *tort*, which means a civil wrong. The tort of negligence arises from the common law and is a means by which a person who suffers injury through a negligent act or omission can obtain compensation from the person responsible for the injury. The onus of proving the negligence lies upon the plaintiff, the person alleging the negligence. To succeed in an action of negligence against a nurse, the plaintiff must prove, on the balance of probabilities, that the nurse was negligent. The plaintiff must prove that the nurse owed the patient a legal duty of care, that the nurse breached this duty of care, and that the patient suffered harm as a result of that breach. Any act or omission that is not found to be negligent is referred to as an unavoidable accident.

In determining whether or not a legal duty of care exists, the courts resort to a test of foreseeability. Thus a duty of care can be shown to exist when a person can reasonably foresee that his or her acts or omissions are likely to place another at risk (see the case of *Donoghue versus Stevenson* [1932] AC 562). This is an objective test and the defendant's conduct is measured by a 'reasonable man' test. The fact that something is foreseeable is not sufficient—the test is 'reasonable foreseeability'. Thus it is reasonably foreseeable that a patient may suffer harm, such as nerve damage, if an injection is given incorrectly. On the other hand, it may not be reasonably foreseeable if the patient suffers some reaction to a drug which is idiopathic that could not have been anticipated with all proper care and history taking.

The duty of care is to avoid unreasonable risk of harm to another. All persons living in a society are expected to take some care for themselves and cannot complain if they suffer loss or injury from an accepted risk of harm. The law will often determine an unreasonable risk of harm by looking at the harm that is likely to be caused and/or the frequency of its occurrence. For example, if a particular harm is known to occur frequently as a result of particular acts or omissions, then the law is likely to hold that these will give rise to a duty of care. Likewise, the law will hold that a duty of care exists in any case where the foreseeable risk can result in serious disability or death, however infrequently such harm is likely to occur.

In some cases the law will hold that a particular risk, which may normally be considered 'unreasonable', may be taken to avoid a greater risk of harm. This is sometimes referred to as 'balancing the risks'. Thus it may be reasonable to do something that clearly poses a risk of harm to another, where the act is intended to avert a greater risk of harm. In one American case it was held that burns resulting from the application of hot water bottles in an emergency were not caused by negligence, as they arose from a calculated risk to avoid a grave risk of harm to the patient. The patient was suffering from severe shock caused by severe postpartum haemorrhage and the hot water bottles had been applied as a part of emergency treatment (*McDermott versus St Mary's Hospital* 133 A 2d 608 (1957)).

Clearly, a duty of care will exist to avoid unreasonable risk of harm to patients receiving nursing care. However, the law does not require that there be an identified person in existence at the time that a negligent act or omission occurs. The law can impose a duty of care in circumstances where a class of persons is likely to be affected now or in the future. Thus, a duty of care can arise to avoid harm to an unborn child, as well as to one that is not even conceived at the time of the negligent act or omission. In such a case, the child must be born alive and prove that any injury present at birth resulted from a breach of duty to take care not to injure it while it was unborn (*X & Y (by her tutor) versus Pal and Ors* (1991) 23 NSWLR 27).

Whether or not a breach of the duty of care has occurred requires consideration of the standard of care required in the circumstances. The standard of care is not perfect care, but reasonable care. It is an objective test and therefore is not dependent upon the particular skills and knowledge of the practitioner. The standard expected of the healthcare worker is that which is attributed to the class of healthcare workers to which the defendant belongs. Thus the conduct of a nurse will be measured against that of the 'hypothetical reasonably competent nurse'.

Persons who claim to have special skills will be required to exhibit a higher standard of care. Thus the clinical nurse specialist will be measured against the standard of the reasonably competent clinical nurse specialists, while the general ward staff will be measured against the standard expected of the reasonably proficient general ward nurse.

The standard of care required can vary according to the condition of the patient and the patient's capacity for self-care. In considering the standard of care required, the nurse must take into account characteristics of the patient that may pose an additional risk for that person. Thus a higher standard of care will be required for a patient recovering from a general anaesthetic following surgery than for a patient who is fully conscious and has been returned to the ward.

The circumstances in which care is being provided can also be a relevant consideration in determining the standard of care required. A nurse involved in resuscitating a person at an accident site away from a well-equipped hospital with trained staff at hand can only be expected to provide the standard of care that is reasonable in the circumstances. Provided the nurse exercises reasonable care and skill in the circumstances, there would be no breach of the duty of care.

Damage is the gist of the case in an action of negligence; a plaintiff must prove that foreseeable damage resulted from a breach of duty by the nurse. Damage may be physical, mental, financial, or a combination of these. Once the plaintiff has proved that the nurse's breach of duty caused damage that was reasonably foreseeable, the defendant will be held liable to compensate for that damage and any further loss that flows reasonably and naturally upon the initial injury. Pain and suffering, loss of enjoyment of life, loss of expectation of life, loss of opportunity in life, and financial consequences are examples of accepted heads of damage (categories of damage recognised by the courts) for which compensation can be sought in a negligence action.

If death occurs as a result of negligence, legislation provides that prescribed persons, usually close relatives, can bring an action against the person whose negligence caused the death (e.g. *Compensation to Relatives Act 1897* (NSW)). For example, a man and his children may commence an action to be compensated for nervous shock suffered as a result of the death of the wife and mother caused by a negligent nursing act or omission.

Finally, the plaintiff must prove causation—that is, that the breach of duty caused the alleged harm. To prove a direct causal connection the 'but for' test can be applied. But for the act or omission of the defendant, would the plaintiff have suffered the alleged harm? Even when an act or omission can be shown to have been negligent, a claim for damages will fail if the plaintiff cannot prove that the alleged harm was caused by the defendant's negligent conduct.

There are three main defences to an action in negligence. These are contributory negligence, *novus actus interveniens* and *volenti non fit injuria*. A defendant can claim contributory negligence where the plaintiff can be shown to have been partially responsible for what happened. The court will award damages in proportion to the extent it accepts that the plaintiff was negligent (*Kalokerinos versus Burnett* CA 40243/95).

Novus actus interveniens is applicable when a second negligent act results in increased harm to a person who has suffered harm from a prior negligent act. However, the second negligent act must be such that the chain of causation flowing from the first negligent act is broken. For example, if a nurse's negligence caused brain damage to a child, necessitating intensive care, and the negligence of a second nurse in the intensive care unit exacerbated the harm to the child, then the first nurse could still be held liable for the increased harm. However, if the child were discharged from hospital following the maximum care that could be given, then dies from other injuries sustained in a motor vehicle accident caused through another's negligence, then the first nurse is unlikely to be held responsible for the death.

Volenti non fit injuria applies when a plaintiff can be shown to have knowledge of risks and voluntarily undertakes those risks. As such, this defence has not been a major factor in cases involving the provision of healthcare services. Its main application is to cases involving sports and dangerous occupations. It cannot be argued that a patient voluntarily agrees to accept all known risks in healthcare.

When a plaintiff has suffered harm as a result of another's negligence, the plaintiff is required by law to minimise (mitigate) any loss. Thus an injured person is required to take reasonable steps to reduce the effects of (ameliorate) the harm caused. To the extent that there is an unreasonable failure to mitigate, a court will discount the amount of compensation that the plaintiff would have received.

Negligent advice

During the course of professional practice, patients ask nurses for advice on a whole range of matters such as diet and how to care for themselves after discharge from hospital. In giving advice, nurses must exercise a reasonable standard of care where the patient could suffer harm as a result of following the advice. Failure to exercise reasonable care in giving advice could leave a nurse open to an action of negligent advice.

The tort of negligent advice is a negligence action that is brought for damage caused by the giving of advice rather than by a defendant's act or omission. Liability for the tort is also applicable to the giving of information where the defendant has a sufficient interest to see that the information given is correct. For an action in negligent advice to be successful, the plaintiff must prove that the advisor is a professional (or claiming to have equivalent skills) and that the advisor was willing to use those skills to advise the plaintiff, in the knowledge that the plaintiff intended to make a decision in reliance upon that advice. It must be reasonable for the plaintiff to do so.

The plaintiff cannot succeed simply because the advice was wrong. The plaintiff must prove that the nurse owed a duty of care, failed to exercise reasonable care in the giving of the advice—according to the standards of a reasonably competent nurse—and that the plaintiff suffered harm following the advice (see *Hills versus Potter* [1983] 3 All ER 716). A disclaimer of responsibility is effective; however, disclaiming responsibility for any advice given in the context of nursing care would be inappropriate given that a nurse's role involves giving advice to patients.

In order to avoid being sued for negligent advice, nurses should ensure that their nursing knowledge remains up to date and never give an impression that they have particular skills when they lack the capacity to give advice. When asked to give advice on a matter about which they lack knowledge, a nurse should either make it clear to a patient that they are not skilled in giving particular advice, or not give the advice and refer the patient to another experienced and competent practitioner. In so doing, a nurse will be exercising an appropriate standard of care.

Patient consent

Most nursing practice involves touching patients. In accordance with common law principles, all persons have the right to determine what treatments or diagnostic tests they will be subjected to, unless there is some overriding law which allows treatment without consent. When a competent adult patient is treated without consent, that patient has a right to sue for assault. If a patient claims that treatment was carried out without sufficient information being given, then the patient must 'sue in negligence'.

Assault is a tort, which serves to protect an individual's right to autonomy and self-determination. Assault consists of intentionally creating in another person an apprehension of imminent unwanted and unlawful contact. Although the actual touching of another without lawful authority is technically known as battery, the term assault is now in use to represent both the apprehension of and the unlawful contact itself.

Touching in anger, even if slight, is an assault. However, an assault may also be committed where a person is touched without consent and the touching is not an accepted incident of everyday life, for which a person is deemed to have given consent.

An assault is complete once touching has occurred without lawful justification; therefore, there is no need for a patient to prove that damage occurred as a result of the touching. It is not a defence to assault that treatment was carried out in good faith for the benefit of the patient when the patient is capable of giving consent and has not done so.

The law acknowledges that there are a number of ways in which consent can be sought. Consent may be obtained orally by asking the patient's permission before commencing treatment, and receiving an affirmative response. Consent may also be implied by the patient's overt physical response to suggested treatments. For example, the patient turns over and exposes a buttock when the nurse approaches with an expected injection. Consent in writing, and witnessed, is usually sought for major intrusions of the body, such as surgery. However, consent in writing cannot be taken to be absolute evidence of consent. In an emergency where a person is unable to consent, a nurse is entitled to proceed to carry out measures that are aimed at saving life or avoiding severe injury.

A patient's consent must be valid. A valid consent is one that is voluntarily given, covers the treatment to be carried out, and is given by a legally competent person who has been given sufficient information about the procedure to be performed. A voluntary consent is one that is given freely by the patient in the absence of fraud or duress (see *Beausoleil versus Sisters of Charity* (1966) 53 DLR 2d 65). The consent must cover the treatment to be carried out, and any treatment that is related to the initial treatment.

In order to give an informed consent, the patient must have a good understanding of what is to be done and the risks involved. Any issue relating to the degree of information given is a matter for the general law of negligence and is determined by what a patient should be told. In short, all patients should be told all material risks inherent in a procedure, together with any risks that are of particular importance to the patient (see *Rogers versus Whitaker* (1992) 175 CLR 479).

Legal capacity covers mental capacity and children. Persons who are mental health patients have issues involving consent to treatment covered by legislation in the various states/territories. Where a patient is unconscious or otherwise mentally incompetent, the defence of necessity applies and treatment may be carried out that is necessary to avoid a severe risk to the life of the patient or others (e.g. sedating a psychotic patient who is a risk to self and others). Legislation may provide for a guardian to be appointed to give consent for medical procedures on behalf of a person who is mentally disabled, or a court may make such an appointment.

A combination of common law principles and legislation applies when treating children. At common law a child may consent to treatment that is therapeutic, provided he or she has sufficient mental capacity to understand the nature and consequences of the proposed treatment. The application of this principle requires a balance between the intellectual and emotional maturity of the minor and the complexity or seriousness of the proposed treatment (see *Gillick versus West Norfolk and Wisbech Area Health Authority* [1985] 3 All ER 402). Presumably, a child of a quite young age could give a valid consent to a simple procedure that does not involve a great risk of harm. For example, a child who falls over and suffers a graze in school grounds could be expected to have the capacity to consent to the wound being treated. In all other cases, parental or guardian consent should be obtained.

Legislation can modify the common law. For example, legislation in New South Wales provides that consent to medical treatment given by a parent or guardian of a minor aged less than 16 years, or by a minor aged 14 years or upwards, is a defence to an action for assault and battery in respect of that treatment. Below the age of 14 years, the consent of the parent or guardian is required (except in an emergency to save the life of the child). The definition of medical treatment includes treatment carried out by persons following the orders of a medical practitioner, and this would apply to nurses (see section 49 of the *Minors (Property and Contracts) Act 1970* (NSW)).

When a parent or guardian has not given consent, most states/territories have legislation that enables doctors to perform life-saving treatments on children without consent (e.g. section 174 of the *Children and Young Persons (Care and Protection) Act 1998* (NSW)). The matter may be referred to the Supreme Court of a state/territory in its *parens patriae* jurisdiction, or the Family Law Court can make a decision consistent with the best interests of the child where parents or guardians refuse consent to non-urgent treatment for a child, or there is any dispute regarding consent. Children who are wards of the state/territory have issues relating to consent to medical treatment covered by relevant child welfare legislation in each state/territory.

There are a number of defences against an action in assault that are relevant to the provision of healthcare. The defence of necessity permits a health professional to carry out treatment without consent, provided the treatment is intended to avoid a greater risk of harm to the person. The defence operates in those circumstances when patients are unable to give consent and the treatment is necessary to preserve them from a serious danger to their life.

Legislation may authorise particular acts without consent. For example, mental health legislation provides the rules for non-consensual treatment of mentally ill patients.

Finally, the defence of self-defence is applicable in the event that a patient or others assaults a healthcare worker in anger or vice versa. Persons who are assaulted are legally entitled to defend themselves, but the force used must not exceed what reasonably appears to be necessary to repel the attack.

Patient freedom of movement

During the course of clinical practice, a nurse will encounter patients who wish to leave a healthcare institution against advice. Unless there is some law that allows for the detention of patients without consent, then patients do have the right to leave.

The tort of false imprisonment compensates a person who has been subjected to an intentional and total restraint of movement without lawful justification. Restraint is either by total confinement or by preventing the person from lawfully leaving the place in which he or she is. The tort can be committed where a patient is too ill to move, or is unaware of the fact that he/she was imprisoned by reason that he/she is in a state of drunkenness, while asleep or while they were a lunatic (see *Meering versus Grahame-White Aviation Co Ltd* (1920) 122 LT 44).

147

The plaintiff must prove the confinement was total. If the person can leave by some reasonable alternative exit, there is no false imprisonment. To lock a patient in a room with no reasonable avenue of escape, or barring a patient from lawfully leaving a healthcare institution, could amount to false imprisonment in the absence of lawful justification.

Using bed rails, manacles and chemical restraints can also be regarded as false imprisonment if they are used without lawful justification and totally confine the patient. It can also amount to false imprisonment if a patient reasonably believes that any attempt to leave a healthcare institution will be prevented by a nurse, even if there are no physical restraints. However, the patient would have to prove the submission to the nurse was complete and was reasonable.

Hospitals develop policies requesting patients to see a doctor and to sign a release form in the event that a patient wishes to leave hospital against medical advice. There is no problem if a patient voluntarily agrees to the request. Some doubt exists as to whether hospital staff could detain a patient without consent in order to fulfil the hospital requirements. In the event that a patient leaves without advising staff, or refuses to stay to sign a release form and see a doctor, the patient should not be prevented from leaving and the events should be clearly documented in the nursing notes.

The fact that a patient wishes to leave hospital against medical advice does not relieve the staff from fully advising the patient of any deleterious effects a premature departure from hospital could entail. Wherever possible, staff should ensure that the patient fully appreciates the risks involved in leaving against medical advice.

Defences that can be raised against an allegation of false imprisonment include the common law defence of necessity, which permits the restraint of persons who are a danger to themselves or others. However, restraint is not justified if it is merely for the convenience of staff; there must be a real necessity to protect the patient. The restraint of a patient attempting to jump off the roof of a hospital, or threatening staff and other patients with violence, would be justified on this basis.

A second defence exists where legislation authorises the detention of persons (e.g. mental and public health Acts). A third lawful means of detaining patients is where a court authorises the detention of a person for treatment. Such orders are usually reserved for the detention of children where parents wish to remove a child in need of care from a healthcare institution. Finally, detention without consent is permissible to affect a lawful arrest.

Patients' property

During the course of clinical practice, nurses will be faced with the prospect of taking charge of a patient's valuables, particularly when the patient is to be temporarily away from the ward to undergo surgery. When a patient's valuables are handed to a hospital for safekeeping, the law of bailment governs the relationship. The law of bailment is a contract and applies when one person (the bailor) delivers goods to another (the bailee) so that they may be used or stored until they are to be delivered back to the bailor.

Bailment may be for reward or gratuitous (free). When bailment is for reward, the bailee will be held liable to compensate for the loss of the goods according to the ordinary rules of negligence, whereas the bailee is only liable if gross negligence is shown in cases of gratuitous bailment. With respect to patients' valuables handed over to a hospital for safekeeping, the hospital is legally regarded as a bailee for reward and therefore has an obligation to exercise reasonable care in securing the safety of the valuables.

A hospital can become an involuntary bailee for patients' property. A hospital in New Zealand was held liable to compensate the estate of a deceased woman for a ring that disappeared from a woman's hand at the time of her death (*Southland Hospital Board versus Perkins Estate* [1986] 1 NZLR 373). The woman's personal control over her property ended with her death, and the hospital was held to be involuntary bailee for the ring.

Where a patient dies in hospital, any valuable property should be removed and kept in safekeeping to be handed over to the deceased patient's legal personal representative. Non-valuable items such as clothing and toiletries can be sent home with a relative or friend. Police usually deal with the property of a person who is brought in dead on arrival.

Healthcare institutions draw up policies and procedures in order to fulfil the duty of care to protect a patient's valuables and nursing staff should follow these. The valuables should be recorded in a document that is signed by the patient. When the patient is unable to sign, the valuables should be recorded by one nurse and witnessed by another.

The valuables must then be stored in a safe place. For short-term care the valuables may be stored in a locked cupboard at ward level (not the dangerous drugs cupboard). If the valuables are to be cared for on a long-term basis, they should be stored in a hospital safe. Patients are generally required to sign for the goods upon return to them. In the case of a deceased patient, the person legally entitled to deal with the patient's property after death would sign for receipt of the valuables.

In the event that the goods are lost, the patient has the onus of proving negligence and the value of the property. Nurses are not trained in evaluating the quality of valuable goods such as jewellery, and should not attempt to describe such goods as being of any particular kind and value. For example, a sapphire and diamond ring in a gold setting should be described as a ring with blue and clear stones set in a yellow coloured band, even if the patient states that the stones are a sapphire and diamonds, and the metal is gold.

Where theft of valuables is suspected the police should be notified. The police can undertake an investigation and lay criminal charges where they reasonably suspect a member of the nursing staff or other person is responsible.

CRIMINAL LAW

During the course of practice a nurse may cause serious bodily harm or death to patients. As well as providing facts that may be the subject of a civil action, such events may result in charges of criminal negligence, manslaughter or homicide.

Criminal negligence

Nurses can be charged with criminal negligence where an act causing serious bodily harm or death shows such a disregard for the life and safety of another that it goes beyond a mere matter of compensation at civil law. The death of a patient resulting from treatment by a nurse would amount to manslaughter where the nurse's negligence was gross and the nurse did something no reasonably skilled person would have done.

A charge of murder could be laid where the nurse intended the patient to die or was grossly reckless as to whether the patient died. Criminal charges may result from a referral by a coroner to the relevant Crown law authorities following a coronial inquiry into the death of a patient.

Charges of criminal negligence against healthcare workers are rare and are difficult to prove to the requisite standard required in criminal law (i.e. 'beyond a reasonable doubt'). The prosecutor must prove both *mens rea* (guilty mind) as well as *actus reus* (an unlawful act). The *mens rea* element can be satisfied by proving that the accused committed an unlawful act, either with intent or could have foreseen that someone could suffer harm but nevertheless proceeded to commit the act.

A further issue is causation. The prosecutor must prove that the act led to the serious injury or death of the victim—a 'but for' test. This is not always easy to do. For example, if a person suffers brain damage as a result of an act and is placed on a life support system, then it cannot be said that the act has caused the death of the person. If the life support system is disconnected because the victim is brain dead, the question arises as to whether the defendant caused the death of the victim. Where the initial act was the operative factor in causing the brain damage, then turning off the life support system does not break the chain of causation.

Criminal assault

Assault can be the subject of a criminal charge as well as a tort. In addition to the elements required to prove civil assault, there must be proof of a forcible or hostile act of the accused, without the consent of the victim. If a patient is criminally assaulted, the matter should be reported to administration and to the police, who can charge the responsible party with criminal assault. The same legal redress is available to nurses who are assaulted by others.

Two defences to a charge of assault are misadventure and self-defence. To constitute misadventure, an assault occurs by accident. For example, a nurse slips on a wet floor and accidentally strikes a patient. Self-defence involves the use of force by one person to repel an attack on him or her. A person may use reasonable force to repel attacks, but must not use more violence than is necessary to repel the attack. The right of self-defence only lasts as long as any danger exists. A nurse would be entitled to exercise the right of self-defence if attacked by a patient or other person provided the nurse used no more force than was necessary to repel the attack. The onus of proving the reasonableness of the self-defence lies with the person relying upon it.

VICARIOUS LIABILITY

When a nurse's act or omission has caused harm to a patient and the patient has successfully sued to recover compensation for that harm, the question arises as to who is responsible for providing the compensation. Under the law of vicarious liability, an employer can be held responsible for the acts of its employees carried out in the course of their employment.

An employer's responsibility is limited to an employee's acts performed during the course of employment. However, this term is fairly broad and encompasses all acts, authorised or not, which are reasonably within the scope of the employee's duties. Thus a healthcare employer can be held legally responsible to compensate an injured patient whose injuries resulted from an employee's negligence. Vicarious liability merely means that the healthcare employer will generally be the party that will be held responsible for compensating a successful plaintiff and does not negate the nurse's personal liability. Responsibility under vicarious liability applies with respect to civil wrongs, but normally does not apply to criminal acts.

An independent nurse practitioner is solely liable for harm caused by that practitioner's practice. An independent practitioner in turn becomes vicariously liable for harm caused by a person employed by the practitioner to assist in the practice.

It is usual practice for a healthcare institution or an independent practitioner to secure insurance cover in the event of successful litigation by a patient. This cover should be sufficient to pay the highest amount that could be awarded from time to time.

Even when an employer cannot be found to be vicariously liable because a person committing a wrong is not an employee, the courts have been prepared to find that an institution such as a hospital has a personal duty of care towards patients and others. A hospital can be found negligent for harm caused to a patient by reason of its personal liability, when the act or omission of a visiting medical officer caused the alleged harm. When a hospital's policies and procedures could expose a patient to an unreasonable risk of harm, a duty arises to avoid that harm.

PATIENT RECORDS

Patient records are legal documents; therefore it is important to keep accurate and complete records of all treatment and care administered to patients. The documents record the progress of patients admitted to healthcare facilities for the period of time that they are in care. Accurate and complete documentation can provide a good defence for a nurse who is faced with an action by a patient when the patient's record discloses that adequate and reasonable nursing care was delivered.

Even when adequate treatment may have been administered, failure to keep adequate patient records can lead to a finding of liability on the part of a nurse. Failure to record treatment may be accepted as evidence that such treatment was not in fact given. Overall failure to keep complete and adequate records can be regarded as a negligent omission, since a reasonable nurse would be expected to keep all patient record notes in order and up to date. It is reasonably foreseeable that a patient may suffer harm from failure to record a treatment given (e.g. a patient may be given two doses of a drug because a first dose was not recorded).

Although it is important that a patient's records be complete and up to date, a nurse should not write more than is necessary since this can lead to excessive questioning in evidence. In circumstances where a nurse offers treatment or advice, and a patient refuses, it would be prudent to include a notation to this effect in the patient record.

Patient records should be objectively written, and those responsible for writing records should avoid making value judgments. 'Patient has a headache' is a subjective statement and should be recorded as 'patient complaining of headache'. A description of the nursing action taken and the outcome of that action should follow this statement.

Records should be as near as possible contemporaneous with the event if they are to be accepted as reliable evidence in a court action. Delays in recording make the record less reliable as a true description of an event. In fact, a record made days after an event can be made to look as though it was an afterthought. Interlineations and notes made in margins should also be avoided, as they can suggest that information has been added to a record at a later date. It is for this reason that nurses are advised not to leave lines between individual reports.

Errors in recording should not be completely erased since this can appear suspicious in the event that a patient is suing on the basis of delivery of healthcare. Mistakes should be ruled through in a manner that enables others to be able to read what was initially written. A notation that the recording was made in error, signed by the person making the error, should be added to the record.

Nurses should recognise the fact that personal information given by patients in the course of administering care is to be kept confidential. Patients are entitled to expect that nurses will maintain a high degree of confidentiality. Should a nurse breach a patient's confidentiality, the legal rights of the patient are limited; nevertheless, the nurse should aim to preserve confidentiality to the maximum extent possible. A patient may be able to sue in defamation for unlawful disclosure if their reputation has been harmed, in negligence if they suffer foreseeable nervous shock, or in breach of contract.

Access to a record can be granted to third parties with the consent of the patient. For all other purposes, access should be denied to all others except other health professionals on a 'need to know' basis (i.e. those who have a genuine need to access the information in order to provide adequate care). Confidentiality may be legally breached by virtue of legal process, statutory authority, necessity and the criminal law.

Despite the fact that patients have a right to expect that their records will be kept confidential, there is no legally enforceable right, in the absence of statutory authority, to access the records themselves (see *Breen versus Williams* HC FC 96/025). The Commonwealth government and various state governments have enacted freedom of information legislation that gives people a right to have access to various documents including personal documents. These Acts also provide for requesting that the documents be amended if there is any material that is false or misleading. However, the legislation applies to government departments and agencies only, and is not applicable to private agencies. A presumption that arises from this limitation is that patients in public hospitals could seek access to their records, but patients in private hospitals presumably could not. Alternatively, state legislation can provide access to healthcare records held by private practitioners (e.g. the *Health Records and Information Privacy Act 2002* (NSW)).

As a general policy, patients should be given access to their records as freely as possible. A healthcare practitioner should be available when a patient is accessing their record in order to ensure that the patient understands the nature of what has been written and why it was written. When a patient could suffer some foreseeable harm, such as nervous shock, when faced with a particular diagnosis or other information contained therein, the patient's practitioner could make a decision as to whether access should be granted.

REGULATION OF DRUGS

Each state and territory has specific legislation that regulates the supply and use of drugs and poisons within its jurisdiction (e.g. the *Poisons and Therapeutic Goods Act 1966* (NSW)). The rules and regulations in relation to the drugs that nurses routinely administer to patients can be found contained within each relevant state or territory Act. While an Act may specify in broad terms the rules regarding the control of drugs and poisons, regulations formulated under the power of the Act set out in greater detail the specifics of the obligations of individuals under the Act.

Drugs and poisons are usually classified in Schedules according to the manner in which they may be supplied. Changes in the Schedules take place when new drugs come into use or there are changes in the manner in which a particular drug may be supplied. For example, a drug that formerly required a doctor's prescription may be moved to a Schedule that permits the drug to be purchased over the counter from a chemist.

All nurses should become familiar with the relevant Act operating in the state or territory in which they work.

REGULATION OF NURSING PRACTICE

Legislation in each state and territory governs the registration of nurses within its jurisdiction. Each Act provides for a nursing board or council to regulate and control the profession. These boards and councils have a responsibility for promoting and maintaining professional standards of nursing practice. Federal legislation provides for mutual recognition of a nurse's state or territory registration upon application to the board of another state or territory when a nurse wishes to work in that other state or territory (*Mutual Recognition Act 1992* (Cwlth)).

Each Act also provides for penalties for breaches of the Act, and for the discipline of nurses who have been reported for acts or omissions bringing into question their professional competence. Major failures to exercise appropriate standards of patient care can lead to deregistration. In other cases, a nurse may be suspended or have conditions placed on their practice. Other powers include a reprimand or caution. A nurse who suffers any physical or mental impairment, alcohol or drug addiction which affects or is likely to affect the nurse's physical or mental capacity to practise nursing may be dealt with as a disciplinary matter, or may be dealt with in a non-disciplinary manner by Impaired Nurses Panels depending upon provisions in state/territory legislation (e.g. the *Nurses and Midwives Act 1991* (NSW)).

All Acts have provisions for a right of appeal against a decision of a disciplinary body to an appropriate judicial body as nominated in each Act. All nurses should familiarise themselves with the provisions of any Act applying in the state or territory in which they are practising as a nurse.

CONCLUSION

A knowledge of the law and its application to nursing practice has become a necessary component of a nurse's knowledge base. Nurses must be aware of and respect the legal rights of patients and the corresponding obligations of nurses in nursing care.

Failure to appreciate the legal rights of patients can lead a nurse to face a legal action mounted by a patient, or some disciplinary action taken by a nursing board or council under a relevant state/territory Act. Acknowledgment of, and adherence to, the legal rights of patients also goes a long way in maintaining the quality of nursing care delivered and the respect to be accorded to the profession. It is a professional obligation of all nurses to acquaint themselves with current legal issues touching upon the profession, and to do so by remaining up to date with their legal knowledge.

REFLECTIVE QUESTIONS

1 To what extent do you believe that the common law adequately provides for the resolution of complaints by patients allegedly harmed by healthcare?

2 What resources could you draw on in preparing to face court proceedings in relation to your professional practice?

3 How can you ensure that you remain up to date with the legal issues associated with the practice of nursing?

RECOMMENDED READINGS

Bos M A 2005 Ethical and legal issues in non-heart-beating organ donation. *Transplantation* 79(9):1143–7.

Chiarella M 2002 *The legal and professional status of nursing*. Churchill Livingstone, London.

Irving K 2002 Governing the conduct of conduct: are restraints inevitable? *Journal of Advanced Nursing* 40(4):405–12.

Staunton P, Chiarella M 2003 *Nursing and the law*, 5th edn. Churchill Livingstone, Sydney.

The author acknowledges that material for this chapter was drawn from a previously published work: J Mair & K Blackmore 1992, in M Cuthbert, C Duffield & J Hope (eds) *Management in nursing*. W B Saunders/Balliere Tindall, Sydney.

CHAPTER TWELVE

The gendered culture of nursing

Sandra Speedy

LEARNING OBJECTIVES

On completion of this chapter, readers will:

- ▲ understand and appreciate the historical development of feminist thinking on concepts such as nursing work and science;

- ▲ have examined the role that gender plays in defining the world of nursing work;

- ▲ develop an enlarged perspective about how the healthcare system and health professionals are impacted on by the issue of gender;

- ▲ have briefly explored the influence that feminisms have had on the discipline of nursing;

- ▲ understand how feminist theory has influenced nursing research; and

- ▲ have considered the debate about the relative advantages and disadvantages that gender provides for nurses.

KEY WORDS

Gender, nursing work, feminism, patriarchy, power, organisational culture

INTRODUCTION

In order to consider a range of gender issues—which are of increasing interest and relevance to nurses all over the world—this chapter will consider the gendered nature of nursing work. This will involve discussion about the nature of women who provide the majority of the nursing workforce. It will also require some analysis of the nature of nursing work, as it is performed by women and men. Inherent in this discussion will be consideration of the role of science in determining views of the concept of woman, as well as the work they undertake. The chapter will also consider briefly the influence of the feminisms on nursing, and the influence of nurses and nursing on feminism. Finally, the chapter will also examine the increasing role played by men in nursing, a gender issue of utmost importance for the future of nursing.

THE GENDERED NATURE OF NURSING WORK

A consideration of the gendered nature of nursing work must examine the concept of woman, since the majority of nurses are women. Whatever views are held regarding women will influence perception of women's work—in this case, nursing work. Perspectives on women are influenced by 'scientific' views about the nature of women, although it might also be argued that perspectives on women influence beliefs about the nature of science.

There is a burgeoning literature that demonstrates a range of approaches and various viewpoints on woman as object and subject. Women can be examined from sociological, psychological, biological, philosophical or political perspectives—and other viewpoints as well. Many of these viewpoints feature devaluation of women, as any examination of the concepts of essentialism, biologism, naturalism or universalism will demonstrate. In an insightful work, Grosz (1990) suggests that all of these terms, which argue the nature of women (and men, incidentally), do fix and define the limits, because they 'are commonly used in patriarchal discourses to justify women's social subordination and their secondary positions relative to men in patriarchal society' (Grosz 1990:333). In their work, both David (2000) and Gherardi (1994:591) argue the similar point that '. . . masculinity and femininity are symbolic universes of meaning socially and historically constructed'. Gherardi suggests also that that the way we 'do gender' in our work '. . . helps to diminish or increase the inequality of the sexes: we use ceremonial work to recognize the difference of gender, and remedial work socially to construct the "fairness" of gender relationships' (p 592). Ceci (2004a) asserts that genders are identified by specific traits, virtues and behaviours that place us as either feminine or masculine—that is, identifiable and named as such. There is no question that in nursing each gender experiences 'cross-over', necessitating the management of dual presence in what are essentially separate symbolic contexts.

There are problems with constructing a 'universal feminism', since allowance must be made for difference and diversity between women, just as there is between women and men. What is worthy of exploration are some of the views about women and nurses within a medical and health professions context, because these views are influenced by the concepts mentioned above. The issue of how women are constructed by science is also relevant here (Kane & Thomas 2000).

Feminist literature argues that the masculinity of science is an image that has been perpetuated for centuries. This image creation is affected by textbook representations, curriculum organisation, classroom behaviour, and stereotypical beliefs and attitudes. It distorts science, yet scientific method has not been successful in filtering out patriarchal bias in the scientific construction of women. In the early 1990s, Lather wrote with clarity regarding this. She says:

> The claim of positivistic researchers that their method is sufficient protection against ideological incursion is debunked by feminist critiques of the conceptual and methodological orientations that reflect and reinforce sex-based inequality. Hence the construction of women brings into question that which has passed for knowledge in the human sciences (Lather 1991a:17).

The masculinity of science is only an illusion (albeit a powerful one), not an intrinsic part of its nature. Science is a social construct, and 'its development is inextricably linked with social relations, not least the relations between men and women' (Kelly 1985:76). This leads, of course, to using male as the norm and female as the referent, a strategy that has been exposed and rejected in a wide range of disciplines, including psychology, sociology, psychiatry, medicine, education and biology. As long ago as the 1970s, it was pointed out that 'male' medicine misunderstood the female body, and these debates have now extended to cover all aspects of women's health, not just those of childbirth and reproduction.

In nursing and medicine, the presence of increasing numbers of women at all levels of authority indicates a modicum of success in producing women-friendly services and conditions. This has come about only because women have been forced to reclaim their healing role, which was given a boost by the knowledge and insights in the classic treatise written by Ehrenreich and English (1979), documenting the exclusion of women-as-healers from professionalised, modern medicine. There has long been 'increasing institutional awareness of the deficiencies and sexism of specific institutional practices' (Evans 1997:42). This has had both positive and negative effects. For the latter, it has resulted in some feminists 'beating up' on nurses, thus earning the title of 'anti-nurse'. This is:

> ... predicated on the belief that nurses willingly capitulate to male (and/or medical dominance), thereby making it difficult for 'real feminists' to achieve their goals. This ... 'complicity hypothesis' ... sees nurses as compliant with patriarchal demands to remain oppressed (Buchanan 1997:82).

Using this argument, nurses can be viewed as either the embodiment of the 'ideal' or 'good woman' (Fealy 2004:653, David 2000), conforming to masculine desires, or as the 'bad mother', 'thwarting women in their endeavours and assisting the medical profession in torturing women patients' (Buchanan 1997:82). In some ways this analysis, awareness and critique could be viewed as hostile criticism; however, it provides us with alternative views and insights that can be growth enhancing for women and nurses should we objectively and critically consider all perspectives.

Of course, we do not need feminists to 'beat up' on nurses—nurses do that very well to each other, whether they are feminists or not (Briles 1994, David 2000). Horizontal violence has long been recognised by a range of authors, who suggest that nurses' self-hate and dislike of other nurses (which is very common in oppressed groups), is demonstrated by the lack of cohesion in nursing groups, as well as the phenomenon of 'eating our young' (Kitson 2004, Roberts 2000, Bent 1993). The systematic oppression of women can assist nurses to recognise the oppressive structures in which they practice, which:

> ... includes recognising that nurses are placed in a culture that does not value their attributes, rather than 'blaming' them for ranking lower on self-esteem and higher in submissiveness in job-trait studies than do people in other occupations. Nurses must no longer assume that they are inherently inferior to the systems that surround them (Bent 1993:298).

Awareness of the social construction of women and nursing and its oppressive nature may change the way nurses relate to each other, and even refrain from 'horizontal violence'. As David makes clear:

> Nurses will never be able to expunge gender politics without first developing an understanding of how many use self-deception and how that action perpetuates nursing's professional mediocrity, limits freedom of thought and action, and preserves nurses' borderline status (David 2000:85).

This brings us to the work of nursing.

THE WORK OF NURSING

The role and function of nursing cannot be separated from those who undertake this activity. It is quite clear that there are particular views held about women and nursing that then create the definitions of women's work and nursing work, and by implication, men's work (Fealy 2004, David 2000, Meadus 2000). Cheek and Rudge point out that the:

> ... the low status of nursing and the way in which the work of nurses is devalued, especially when compared to other health professionals, can at least in part be explained by its gendered nature (Cheek & Rudge 1995:312).

Labelling nursing as 'women's work' creates a deterrent that '. . . inhibits recruitment of men into the profession and aids promotion of the sex imbalance in the nursing workforce' (Meadus 2000:9). Nursing is thus viewed as a natural extension of the female role, valuing nurturance, caring, support, care and concern (Bent 1993, Brykczynska 1997, Evans 1997). These characteristics have been described as encompassing a 'tyranny of niceness' (Street 1995). Nevertheless, researchers have found that these characteristics are selectively eliminated during the educational and socialisation process (Doering 1992). For example, Treacy noted that current 'nurse training' endorses 'compliance, passivity and ladylike behaviour, but it negatively sanctions other female traits such as intuition, empathy, and emotional expression' (Treacy 1989:88).

The descriptors 'compliance, passivity and ladylike behaviour' are words which, it could be argued, are suggestive of 'powerlessness' and 'intuitiveness, empathy and emotional expression', and are often viewed as unscientific and hence unacceptable in the world of science. The social construction of women as emotional beings is also used to undermine their credibility as nurses (Ceci 2004a). As David (2000:86) also points out '. . . the gender dialectic is still so fundamental to gender politics that it permeates the traditions of nursing, such as the belief that nursing is woman's work'.

Because of this, it can be argued that women and nurses are on shaky ground, while men are inhibited from entering the nursing profession. According to Evans (2004:321), the 'ideological designation of nursing as women's work have excluded, limited, and conversely, advanced the careers of men in nursing'. The issue of male advantage will be addressed later in this chapter.

Evans (1997) notes that nineteenth century science and rationality perceived the 'feminine' as an abstraction, which assisted in marginalising women within institutional practices. Women, as we have seen, were constructed as hysterical and intellectually inferior, while men were expected to conform to the stereotype of masculine behaviour. Thus, 'the "soft" feminine and the "hard" masculine then received institutional recognition and confirmation in particular practices' (Evans 1997:39). Feminists have sought to demonstrate the disjunction between supposed institutional objectivity and actual institutional practice. Specifically, the institution of medicine, for example, defines its values as non-gendered, while in practice they are deeply gendered (Evans 1997). This has been exposed in many areas—for example, in the management of childbirth and women's sexuality (Erturk 2004).

Because the values that dominate our health system are so pervasive and reflect the values of society at large, 'it is a struggle for nurses to remain aligned to the person rather than the institution' (Huntington 1996:170). This creates difficulties in nursing work, as the dominant discourses that shape health, illness and perceptions of what it is to be a woman (and a man, incidentally) can disadvantage the individual. As Huntington (1996:170) points out, 'we have been left with only male language to explain the fundamentally female practice of healing bodies'. The only solution to this problem is to develop an alternative discourse to that constructed and dominated by orthodox scientific discourse characteristics of the medical world.

Clearly too, feminist thinking has challenged the cultural code of organisations, designed around masculinity and femininity, which suggests that 'gender is deeply embedded in the design and functioning of organisations' (Davies 1995:44). These workplaces are socially constructed, as is the position of 'nurse' (David 2000), neither of which are gender-neutral, and operate on masculine values for their legitimation and affirmation (Gherardi 1994). Nurses therefore find it difficult to function within such gendered organisations, and frequently resort to 'blaming the victim', who are usually other nurses struggling with their day-to-day functioning within a hostile environment. Alternatively, they may adopt a victim mentality, rather than recognising the dysfunctionality of their workplaces (Kitson 2004). Thus:

> [W]omen, in a very important sense, cannot be 'at home' in the public world—it is constructed in such a way that assumes home is somewhere else, somewhere far away and different' (Davies 1995:62).

However, Kane and Thomas (2000) remind us that nursing has historically provided a haven for women who seek to control their lives within a professional context, although there are significant limits to what can be achieved. In fact, David (2000) suggests that this is delusion, because power does not belong to women in a male-dominated system.

There is a range of other historical scholarly work that demonstrates the further weakening of nursing's value. For example, Gamarnikow (1978) linked nursing to domesticity; Treacy (1989) suggested that the invisibility of nurses' contribution to care reflected the invisibility of much of the work contribution of women in society. Other scholars have pointed out that the sexual division of labour in the home disadvantages women in the workplace, which creates enormous stress for working women, and, in this case, nurses. This taps into the work of feminist scientists who have 'identified "women's work" the "caring professions", "unpaid domestic labour", "the double shift" and other manifestations of the apparently "natural" social division of labour' (Evans 1997:59).

It has been pointed out by many scholars that caring itself is a gendered construct, since notions of professional caring are derived from traditional concepts of caring as a feminine obligation (Caffrey & Caffrey 1994, Falk Rafael 1996, Wuest 1997, Ekstrom 1999). Caring in nursing has in the past been constructed as an inherently feminine pastime, and traditionally has received little social or economic recognition; it has been perceived as women's work, as unintellectual, unskilled and emotional, and thus likely to perpetuate gender exploitation (Bubeck 1995, Ceci 2004a). It was long believed that the work nurses undertake in order to provide care does not require any particular skill or knowledge; it has been viewed as a quality that women possess 'naturally' (Falk Rafael 1998, Henderson 2001, Zebroski 2001).

However, this view has been challenged. For example, Meadus (2000) cites research that demonstrates that men enter nursing because of their desire to care for others, thus challenging the stereotype that only women nurses care. He also notes that such men run the risk of being perceived as 'gay' because of this role violation. This viewpoint is challenged by Bubeck (1995:114), as she notes that 'part of the practice of care is to focus on the needs of the other, to become attentive, to be selfless'. By the construction of masculinity, caring is very difficult for men; they also escape from the care burden through the 'public/private' split in responsibilities of women and men (Tronto 1999).

Nursing's detractors have long promoted the idea that nurses are 'doers' rather than 'thinkers'; that is, nurses do not need to 'think' to do nursing, as long as they can 'do' certain tasks. This has resulted in an anti-intellectual bias, which creates the perception that the 'intelligent nurse was not a good practical nurse' (Fealy 2004:652), a myth that then threatens the academic preparation of nurses (Liaschenko & Peter 2004). This has, in no small measure, led to a significant devaluation of nursing, assisted by the unequal power relations that characterise the position of nursing vis-a-vis medicine (David 2000). For many years this view was used to justify the low-level education provided to nurses prior to their entry into the higher education system.

That caring is assumed not to require knowledge is not without practical consequence. The replacement of registered nurses with less skilled personnel is considered less of a reflection of economic rationalism than a reflection of the idea that caring is unskilled activity intrinsic to domesticity and womanhood. To engender nurse caring as feminine, therefore positioning it as innately instinctive to women, is to deny the advanced knowledge and skills that lie within the therapeutic caring acts of nurses. Despite the fact that 'emotional labour' is a vital and necessary part of the nursing labour process, it 'tends to be marginalized as a skill that a predominantly female nursing workforce would naturally possess' (Bolton 2000:580).

Emotional labour can be conceived as a 'gift in the form of authentic caring behaviour' (Bolton 2000:586), which truly reflects the state of 'being a nurse'. The fact that it is undertheorised and not appreciated is of serious concern (Henderson

2001). Emotion work can be hard labour, and relief measures are sought to cope with this continuous labouring. Relief can be found in 'backstage regions', such as the nurses' station, where profound irritation with patients or emotional anguish can be expressed, where nurses can 'drop their public mask' and express their true feelings. As Fineman (1993:21) indicates, 'off-stage settings are not emotion-free ports'. Here, implicit feeling rules can come into play; colleagues can express emotion to a degree that will be cathartic for them, but will also maintain organisational order.

Despite the fact that it is now acknowledged that emotional labour occurs in organisations, and that employers have expectations about what sort of emotion one should feel in particular contexts, emotion work tends to be privatised and moved out of the realm of organisational responsibility (Boyle 2002a, 2002b). Emotional labour work involves remaining continually vigilant and sensitive to the environment, constantly noting and responding to others' emotional states, alleviating resultant distress, and assisting those who are 'inappropriately emotional' to regain their stability (Lupton 1998). The fact that this creates workplace stress for nurses is rarely acknowledged (McVicar 2003).

Emotional labour work can be emotionally and physically demanding, but requires interpersonal and intrapersonal skills and competencies that are not acknowledged (McQueen 2004, Myerson 2000, Nicolson 1996). They assert that this lack of acknowledgment occurs for three reasons. First, emotion work remains largely invisible. Second, it requires the development of awareness and of a vocabulary to describe this work as a competency. Third, this work is predominantly done by women. Women tend to be more involved in the caring and service industries than men (as in nursing), and also perform much of the 'backstage' or behind-the-scenes work (Goffman 1959). While this work may be perceived as trivial, it is usually of a supportive nature, enhancing the intellectual capability or productivity of organisations (Lupton 1998). This is not to say that men do not 'do' emotional labour; some do. However, management is still predominantly done by men, and their power to demand emotional labour from both women and men is maintained by management, although is 'often constructed as (non)emotions' (Hearn 1993:161).

It is important not to forget the value of relationships that nurses develop with their patients, with relatives and carers, all of whom are part of using the self in caring mode, often critical to recovery, and which can be very demanding. Sandelowski makes the point that those who engender nursing as female:

> . . . inadvertently minimise or deny nursing its record of expertise and innovation within technology, the primary roles nurses have played in the deployment of technology and the power and remuneration that comes with technological knowledge and skills in a high-technology culture (Sandelowski 1997a:172).

Traditional expectations that surround caring as a feminine and nursing activity involve subjugation of the self and selfless devotion to duty (Caffrey & Caffrey 1994). In some circumstances nurses may experience feelings of powerlessness and eventually burn out, as a result of suppression of their own feelings and needs (Demerouti et al 2000).

For Benner (1984), caring may be experienced as an empowering, enabling process. Power and caring are gendered concepts—power as 'male' and caring as 'female'—and though relatively few studies examining gender-related differences in nurse caring have been undertaken, there is some evidence to suggest that nurse gender has an influence on how nurse caring behaviours are demonstrated (Greenhalgh et al 1998, Ekstrom 1999, Jones 2001). Because of the gendered nature of power and caring, these two concepts may thus appear as oppositional. Benner (1984) associates power with caring by identifying power characteristics related to the caring dimensions of nursing practice, specifically transformative power, integrative caring, advocacy, healing power, participative/affirmative power and problem solving.

Transformative power refers to power that patients claim for themselves in order to take control of a situation, but which is only possible because of the particular way nurses choose to care for such patients. Integrative caring refers to the care nurses provide which enables the patient to be integrated into his or her social world, despite the limitations that illness may impose. Participative/affirmative power refers to the power nurses gain from engagement and involvement with the patient by using the meanings and resources that flow from the specific situation.

Davies (1995:183) argues that femininity itself is what provides the threat in caring. Nursing stands for a set of qualities that are unacceptable, since they are the 'vulnerabilities and dependencies that are edited out of masculinity'. She continues:

> . . . femininity—with its stress on dealing with dependency, acknowledging emotions and intimacy and nurturing others—comes to represent qualities that are feared and denied in masculinity, qualities that at best are seen as to be contained and allocated to a different sphere, and at worst are repressed or treated with contempt (Davies 1995:183).

Jones (2001) points out that claiming caring as nursing's unique essence creates serious vulnerability for nursing, particularly as caring has such widespread currency within the profession (Traynor 1996, Snellgrove & Hughes 2000).

Peacock & Nolan (2000) have expressed concern that the 'spread of outcome-oriented health services has led to care being redefined as the provision of the finest form of treatment that is financially viable' (p 1066), or as part of a 'business model' of healthcare (Bolton 2000), or 'mangled care'—a term used to describe 'managed care' that is perceived as economically, rather than 'caring', driven (Georges & McGuire 2004). This immediately places the concept and practice of care at risk, since it creates considerable tension for the delivery of modern healthcare. As Gattuso and Bevan (2000) point out, the caring relationship is hard to measure, but to not do so in the outcomes context may be dangerous for the future of nursing.

THE INFLUENCE OF FEMINISMS ON THE DISCIPLINE OF NURSING

'The feminisms' refers to the variety of theoretical approaches to the advocacy of equal rights for women, accompanied by a commitment to improve the position of women in society. They are informed by a range of theoretical propositions, which include liberal feminism, socialist feminism, postmodern feminism, postcolonial feminism (Rancine 2003), feminist ethics (Peter et al 2004) and other forms.

This chapter has developed the argument that women and nurses are devalued in general, notwithstanding that gains have been made in recent years. Feminist nurses, and others, have provided feminist analyses of their clinical practice, their educational understandings and their research. It is most notable that the feminisms have been promoted more by nursing scholars than practitioners, which has led to some uneasiness between the two groups. This may have arisen because the feminisms have an 'image' problem due to stereotypical views of what constitutes a feminist.

In reality, the feminisms are political perspectives, which seek to balance societal power, to gain equalities and autonomies for women of all races, classes, ethnicities, ages, disabilities, sexualities and professional status (Peter et al 2004). These feminisms offer the opportunity for nurses to recognise and analyse the unequal power relations that have been discussed earlier in this chapter, and to develop a raised consciousness about gender issues (Dendaas 2004, Valentine 2001, Meadus 2000). Feminist analyses have been extended to clinical practice to examine nursing and healthcare contexts, particularly 'managed care' from the 'feminist philosophical assumption that "the personal is political"' (Georges & McGuire 2004:11).

It is noteworthy that the feminisms have been eschewed by a large number of women, particularly younger women (Baumgardner & Richards 2003). This may be partly attributed to (mis)understandings of the meaning of feminism. Those who seek to denigrate feminism and what it can offer suggest that feminists are 'man-haters' and therefore have an inappropriate sexual orientation; a number of other jaundiced and inaccurate epithets are hurled at them.

In reality, one can espouse feminist philosophy or be driven from a feminist perspective while celebrating womanhood, whatever individualistic form it takes. Thus, women can enjoy male company and be interested in fashion, and enjoy their youth and femininity.

The key point is that feminism can be individually practised, which includes making choices about life. This can range, for example, from career choice and relationship definition, to shaving whatever parts of our body we wish, wearing nail polish and make-up, and even enjoying relationships with males. Feminism is thus about taking control of one's life, respecting one's womanhood as well as men; feminists can (and do) enjoy male company. The radical left of the 1970s view was that all men were rapists and perpetrators of violence. The reality is that some are, but the majority are not. So adopting a feminist perspective does not mean rejecting relationships with men; there can be (and often is) a natural and harmonious coexistence between women and men.

So while it is true that the feminisms have not been adopted wholeheartedly by nurses, they certainly have had an impact. Some feminists have been hypercritical of nursing and nurses because of the latter's inability to embrace feminist theories: they believe that nursing as a women's field needs 'rescuing'—that it is a victim of patriarchy and needs help in recognising this. As previously noted, some feminists place the blame for the continuance of nursing oppression at the feet of nurses who collude with their oppressors to prevent change in the system (David 2000). In this way, nurses are viewed as weak and compliant with the dominant forces that seek to retain the status quo or as deceiving themselves. This may be a deliberate act, but it is more likely that insight and awareness has not been developed, thus disadvantaging nurses and nursing.

Nursing has, however, provided fertile ground for the development of feminist theories, as these provide useful perspectives for nurses who work with disempowered and marginalised groups in their practice. Many nurses have recognised that they are also disempowered, marginalised and disadvantaged within the healthcare system (Ceci 2004a), and are developing understandings of these processes in order to action change. But while this is an ongoing movement, it certainly is no easy task.

One example of the way feminist theory has influenced nursing will now be explored. While feminist theories have focused on nursing and the development of nursing research, there is a significant 'halo effect' that works against the valuing of nursing research. In accepting the premise that women and nurses are devalued in general, by 'scientific' researchers in particular, nursing research itself is devalued, because it is done by women and nurses. The qualities that define a 'good nurse' are quite distinct from those defining a 'good researcher'. Hicks (1997, 1999) argues that 'research has fundamentally masculine connotations and nursing is quintessentially feminine' (Hicks 1999:130), which in itself contributes to the relative paucity of nursing research output. Clearly, two cultures are in collision: nursing and research (Valentine 2001, Neuman 1999).

There is a long history of males who, in the past, were the academics and intellectual and political gatekeepers of Western thought. They constructed and reproduced knowledge. But with the deconstruction and reconstruction of knowledge by feminists who have challenged the 'received view', nurses can take advantage of the liberalising approach inherent in the scholarly work published since the 1970s and 1980s in academic feminism and nursing. Since this time, feminist critics of science have exposed the history and assumptions of science and identified its masculinist practices.

Evans (1997:54) argues that 'women then had to fight and argue their way back into science—and a scientific epistemology and community that they had had little or no part in constructing'. Not only were they literally absent from science, there was also a wider absence of the 'feminine' and an absence from the findings and conclusions of science. This was not surprising because 'the *questions* that science identified as important were determined by the construction of the social world in which men occupied the public, and women the private, space' (Evans 1997:54).

According to Huntington (1996), this created an opportunity for scientific knowledge to maintain the control of women (primarily through their bodies), as men have constructed a knowledge base that is able to be extrapolated to women. She continues: '. . . nurses . . . have not addressed the issue of the place of science in nursing nor the impact this has had on nursing generally, and the nursing of women in particular' (p 168). This, of course, has implications for nursing work and nursing research, as it suggests that nurses may be instrumental in maintaining a medical ideology for women patients, calculated to be negative and oppressive (Buchanan 1997).

Part of the rejection of masculinist science was fostered by scholars, intellectuals and researchers who adopted the 'emancipatory science' perspective promulgated by the Frankfurt School of Sociology and Philosophy. The inaugural address given by Habermas in 1965, entitled 'Knowledge and interest', defined emancipatory science as 'one which reveals the relationship of knowledge and interests which the objectivist attitude conceals' (Hagell 1989:227). This included a rejection of logical positivism as the only or most appropriate approach to research; interpretive and other qualitative forms were deemed by many to be superior for the task at hand in a range of disciplines, including nursing.

In the 1960s, the nursing discipline was given opportunities for development by a nursing science that was driven by an empiricist or logical positivist philosophy. Edwards (1999) suggests that nursing was driven to claim its science base for reasons of prestige and status, as well as a need to be perceived as a 'successful' profession. He concludes that nursing does not qualify as a legitimate science, since it must be empirical (and is not). Nurse researchers and scholars have long acknowledged the inappropriateness for *all* nursing research to be undertaken using the empiricist model, because many of the questions framed were not valid for nursing knowledge development (Whittemore 1999). Winters and Ballou (2004:533) argue that 'legitimate science includes both empirical and non-empirical scientific methods'.

However, if we return to the argument that has been developed, given society's attitudes to women, and hence nurses, there may be more value in conforming to the dominant culture (i.e. 'scientific research' that is acceptable to masculinist science). This is not appropriate, however, because it will not answer many of the questions nursing asks. Thus, Winters and Ballou (2004:533) propose that nursing should work towards integrating 'all applicable modes of scientific inquiry into the discipline'.

An alternative approach for the development of nursing knowledge underpinned by feminist principles can provide nurses with understandings of what it is that they know, and what it is they experience, which involves reclaiming and renaming nursing's experiences and knowledge of the social world lived in and daily constructed. Rancine (2003:91) contends that there are other promising and more appropriate ways of developing knowledge that support social activism, including that deriving from nursing research. These include the use of critical and feminist approaches to explore 'health issues related to race, gender, and social classes'. This builds on the work of Doering (1992:25), who suggested that feminism and poststructuralism were particularly relevant to nursing because they incorporate the concepts of the female experience and of power. These concepts reflect the historical, social and political dynamics in which the discipline of nursing operates. They encompass a theme central to nursing—that of powerlessness, characterised by oppression, submission and male domination.

It is important to note that feminist research 'permits the recognition and exploration of socio-cultural factors that transcend gender' (Jackson 1997:87), which signals that, while the concept of oppression is central to feminism, it is clearly shared with other groups (Evans 1997). Thus:

> Accepting that experiences around oppression and struggle are not exclusive to women permits recognition that institutionalised patriarchy and androcentricity are oppressive to all but those of the dominant class, race and gender (Jackson 1997:87).

This insight attempts to deal with the charge by Allen et al (1991) that feminist research marginalises men. These authors raised the question of whether research involving only women simply 'supports a conceptual scheme that reinforces the material subjugation of women' and thus 'perpetuates problematic social categories' (p 50). They concluded, somewhat controversially, that 'a better strategy is to deconstruct the dichotomy itself and to expand awareness of the diverse contemporary and historical forms of gendered existence' (Allen et al 1991:56), which has subsequently occurred.

It may be reasonable to support the view that the value of feminist research is that it 'empowers women and addresses issues that can make a difference to the quality of life for all humankind' (Parker & McFarland 1991:66). There are those who believe that nursing research should be approached from a much broader perspective and incorporate a range of paradigms. The method used is defined by the questions being asked. Unfortunately, too, the method may be driven by other motives, such as economic rationalism, and the need to obtain research funding, regardless of the ethical and moral imperatives that would normally guide research behaviour. But it is clear that the research approach must take into account the context in which it is conducted, and for nursing this has political and power implications. There is no question that gender is a critical and all-encompassing variable to be acknowledged. And it is feminist theory that has largely been responsible for raising nursing's consciousness in this domain.

MEN IN NURSING

It has long been noted that men are a minority in nursing, despite the fact that their numbers have increased over the decades. In 1996 the nursing workforce in the United States consisted of 5.9% men (Janiszewski Goodin 2003), while in 1998 they comprised 4.4% of the Canadian workforce (Meadus 2000). This compares to statistics from Britain, where men have constituted less than 10% of the qualified nursing workforce, while in Australia it is around 8%. More specifically, analyses of gender breakdown of the UK registration authority indicate that, in 1990, 8.37% of registrants were male; in 2000, this figure had increased to 9.75% (http: www.ukcc.org.au). In the United States, males comprised 8.6% in bacculaureate programs, 9.6% in masters' programs, and 6.7% in doctoral programs (American Association of Colleges of Nursing 2002). The proportion of male nursing undergraduate students in Australia increased from 11.9% in 1987–90, to 15.9% in 1995 (Brown 1998).

Nursing school faculties in the United States comprise 96.3% females and 3.7% males (American Association of Colleges of Nursing 2002). In a national survey which examined numerical representation, seniority status and experiences of men compared to women in the university-based nursing education workforce in Australia, men were found to be overrepresented at the highest levels. Fifty-two per cent of deans having control of nursing were males, 19% were professors and associate professors, and 26% were at the next level of senior lecturer (Sharman et al 1996:308). The study indicated that women were supporting men in the workforce and the home, often at the expense of their own career advancement.

This is a finding that has previously been highlighted in other traditionally female occupations, such as teaching, physiotherapy, occupational therapy, librarianship and social work (Williams 1992). What it demonstrates is that males are moving into powerful positions over the largest occupational group in the health workforce, nursing, an occupational group that has traditionally been 'managed, taught, disciplined and organised almost entirely by women' (MacGuire, cited in Sharman et al 1996). There is little doubt that 'the ideological climate, socialisation processes and women's family and domestic responsibilities underlie a glass ceiling for women and a glass elevator for men in non-traditional occupations' (Sharman 1998:56). Nevertheless, males continue to be viewed as increasingly disadvantaged and reduced to 'lifting machines' (Shakespeare 2003:53).

While men in some numbers are relative newcomers to nursing, they are increasingly being promoted to higher levels than women, despite their disproportionate numbers; furthermore, they seem to have less experience and fewer qualifications (Evans 2004). This appears to have been due to a recruitment campaign, which attacks the negative stereotype of men in nursing, and highlights the fact that management positions were 'made ripe for male capture', thus positioning men with 'poor formal educational qualifications' (Evans 2004:326) for leadership positions.

Brown's study (1998) found that men were overrepresented in senior nursing administrative positions. Although men comprised only 8% of the registered nurse workforce, they held 22% of senior nursing positions. Poliafico (1998) indicates that this comparative figure is only 6% in the United States, and suggests that there is a common misconception that men hold a disproportionate number of administrative positions. Brown (1998:21) considers a range of explanations as to why this is happening in Australia. One of the most compelling is that women are seen to be invading the workplace, since workplaces are constructed by men. So it is that even in 'women's occupations', such as nursing, where it may be expected that men would be perceived as not fitting in, the overriding culture of the workplace turns this disjunction into a benefit for men.

Thus men who enter nursing are seen to be 'lowering themselves, losing status by undertaking "women's work"' (Brown 1998:21), yet are expected to be better workers than female nurses. They retain the benefits of their ascribed gender role: they are seen to be the 'breadwinner', to have leadership qualities, to be worth mentoring (since they are more likely to be serious about their career), and they are more likely to be assisted in accessing 'power networks' in nursing. Hicks (1999) argues that if men in these top positions behave consistently with the findings of research studies, then they are most likely to reproduce themselves at these top-level positions. This will then serve to widen the gender/power divisions in nursing.

Further evidence that men are being promoted to the highest levels of service in nursing, despite their numerical minority, is provided by Boughn (2001:23) who notes that 'men who go into nursing rise like cream in milk' because they expect practical rewards and set up their lives to achieve and retain these, whereas women fail to recognise their economic and political power.

A study which examined senior nursing administrative positions in the United Kingdom found that, in 1987, 8.6% of registered nurses were men, but 50.3% held chief nurse/advisor posts, and 57.8% were Directors of Nursing Education (Gaze 1987). There has been a disproportionate increase of males in senior nursing positions in the United Kingdom, which has also occurred in the United States. It should be noted, however, that there was a concerted effort in the United Kingdom to 'defeminise' management within nursing, enabling men to be more easily promoted into these positions (Carpenter 1977).

Jenkins (1989) notes that Florence Nightingale had a vision that nursing would always be under the control of women; she saw no place in nursing for men, just as there was no place for men in controlling nursing. Mackintosh (1997) and Meadus (2000) believe that the contribution of men to nursing has not been recognised and that it is time for affirmative action in favour of men for nursing to survive the twenty-first century. This means 'that the Nightingale image must be counter-balanced by the entry and acceptance of larger numbers of men into the profession' (Meadus 2000:10).

This view is rejected by other researchers who suggest that nursing, rather than increasing male numbers, should introduce feminist strategies to enhance the power of women nurses, since their lower disproportionate voice in academic writing and actual power in practice requires improvement (Ryan & Porter 1993:43). Other research that focuses on the experience of male nurses suggests that attrition is a major issue, due to the treatment given to males (Morin 1999, Kelly et al 1996).

To counteract the inequities experienced by men in nursing, the American Assembly for Men in Nursing was formed in 1971 (Evans 2004). Its aims were 'to recruit more men into the profession, to provide support to those men who already are nurses, and to increase the visibility of men in nursing' (Poliafico 1998:43). Evans (2004) documents how nursing associations have acted as gatekeepers of change, limiting men's participation in nursing, including the refusal of approval to employ male nurse educators, on the grounds that it was inappropriate for men to teach women how to nurse. Nevertheless, gendered attitudes, which are 'reinforced and perpetuated by patriarchal societal institutions and processes' (Evans 1997:231), continue. The solution lies in challenging our stereotypes of femininity and masculinity, and addressing structural relations.

CONCLUSION

The aim of this chapter is to bring into sharp focus the gendered culture of nursing. Quite clearly there are inequities at work that can be documented with respect to control, management and leadership in nursing. Additionally, there are more subtle ways that gender impacts on nursing. This chapter has argued that nursing work in all its forms (including clinical practice, education and research), mostly undertaken by women, is affected severely by gender because of its construction and the context in which nursing is carried out (Valentine 2001). Becoming aware of such systematic oppressions is the first step in changing paternalistic structures and systems that operate to disadvantage nurses, their patients, and the overall healthcare system.

David (2000:90) suggests that nurses 'must reframe the sociopolitical reality and give it back', otherwise they will continue to be '. . . shackled in servitude, denied freedom to acknowledge the full benefit of their health and healing practices'. Failure to challenge the stereotypes rife in nursing effectively results in collusion 'with nursing's power brokers in maintaining for the nurse the status of "trained worker" as opposed to that of "learned professional"' (Fealy 2004:654). And such challenges are part of that which the feminisms seek to contribute to the nursing profession.

REFLECTIVE QUESTIONS

1 What do you think the feminisms have to offer the discipline of nursing?

2 Do you believe that the role and function of nursing cannot be separated from nurses who undertake it? If so, why is this? If you disagree, outline your arguments to support your position.

3 What do you think of the fact that men in nursing, despite their numerical minority, have the majority of leadership positions? Why do you think this is? What implications does this have for nursing as a profession?

RECOMMENDED READINGS

Barrett M, Phillips A eds 1992 *Destabilizing theory: contemporary feminist debates*. Polity Press, Cambridge.

Davies C 1995 *Gender and the professional predicament in nursing*. Open University Press, Buckingham.

Horsfall J 2000 Feminism in nursing. In J Greenwood (ed) *Nursing theory in Australia: development and application*. Harper Educational Publishers, Sydney.

Lumby J 1997 The feminised body in illness. In J Lawler (ed) *The body in nursing: a collection of views*. Churchill Livingstone, Melbourne.

Speedy S 1991 The contribution of feminist research. In G Gray & R Pratt (eds) *Towards a discipline of nursing*. Churchill Livingstone, Melbourne.

CHAPTER THIRTEEN

Power and politics in the practice of nursing

Annette Huntington & Jean Gilmour

LEARNING OBJECTIVES

After completing this chapter, the reader will:

▲ understand the nature of power and politics;

▲ have an awareness of different theoretical conceptions of power;

▲ understand the way in which nurses possess power individually and collectively;

▲ understand the advocacy role and how it relates to power; and

▲ appreciate the complexities of whistleblowing and its consequences.

KEY WORDS
Power, politics, agency, influence, whistleblowing

NURSING AND POLITICS

Nursing is a political activity. Politics, in the broadest sense of the word, is part of all nurses' lives, especially in the large institutions within which many of us work. It is thus important for us, as nurses, to think about power and politics. At the very least we need to understand that the health sector is a highly politicised environment at the micro and the macro level, and that the health sector is not an apolitical or neutral site. As nurses, we are both active in this highly political arena, and also have considerable power within it.

Healthcare is fundamental to life, and nurses are intimately involved in caring for the sick and supporting the healthy, either directly or indirectly, wherever they are working. Nurses are in a privileged position in that millions of people every day put their trust in us and assume that we will always work on the public's behalf. When you become a nurse you accept the obligations and expectations that go with being in that highly responsible and highly respected (particularly by the general public) role. When you become registered you also accept all that registration carries with it in terms of commitment to a code of ethics, at the centre of which is the safety and wellbeing of those for whom you care. Key to this is using the power that you have wisely, and being aware of the moral and ethical obligations you have because of this position of trust.

Every nurse has a degree of power. Even as a newly registered nurse you immediately have power over patients/clients, who are nearly always in a less powerful position due to your knowledge of both health and illness, and the healthcare system. Knowledge is power, and just the ability to impart or withhold information puts you in a privileged position in relation to the people and/or communities you work with. Henderson's (2003) research in Western Australia exploring the power imbalance between nurses and patients clearly highlighted this, as the nurses in the study showed a reluctance to share any meaningful power with the patients. As the author says: 'This imbalance of power was most evident in information-giving and during nurse–patient interactions, where nurses used their power to maintain control' (Henderson 2003:504).

In addition to an individual nurse's power in the patient/client relationship, nurses as a collective also have considerable potential power. In many countries, nurses are the largest occupational group in the healthcare sector. In New Zealand, nurses comprise 50% of the health and disability workforce (Health Workforce Advisory Committee 2003) and, in Australia, nearly 60% (Commonwealth of Australia 2002). Many of the reforms and restructurings that have taken place in Western health systems in recent years are focused on controlling and managing this considerable workforce—often due to the perceived cost of providing nurses' services in the health sector. However, these same numbers give nurses power—power that can be used to influence the health system and improve it for both nurses and the public. As Holmes and Gastaldo (2002:563) state: 'Nurses also form a critical group that challenges the status quo and works for a more equitable society'. To be active in such a way, nurses require an understanding of power and its effects, and the way that they can use their power to enhance the health and wellbeing of people.

Power is often considered a negative and oppressive attribute. However, new definitions of the nature of power by philosophers such as Michel Foucault, who will be discussed below, incorporate the notion of power as constructive and constitutive, as well as having the potential to be destructive and oppressive. These new definitions also provide nurses with a new way of considering power, a way that means we can view nurses as being 'powerless' in certain situations but very powerful in other circumstances. This frees us from the idea that we are inherently powerless through being nurses. This rethinking and reshaping of nurses' positioning can be particularly valuable in the current climate of global nurse shortages and shrinking health sector resources, which can result in a highly stressful environment in which nurses can feel they have little power to influence or change practices or structures.

In this chapter we firstly explore the concept of power and its multiple meanings and understandings. We then discuss nurses' political power, followed by a discussion of power in practice, including issues of advocacy and whistleblowing.

UNDERSTANDING POWER

Power is a concept that has many meanings and definitions, and different perceptions of power will influence both people's actions and the outcomes of these actions. Simple definitions consider power to involve something one person has over another (Poggi 2001), creation of causal effects (Scott 2001), and the potential to be influential—that is, make your ideas known to others and gain their support (Sullivan 2004).

Dye and Harrison (2005) offer a more complex definition of influence, suggesting that it is a form of power where particular effects are produced through a system of reward and punishment. They argue that power is based on access to intertwined resources such as wealth, education, political influence and economics. Resources are not evenly distributed through society, and those with 'power' control resources through rewards or the threat of deprivation of resources. An example related to nursing is when managers or clinical leaders control nurses' workload and conditions through processes such as rostering. The management role can be enacted in a range of ways, from an autocratic top-down directive with no space for personal preferences to be voiced, to a participatory style of management where the staff nurses in a ward manage their own roster and the allocation of patient care. Ultimately, however, the manager or clinical leader has the ability to choose how they will organise work and shift allocations, and therefore has the power in this situation.

Michel Foucault (1980), a French philosopher, has another viewpoint on power. He suggests that power is exercised rather than possessed, is productive rather than mainly repressive, and furthermore emerges from below. This means that people traditionally constructed as powerless and oppressed can be seen as actually having agency—defined as the capacity to act and exert power, and therefore affecting the way it is enacted. Power circulates, rather than being localised 'never in anybody's hands, never appropriated as a commodity or piece of wealth' (Foucault 1980:98). People are simultaneously affected by power relationships and participate in those relationships.

Foucault's definition highlights the flow of power in everyday practices and relationships, and the inherent potential for the exercise of power as a productive force in social relationships. He also differentiates power relations from relations of force or violence where there is no choice and where possibilities are curtailed. The significant factor for nurses in this representation of power is that power relationships involve the possibility of resistance—the person over whom power is exercised has the capacity to react and respond in a range of ways (Foucault 1983).

Feminist writers also focus on power, as it is a central concept in any discussion of agency and/or oppression. Many feminist scholars engage with postmodern thought that considers power, in a similar way to the work of Foucault, as being a discursively constructed relationship, rather than an oppressive force requiring a victim (Peter et al 2004). As Shildrick states:

> . . . what becomes possible is to speak of power, not perhaps in the sense of monolithic structures, but as a field of forces held together in shifting but temporally analysable contestable configurations (Shildrick 1997:115).

While many feminist scholars consider concepts from the work of Foucault and postmodernism to be useful for feminist thinking related to power (Weedon 1997, Lupton 2003), others critique the lack of acknowledgment of the gender dimensions in such constructions of power—gender obviously being a central tenant of feminist thinking around power (Huntington & Gilmour 2001).

POLITICS AND POWER

Politics permeates all aspects of life. Mason et al (cited in Sullivan 2004:60) define politics as 'the art of influencing others to achieve desirable goals, usually by aquiring resources'. As to who is influential, Lasswell (1958) describes them as those who get the most of what there is to get. If success in politics is judged by control over resources, nurses historically have been unsuccessful in the political arena when judged by such factors as pay parity with equivalent professional groups or satisfactory working environments. Sullivan (2004) argues that historical factors still impact on nurses' degree of influence in contemporary healthcare. The origins of formalised nursing in military and religious organisations permeate the profession, with values such as personal discipline, a focus on service and obedience being seen by some as fundamental characteristics of nurses.

While many nurses have effectively engaged in politics at all levels, these values, along with the issues around the gendered culture of nursing (discussed in Ch 12), have limited the full realisation of nurses' and nursing's potential for political action, influence and advocacy. Takase et al (2001) also argue that nurses have been historically disadvantaged by their close relationship with medical colleagues. This has positioned the practice of nursing as subservient to the practice of medicine, and impacts negatively on nurses' perception of themselves. This perception can inhibit nurses from seeing the power that their increasing professionalisation confers.

Politics at state and national level is often thought of as only involving government. Governments are critical bodies for regulating behaviour in that 'government lays down the "rules of the game" in conflict and competition between individuals, organizations, and institutions within society' (Dye & Harrison 2005:198). But politics, seen as the exercise of power in the form of influence, is also part of everyday life. Engaging in political action—learning to be more influential in relation to matters that count—is therefore a possibility for all nurses. Sullivan (2004) suggests that influence exists through relationships and is more significant than authority. It is gained through position or respect for knowledge and skills. She also suggests that influence is earned through effort and that the skills of influence can be learnt, the most crucial factor being the personal decision to become influential.

Nurses tend to think that because they are good people doing a good job they should be valued and fairly rewarded and, if that does not happen, they blame themselves or the profession (Sullivan 2004). However, nurses may in fact be unrewarded due to not effectively engaging in the underlying political game—engagement, which requires adherence to a particular set of rules that they may not even know exists. Critically, we as nurses must therefore recognise the existence and reality of politics, the legitimacy and necessity of being involved in politics, and learn skills to gain greater influence if personal and professional goals are to be achieved. Sullivan (2004) identifies some possible workplace strategies for developing influence, including:

- reciprocity with other workers (i.e. exchanging favours);

- having a good understanding of the informal information that circulates within the organisation;

- avoiding confrontation;

- compromising when necessary to achieve a more important goal;

- networking;

- accepting responsibility for individual actions, both positive and negative; and

- finding a mentor.

The idea of playing workplace politics may not initially resonate with the cherished nursing ideal of teamwork, but having influence and developing assertive and satisfying interdisciplinary relationships are essential factors in nurses being active in ensuring the provision of high-quality nursing care.

NURSES' POLITICAL POWER

All people have political power as individuals, but nurses also have great potential as a collective body to exercise their power. As noted above, nurses are the largest professional group in the health workforce. Australasian nurses are increasingly well educated at graduate level and have a growing evidence-based body of knowledge to support nursing practice. Nurses also work in wide-ranging roles in healthcare, spanning clinical, management, research, teaching and health policy domains that provide multiple opportunities to exert influence.

A key element of realising collective power is having formal ways to organise collectives of people for a common cause that is well articulated and appeals to broad segments of the population. In nursing, the protection, support and influence derived from the power of the collective is realised through professional organisations. This is shown clearly in situations such as collective salary bargaining or guaranteed nurse–patient ratios, such as those negotiated in Victoria, which have had a major impact on the working environment for nurses. Neither of these would be possible to negotiate at an individual level. There are many professional bodies that primarily serve to advance the interests of the nursing workforce. As nurses, you have the opportunity to be involved and shape the political activity of these organisations through contribution as a member or at governance level.

One of the most important choices you will make as a registered nurse, therefore, is the decision to join your professional body. The particular structures and focus of nursing organisations varies considerably, but their two broad areas of interest are industrial or employment concerns, and what are loosely called 'professional issues'. Some organisations have two arms and encompass both these aspects, while others will focus specifically on one area. The choice of which organisation to join is up to you, but should be given careful thought, considering what each organisation's role is, the focus and achievements of each organisation, and what they can provide for you. An excellent overview of Australasian organisations is provided at: http://www.nurses.info/organizations_australia_newzealand.htm.

While nurses work collectively and are often considered an homogenous group, it is important to accept that nurses are enormously diverse. As a result, while the overall goal of nursing may be shared by everyone in the profession, individual nurses will not always share worldviews at either the macro or micro level. Therefore, using the power that nurses have means being highly skilled at working not only with diverse population groups, but also with diverse nurses and nursing groups. Nursing and its practitioners have widely differing philosophical and political positions, and one strategy for managing this diversity is through the focus that professional organisations can bring. This means that individual difference can be accepted, but organisational power can focus on collective professional issues.

An example of nurses successfully using their collective political power to advance practice through the legislative process is the gaining of prescribing authority for community nurses in the United Kingdom in the 1990s. Prescribing is an area of current political interest for Australian and New Zealand nurses, where we are engaged in advocating for changes in legislation and governmental processes to enable nurses (usually advanced practitioners) to prescribe in their scope of practice. In New Zealand, extending prescribing rights to nurse practitioners has been particularly contentious, with some members of the medical profession, such as general practitioners, concerned with potential competition for funding (Mackay 2003).

Jones' (2004) description of the approach taken by the Royal College of Nursing (RCN) in the United Kingdom notes that the implementation of nurse prescribing required 'political machination, the need to construct an effective case, and deft manoeuvring within the corridors of power' (p 266). Initial elements of the strategy to increase political influence included focusing on a clear objective, taking advantage of an existing opportunity (which in the United Kingdom was the review of community nursing), developing alliances with the British Medical Association and pharmacists, and ensuring a unified professional position by managing internal concerns raised by groups such as practice nurses.

The next level of political activity involved communicating nurses' experiences of prescribing, which showed the positive impact on patient outcomes, to parliamentarians, enlisting patient representative organisations to support the Nurse Prescribing Bill (Jones 2004), and individual RCN members contacting local media to inform the public about the issue. The progression of the legislation through parliament was far from smooth, and considerable tenacity and ongoing alliances with a wide range of supporting organisations were necessary to achieve a successful result. Positive change did, however, occur through the deliberate and strategic use of political influence.

Table 13.1 lists some ways of developing influence through knowledge, communication skills and action.

Table 13.1: Developing influence through knowledge, communication skills and action

Knowledge	Communication skills	Action
Nursing knowledge base		
• Evidence-based clinical practice knowledge • Patient and family knowledge/agendas/issues • Policy/legislation knowledge at government, discipline and organisational levels	• Articulate and assertive verbal communication • Clear and appropriate written communication meeting academic/media/political/popular conventions, depending on context	• Respond in a timely and coherent manner • Document using appropriate channels • Take opportunities to be involved in shaping policy through submissions and committee work • Use information technology competently for communication and information retrieval
Understanding power		
• Relationship of knowledge with power • Power as a circulating force • The capacity for resistance • Differentiation of power relations and force relations	• Professional introductions • Title parity • Adhere to professional code of dress • Prepare accounts demonstrating importance of nursing work	• Take leadership opportunities—formal and informal • Accept responsibility • Use knowledge to inform patients and families • Act as an advocate
The rules of the game for		
• Nursing • Heathcare teams • Organisations • Communities	• Network within and outside the profession • Develop and use relationships with media and politicians	• Develop respectful and communicative relationships within and outside nursing • Be tenacious • Enlist support from broader communities of interest in issues of concern to nursing

POWER IN PRACTICE

Knowledge carries with it power and authority, but not all forms of knowledge are created equal. In the preceding section on nurses' political power, we discussed the power that nurses have as a collective. However, there is ample evidence to suggest that nurses have been conspicuously silent, or that they have been silenced, at times when it has been vital that patients have had vocal, assertive and knowledgeable advocates. Chiarella (2000) argues that within the legal system, nurses are seen as a separate but subordinate group to medicine, which impacts on the authority of nurses' testimony and their opportunities to speak:

> Today or tomorrow or the next day, a nurse may or may not intervene to stop a doctor from making a mistake, which might harm the patient. It will not depend on the law. It will depend on how brave they are. They operate inside (or outside) a legal framework, which insufficiently recognises their work and their presence (Chiarella 2000:198).

One instance of the devaluation of nurses' knowledge and authority by the medical profession with lethal results involved the deaths of 12 children who died during or shortly after undergoing cardiac surgery in a Canadian hospital in 1994. Nurses involved in the cardiac surgery service had made sustained attempts to voice their concerns through the appropriate hospital channels during the preceding year, but these had not been taken seriously (Ceci 2004b). Medical peers of the surgeon dismissed the validity of claims by several nurses that there were competency issues on the grounds that nurses did not have medical expertise.

When nurses themselves feel powerless, however, they may choose not to act, and this can also have dire consequences. One example of this, which also had lethal consequences, was revealed during New Zealand's Cartwright Inquiry into cervical cancer, which revealed unethical medical research practices, such as the lack of informed consent, in the experimental trial. This research, carried out from 1966 until the early 1980s, studied the progression of cervical cancer *in situ* in a group of women, without offering medical intervention, until progression to invasive cancer (Coney 1988). Nurses throughout this period working at the hospital concerned did not openly voice their concerns or ensure the women had been provided with the information necessary to make an informed choice about participation. Judge Silvia Cartwright stated that:

> . . . nurses who most appropriately should be advocates for the patient, feel sufficiently intimidated by the medical staff (who do not hire or fire them) that even today they fail or refuse to confront openly the issues arising from the 1966 trial (Committee of Inquiry into Allegations Concerning the Treatment of Cervical Cancer at National Women's Hospital and into Other Related Matters 1988:172).

Although by speaking out the nurses may not have been able to stop the research, their complicity through silence is something that nurses in New Zealand have to acknowledge. Constructing ourselves as powerless and lacking in agency can lead to nurses behaving unethically and not putting patients' best interests at the centre of our professional obligations.

Buresh and Gordon (2003) have offered a powerful critique of nurses' lack of visibility and voice in the public arena, and suggest many strategies for 'creating a voice of agency' (p 35). Expressing agency is built upon the realisation of the importance of nurse's work and the confidence of nurses themselves. To make this agency explicit requires change at the fundamental level of day-to-day practice. Every encounter with patients, families and other staff members is an opportunity to communicate, verbally and non-verbally, messages about the competency and the knowledge base underpinning our decisions and practices.

Expressing agency begins right at the first introduction to patients and colleagues. For example, status can be reinforced through the use of both first and last names rather than just first name, along with title and role, a professional standard of dress, and non-deferential body language. Buresh and Gordon (2003) have written extensively on the necessity for nurses to take every opportunity to educate people they meet about what they do and why they do it:

> To convey the content of nursing, nurses must describe the complexity of care *they* give and the clinical judgments *they* use. They must take care in their discussions with patients and families, with the broader public, and with media and political representatives not to depict themselves as extensions of the doctor's agency (Buresh & Gordon 2003).

As nurses, we are highly educated practitioners with both formal education in, and considerable informal knowledge of, the culture and processes of the health system within which our clients and patients find themselves. This has important implications for power relationships between ourselves and the people for whom we care.

An example of our everyday exercise of power is the categorisation of people through the practice of assessment and the ensuing allocation of resources to them. Assessment requires recording a range of information and judging whether a person meets certain predetermined criteria for normality and/or abnormality. The distribution of a wide range of resources, including the time and expertise of nurses and other health professionals, medical equipment, pharamaceuticals, and access to the care setting is determined by nursing assessment.

From a Foucauldian perspective, the assessment process therefore needs to incorporate opportunities for patients and their families to exercise some control. This can be achieved by providing information about the purpose, scope and implications of the assessment in clear language, obtaining informed consent, and validating the documented information with the person concerned.

Power can also be used by nurses to improve practice and the experiences of the people and groups with whom we are working. We have chosen to highlight two particular situations or practices where power can be used by the individual nurse. The first of these is the advocacy role that for many nurses is an integral part of day-to-day practice, and the second is what is commonly called 'whistleblowing'.

Advocacy

Advocacy consists of taking action on behalf of a person, or supporting an individual or group to gain what they need from the system. This is now considered a fundamental element of practice at all levels. For example, it is increasingly being included in basic texts, where it is addressed as one of the most important aspects of nurses' work (e.g. Craven & Hirnle 2003). It is also raised as a strategy or technique useful for nurse leaders (Borbasi et al 2004). The increasingly overstretched and changing world of service delivery means that, more than ever before, nurses need to understand and enact our advocacy role at the micro and macro level.

Authors such as Teasdale (1998:1) define advocacy as 'influencing those who have power on behalf of those who do not'. However, this definition could be seen as limiting the empowerment of individuals or groups—as in many instances it may be more appropriate to support a person or community to advocate for themselves. It is important to recognise that acting as an advocate does not involve taking over the situation. This can result in a nurse acting out what he or she feels is best for the person, rather than acting to ensure that the person achieves what they want

(Henderson 2003). This second form of advocacy still involves the nurse in an act of advocacy, but one that reflects a more Foucauldian approach to power, in which everyone *has* power but may need support and information to *enact* that power. If a nurse is not able to act in this way, then the appropriate action is to ensure that the person or group has access to another source of advocacy.

To be able to act effectively as an advocate, nurses need the following:

▲ understanding of the politics, culture and systems of health sector institutions and health service delivery;

▲ respect for the client or community and their rights;

▲ understanding of relevant clinical issues;

▲ understanding of ethical issues;

▲ commitment to the client and/or group; and

▲ understanding of the need for evidence and the way it can be used to support decisions.

Advocacy can be used at all levels in the health system. It can be part of day-to-day practice in relationships with patients and clients, or it can involve influencing service delivery to enhance services for a client group or community as a whole. It is important, however, that nurses understand that there are limits to their advocacy skills, and that in some areas such as mental health, people may prefer external or non-health professional advocates. External advocates can be provided by special interest sector groups, or be paid independent advocates.

Many nurses are also key players in special interest groups working with people with particular health issues. Patient and family representative groups are effective lobbyists often accorded a voice in health policy development. Joint initiatives with these groups offer productive alliances to further nurses', and health consumers', agendas focused on improving healthcare services (Davies 2004). Part of our advocacy role is to be aware of the form of advocacy that is preferred by the clients or patients concerned, and to be able to discuss this in an informed manner.

Whistleblowing

Whistleblowing, like advocacy, requires the nurse to be assertive, but also involves taking a very public stand, something that requires 'conviction, assertiveness and self-confidence' (McDonald & Ahern 1999:12). We would also add that the nurse in this situation is usually motivated by a strong sense of the moral obligation that, as noted in our introduction, comes with being a nurse.

Although authors have defined whistleblowing in a range of ways, according to Greene and Latting (2004:2) there are certain consistencies:

▲ it is an act of notifying powerful others of wrongful practices in an organisation;

▲ the whistleblower is motivated by wanting to prevent unnecessary harm to others; and

▲ it is the action of an employee or former employee who has privileged access to information.

Or, as Dawson (2000:1) says: 'Whistleblowers are those who sound the alert on scandal, danger, malpractice, or corruption'. In situations where resources are stretched in the health sector and nurses as the biggest group are often being targeted in inevitable health cuts, events serious enough to warrant such a step may well increase.

Whistleblowing is an extremely serious action and there are major implications that must be considered by a nurse when he or she decides to take this step. Nurses who take such action must be considered as courageous and need the support of colleagues, friends and family, rather than being subject to hostility and harassment. As McDonald and Ahern (1999) highlight in their research into the coping strategies of those considering whistleblowing, whether the nurses chose to take that final step of actually whistleblowing or not, they experienced fear, anxiety and intimidation.

Jackson and Raftos (1997) found in their research with registered nurses that whistleblowing was an extremely difficult decision, and one that left the nurses feeling exposed and unsupported. However, this study also highlights the way in which these particular nurses put their moral obligation to the residents above the possible harm they may experience themselves. Greene and Latting (2004) provide guidelines for whistleblowing and stress that this is the step taken only when all other avenues have been exhausted. The box below provides a list based on their work that is applicable for nurses in this situation.

Guidelines for whistleblowing (Greene & Latting 2004)

- Assess the situation and one's own preparedness to go forward—how serious is the issue, what are my motives, can I live with myself if I stay silent, can I cope with the results of 'going public'?

- Assume others in the organisation are concerned—discuss the issue with colleagues, and see if there are steps that could be taken that you have overlooked.

- Obtain corroborating evidence and supporters—collect as much evidence as possible, and discuss it with colleagues.

- Keep careful records—keep precise and detailed documentation, as often whistleblowing can result in legal proceedings, and/or internal or government inquiries.

- Use the chain of command—unless urgent and extremely serious, ensure you have exhausted all other avenues within the organisation for addressing the situation first.

- Obtain the advice of dispassionate, expert outsiders—such as your professional organisation, your registration body, a lawyer or employment advisors, and consult websites.

- Obtain emotional support—as this is going to be a difficult time for you, ensure you have someone you can talk to who will encourage and support you.

> - Consider going outside the organisation only as a last resort—keep foremost in your mind that this action is for the benefit of the clients/patients/residents and that the experience of many professionals in this situation is that they do, in the end, leave the institution.

The need and value of whistleblowing is increasingly being recognised. A number of countries, or states and territories within countries, are enacting whistleblowing protection legislation. For example, in New Zealand there exists the *Protected Disclosures Act 2000*, which has been passed with the express purpose of promoting public interest by:

> . . . facilitating the disclosure and investigation of matters of serious wrongdoing in or by an organisations and by protecting employees who . . . make disclosures of information about serious wrongdoing in or by an organisation (section 5(a) and (b)).

In Australia, the existence of such legislation depends on the state or territory, with examples including the South Australian *Whistleblowers Protection Act 1993*, the Queensland *Whistleblowers Protection Act 1994* and the New South Wales *Protected Disclosures Act 1994*. In the United States, whistleblowing legislation came into being in 1978 (Dawson 2000).

Although there is considerable discussion about the extent to which employees are in fact protected by such legislation (Dawson 2000), it is essential for a nurse who has decided that this course of action must be taken to find out whether the state, territory or country has such legislation, and what this legislation provides in terms of protection. This is particularly important given that some legislation only applies to state sector employees, and does not extend to the private working environment. There are also organisations that support those who are contemplating or have already been involved in whistleblowing. The website http://www.uow.edu.au/arts/sts/bmartin/dissent/contacts provides the names of organisations in a number of countries who can provide information in this area.

Another extremely important issue is for nurses to understand and support those who feel that whistleblowing is their only avenue for dealing with an issue. Too often, those who choose to take a stand can feel isolated and be subject to both overt and more subtle forms of harassment. Recognising what is involved for a nurse taking such an action, even if you do not agree with it, and making this known to the person can make a significant difference to their experience in what is an extremely stressful situation. This stress can be due to both ongoing concern for those people who have been subject to whatever practices have led to the whistleblowing, and also a very realistic concern for the fallout that the nurse will inevitably experience.

It also is important to note that *not* doing anything in the face of clearly inappropriate, destructive or neglectful practices can be harmful for a nurse. It can be very stressful not doing anything, and a factor in that stress can be that many nurses feel because they understand what is going on they have a responsibility to react in some way. McDonald and Ahern (1999) note previous studies showing that those nurses who chose not to act as whistleblowers or advocates felt depressed and suffered from fatigue and moral anguish.

CONCLUSION

Nurses have traditionally been constructed as powerless by both themselves and others (Holmes & Gastaldo 2002). However, it is time that we reconsider this and acknowledge that nurses are in a very powerful position in society. More nurses than ever are both prepared at degree level, and are undertaking postgraduate study that enhances their ability to provide care in the increasingly complex health services. Nursing services are pivotal in the provision of healthcare and in enacting the health goals of the international community: 'they form the backbone of health systems around the globe and provide a platform for efforts to tackle the diseases that cause poverty and ill health' (World Health Organization 2002:vii). As nurses, we mediate between healthcare institutions, with their associated mysterious practices, language and technologies, and the person—translating and making the health system understandable for the individual or community.

Nurses are a powerful group, expert in terms of their knowledge base, their practice and their understanding of the impact of health on people and communities. This knowledge and experience places the nurse in a very powerful position in terms of being able to influence people they are working with to make particular decisions regarding their health and wellbeing. Understanding and being consciously political at both the collective and individual levels is central to using the privileged position we have to work on behalf of patients and clients, and improve their experience of healthcare and their health outcomes.

REFLECTIVE QUESTIONS

1   How can nurses as a professional group be more effective in terms of political action?

2   How can power imbalances between you and your patients be minimised in everyday practice?

3   What do patients and families need to know to be effective advocates for themselves and others?

RECOMMENDED READINGS

Buresh B, Gordon S 2003 *From silence to voice: what nurses know and must communicate to the public*. Cornell University Press, New York (first published in 2000 by the Canadian Nurses' Association).

Chiarella M 2000 Silence in court: the devaluation of the stories of nurses in the narratives of health law. *Nursing Inquiry* 7(3):191–9.

Greene A D, Latting J K 2004 Whistle-blowing as a form of advocacy: guidelines for the practitioner and organization. *Social Work*, 00378046, 49(2):1–13.

Jones M 2004 Case report. Nurse prescribing: a case study in policy influence. *Journal of Nursing Management* 12:266–72.

Sullivan E J 2004 *Becoming influential: a guide for nurses*. Pearson/Prentice Hall, New Jersey.

Online resources

http://www.nurses.info/organizations_australia_newzealand.htm
http://www.uow.edu.au/arts/sts/bmartin/dissent/contacts

CHAPTER FOURTEEN

Multidisciplinary teams

Rhonda Griffiths & Patrick Crookes

LEARNING OBJECTIVES

Information in this chapter will assist the reader to:

▲ discuss the advantages of multidisciplinary teams as a model of providing healthcare;

▲ discuss the attributes that contribute to high levels of satisfaction and effectiveness among members of a multidisciplinary team;

▲ outline triggers that may contribute to conflict in a multidisciplinary team; and

▲ describe strategies for managing conflict in multidisciplinary teams.

KEY WORDS

Models of healthcare, organisational culture, communication, role, socialisation, conflict resolution

INTRODUCTION

The health reform agendas over the past decade have transformed the public, and to a lesser extent the private, health systems in Australia. One feature of these reforms has been an emphasis on establishing an effective continuum of care across care delivery systems and, to achieve that, a focus on multidisciplinary and interagency collaborations. The multidisciplinary team approach is well established in healthcare since it first appeared in the 1970s. The approach is promoted as the 'ideal' model for providing holistic care and enhancing outcomes (Jefferies & Chan 2004). Teams initially focused on providing community-based care at a 'one-stop-shop', where patients with chronic disorders could consult various health providers who would be familiar with the history of individuals and who would discuss progress and design ongoing care at formal case conferences (Madge & Khair 2000).

In recent years multidisciplinary teams have been established in acute care settings, and the literature reports establishment of teams in areas not previously associated with that approach. The use of multidisciplinary inpatient records (Baker 1996) and a multidisciplinary protocol for extubation (Chan et al 2001) have been reported, while multidisciplinary teams working in an acute medical admissions unit (Cameron et al 2000), discharge planning (Atwell 2004) and a neonatal intensive care unit (Brown et al 2003) have been evaluated.

We are constantly reminded of the benefits of working in teams, but in reality teams face many challenges, and working collaboratively can be difficult to achieve. According to Dion (2004) the key is collaboration. As a student of nursing, who is preparing to work in a contemporary healthcare system, it is imperative that you recognise the significance and responsibilities of being an active participant in the multidisciplinary team. To achieve this requires not only an awareness of the role of nurses, but also of others within the team.

Members of the team need to understand group dynamics and be cognisant of factors that impact upon the nature of teams and how they form and function (Crowell 2000). In some areas of healthcare, a multidisciplinary approach represents a significant departure from the traditional way the professions have practised; therefore, each member of the team must be committed to assisting the team to achieve its goals (Madge & Khair 2000, Jefferies & Chan 2004).

WHAT IS A MULTIDISCIPLINARY TEAM?

A multidisciplinary team is defined as '. . . a team of professionals including representatives of different disciplines who coordinate the contributions of each profession, which are not considered to overlap, in order to improve care' (O'Tool 1997). Gallagher (1995) draws an interesting distinction between 'groups' and 'teams' in that she asserts that while both are constituted of a number of individuals with some unifying relationship, the two can be differentiated by virtue of the members of a team being '. . . associated together in specific work or activity' (p 276). A team is characterised by common goals, interdependence, cooperation, coordination of activities, division of effort and shared language (Arthur et al 2003, Jefferies & Chan 2004).

The values that healthcare organisations (Lenkman & Gibbins 1994) and individuals (Davis & Thurecht 2001) must demonstrate for multidisciplinary care to be achieved have been described. Organisations must be patient-focused and service oriented, with attention to organisational, technical and professional issues. Staff who feel empowered to 'make a difference', who are also experts in systems thinking, feel involved, and who are dedicated to the achievement of the goals of the organisation, form the basis of effective multidisciplinary teams. Multidisciplinary approaches are more likely to be successful if efficiency and flexibility are valued, there are shared goals, good communications, minimal structure and an holistic view of the patient (Davis & Thurecht 2001).

This type of culture may not naturally evolve in healthcare organisations because of differing allegiances to the various professional groups (Firth-Cozens 2001). We will return to this later when we discuss factors impacting upon the effectiveness of multidisciplinary healthcare teams.

SO WHY DO MULTIDISCIPLINARY TEAMS EXIST IN HEALTHCARE?

If we extend from the earlier Miller-Keane definition (O'Tool 1997), we can say that the purpose of a multidisciplinary healthcare team is to involve professionals from various health-related disciplines, whose contributions do not overlap, in the planning and provision of ever-improving standards of healthcare. The provision of safe, effective care is a goal for health providers of all disciplines, and multidisciplinary teams have demonstrated improved outcomes for patients, optimal use of existing resources, and cost containment. The focus on multidisciplinary teams in recent service frameworks (New South Wales Health Department 2001, 2002) has patient outcome and organisational benefits in mind.

Healthcare needs to be a team effort because no one person or any single discipline can provide the care and services required by the range of clients wishing to access health services, particularly in Western societies (Liberman et al 2001). However, establishing a healthcare team poses particular challenges. Not only do team members have allegiances to their professional groups (Firth-Cozens 2001), but there is also a traditional hierarchy whereby some professions exert disproportionate influence (Gair & Hartery 2001) Teams are likely to be dysfunctional when members continue to work as individuals, with little understanding of the role of other disciplines and little interest in learning what they are (Crowell 2000, Jenkins et al 2001).

MEMBERSHIP OF MULTIDISCIPLINARY HEALTHCARE TEAMS

Research has demonstrated that members of a multidisciplinary team may not be well informed about the nature and scope of practice of their colleagues (McGee & Ashford 1996). An overview of the role of disciplines common to multidisciplinary health teams is presented here.

Nurses

The role of the modern-day nurse is multifaceted, encompassing the promotion of wellness, the provision of curative, rehabilitative and palliative care, and the facilitation of peaceful death—all within a framework of caring practice. Such care takes place in a range of settings, both institutional and community-based.

In the health team situation, nurses work autonomously and collaboratively, performing functions that are independent, interdependent and dependent upon the roles and functions of colleagues. Nurses may work collaboratively when administering prescribed treatments and then independently assess their effectiveness.

Nurses are responsible for much of the care provided in both hospital and community settings, an important aspect of which involves the role of communicator, often acting as a conduit between patients, relatives and staff from other disciplines within the team. Nurses have traditionally assumed the role of advocate for patients and their relatives, and frequently find themselves translating professional language (read 'jargon') into terms that have meaning for non-professionals.

The role of the nurse is challenging, intellectually demanding and diverse. Over the past 15 years, change in health services provision and models of care have required, and supported, increasing autonomy (and responsibility) for nurses who, in some practice settings, have assumed roles previously seen as the domain of the medical practitioner. Nursing careers are moving in new and exciting directions, as evidenced by the formal establishment of the role of 'nurse practitioner' in New South Wales in 1998.

Such a role makes nursing an interesting and rewarding profession to work within. However, it may also act as a source of irritation when colleagues fail to acknowledge or respond to nurses' input (Lenkman & Gibbins 1994). This is discussed further shortly, with regard to the power differentials that continue to exist within multidisciplinary healthcare teams.

All courses leading to authority to practice as a registered nurse (RN) in Australia are tertiary based, with a duration of between 3 and 4 years. You will also find enrolled nurses (ENs) working as part of the nursing team. Such clinicians have a more practical focus to their role than RNs. They are currently prepared within the Technical and Further Education (TAFE) system.

Medical practitioners

Medical practitioners are highly trained individuals (at many universities medicine is now a postgraduate course, with medical students requiring a first degree to enter medical school), with expertise that is in the main directed towards the diagnosis and treatment of disease or injury via the use of medication and/or surgery. Historically, medical practitioners have been central to health service design and delivery, largely as a consequence of their rights under the law to admit patients to hospital, to prescribe diagnostic tests, medications and other treatments, and to make referrals to other health practitioners.

Dieticians

Dieticians are a particular group of professionals within the wider field of nutrition who work in a number of environments and areas of speciality. Clinical dieticians work in acute care or ambulatory settings in both public and private practice, prescribing and advising individuals and groups on appropriate nutritional strategies for dietary management of disease and for health promotion generally. Dieticians also work in the food industry. Dieticians working in public health and health promotion positions undertake diverse roles relating to nutrition awareness, education and policy development at community and government levels. Preparation for the role is currently within the university sector.

Occupational therapists

Essentially, occupational therapists (OTs) focus their efforts on optimising the level of their clients' independence in undertaking everyday tasks, in both the private and public areas of their (clients') lives. For example, after often quite detailed functional assessment, they may prescribe and/or modify work-related equipment to allow an individual to continue in employment. Alternatively, they may be heavily involved in the rehabilitation process of stroke victims. Their work also involves protecting and maximising the function of joints affected by diseases such as arthritis, using splints and other supportive devices. OTs should not be confused with diversional therapists (DTs), whose job is to help clients to occupy their time—not necessarily to be more independent. Currently OTs undertake a 4-year undergraduate degree in preparation for the role.

Physiotherapists

Physiotherapists are currently university-prepared practitioners. They deal with the assessment, treatment and prevention of human movement problems. They work in a variety of settings such as hospitals, health centres and sports centres. Their client group ranges from the very young to the aged, and from the severely disabled to elite sportsmen and women. A popular misconception is that physiotherapists focus only on muscles and joints. In reality, their work is much wider than this, encompassing, for example, cardio-pulmonary functioning in relation to chronic respiratory disorders such as asthma and cystic fibrosis, and in cardiac rehabilitation. They can also often be seen in the postoperative phase of client recovery, aiding in the maintenance of clear airways and effective expectoration.

Social workers

In healthcare, social workers assist people to adjust to the changes which illness and hospitalisation can bring. They do so via the provision of psychosocial assessments, counselling, information, advocacy and referral for clients and their families. Their help can be needed in a variety of circumstances. For example, counselling could be offered following bereavement, the birth of a child, or perhaps to support the relatives of a person with a psychiatric disorder. The help may also be rather more practical; other activities include coordinating community support services, negotiating for hostel or nursing home placement, and linking people from Aboriginal and non-English speaking backgrounds to relevant support agencies. Preparation for this role is currently a 4-year undergraduate degree encompassing sociology, psychology, counselling skills, and the history, economics and politics of welfare.

Speech pathologists

Traditionally speech pathologists have been involved in dealing with clients with speech difficulties, such as stammering, stuttering or following various forms of brain trauma. In doing so, they have become focused on the functions of the mouth and throat. In more recent years the discipline has moved in other areas, such as the assessment and management of clients with swallowing disorders, including post-stroke and babies with ineffective swallowing reflexes. Currently speech pathologists undertake a 4-year undergraduate degree.

Chaplains

Chaplains may not be an obvious inclusion in a multidisciplinary health team; however, we need to recognise that clients and health professionals have spiritual needs as well as those of a physical, psychological, social and cultural nature. Clergy from a range of religions offer their services, not only in terms of 'religious' input, but also as sympathetic listeners. Hospital chaplains also offer great support to staff during times of personal and professional distress. Their importance to the team should not be overlooked.

Nurse practitioners

Nurse practitioners (NPs) are registered nurses who have postgraduate qualifications and extensive clinical experience, usually in an area of speciality practice, to assume an advanced practice role. The procedure to achieving nurse practitioner status varies slightly between countries, as does the focus of their work. In Australia, the nurse-registering authority in each state and territory determines the criteria a registered nurse must meet to register as an NP, and administers the register of registered nurses authorised to use the title of NP and function in that role. The majority of NPs in Australia are employed by public health facilities where they work in inpatient and outpatient settings.

The NP role evolved from unmet needs for health services, and in that environment the advanced practice role enables NPs to provide a service that is innovative, accessible and responsive to the health needs of specific populations. NPs are authorised to order diagnostic tests, prescribe drugs from a formulary specific for their specialisation, and refer clients to doctors and other service providers. Courses at masters' level are being offered by tertiary institutions in Australia to prepare registered nurses to work as NPs.

Practice nurses

Practice nurses are state-board registered and are enrolled nurses employed by general practitioners to provide care for patients in their surgery. The practice nurse role in the United Kingdom is well established, with nurses providing clinical care and specialty services, such as well-women's clinics, diabetes care clinics and asthma clinics, in the surgery.

The practice nurse is relatively new in Australia, and in this developmental stage the role varies between locations ranging from the performance of specific clinical tasks under the direction of the general practitioner to an extended role with high levels of autonomy. Nurses working in general practice are not required to undertake additional education in preparation for their role, although they have formed a professional association, the Australian Practice Nurses Association, which does have professional development of members as a principle function.

DYNAMICS OF MULTIDISCIPLINARY TEAMS

Not all people want to work in teams, even when the benefits are clear, and getting health professionals to work together is not straightforward (Arthur et al 2003).

Successful healthcare teams are usually guided by a clear strategy and defined roles and functions, have an organisational identity that is also recognised externally, and members of the team are aware of objectives and boundaries (Madge & Khair 2000, Arthur et al 2003).

Liberman et al (2001) make the point that smaller teams tend to be the most effective and productive, not least because such teams find it relatively easy to meet together not only to communicate but also to work through to an agreement of what their 'common purpose' should be. The opportunity for direct communication between team members has been identified as a critical factor in the success of teams. These authors suggests that teams of 4 to 12 members tend to be the most effective and productive, because larger teams have difficulty meeting to discuss team issues, including forming and reinforcing the shared vision (Liberman et al 2001). There is a connection between the quality of relationships between members and the success of the team. Managing multidisciplinary teams is a leadership challenge and at times the team experience does not fulfil the workplace expectations of members.

The key features of effective multidisciplinary healthcare teams have been described (Liberman et al 2001). These authors have established rehabilitation teams around the principles; however, the attributes can be adapted and applied to all multidisciplinary healthcare teams. They have found that teams will be most effective when members' roles are clearly defined with clear job descriptions and performance standards. Positive supervision of a team is necessary and competency-based training must be provided for all team members. They also emphasise the importance of providing visible and continuing administrative support appropriate for priorities of the team to enable the goals and outcomes to be realised. The skills and attitudes of team members also need to be considered, with team members selected for their personal skills and attitudes, such as communication, cultural competencies, enthusiasm and eagerness to learn.

In practice, few multidisciplinary healthcare teams meet the ideal (Firth-Cozens 2001). Multidisciplinary teams may begin with high levels of motivation and competence; however, in the absence of clear goals, organisational support, appropriate autonomy and resources, the team experience may not achieve expectations (Liberman et al 2001).

Developing a team culture and commitment is a challenging role for team leaders, and various approaches have been promoted to direct activities. An integrated team-building model is the Team Spirit Model (Crowell 2000), a five-phase model based on organisational development and group process theory. While each phase must be completed prior to moving on to the next, the model is described as a spiral evolving around a core of *Service*, rather than linear, to signify an evolving process. During the developmental process, the team has opportunities to relive earlier stages with members reflecting on times of harmony (consonances) and disharmony (dissonances). The five phases are:

1 *Initiating: getting to know each other*. Sharing and appreciating each other's viewpoint and orientation builds trust, and a sense of belonging is the beginning of team building.

2 *Visioning: sharing meaning and mission*. An effective team has a shared vision and mission. The first step towards that achievement is for the team to be open

about the assumptions they have of their own and other's work. The team can then move to the second stage, which is to be open and accepting of the work mission of individuals.

3 *Claiming: doing the work*. Teams are unlikely to be successful in this stage until a shared vision has been achieved.

4 *Celebrating: recognition, awards, rewards*. Busy teams may overlook this stage; however, sharing success stories and recognising achievement is an invigorating experience for all members of the team.

5 *Letting go: really communicating*. Effective communication is a difficult, but essential, part of team spirit. 'Seek first to understand, then to be understood' is a guiding principle that applies to effective communications between individuals and teams.

THE IMPACT OF TRADITION ON THE MULTI-DISCIPLINARY HEALTHCARE TEAM

Each member of a multidisciplinary healthcare team has expected roles and functions, which are influenced partly by members of the team, and partly by external factors. Health services have traditionally been organised around functional areas of professional expertise (e.g. nursing, medicine, nutrition) with a strong hierarchical structure.

Individuals bring with them expectations associated with their discipline, which coalesce with the established social roles and rules (written and unwritten) associated with healthcare facilities. As a result, multidisciplinary healthcare teams tend to develop along traditional hierarchical lines, partly because of the varying skill levels of members, but also reflecting organisational norms. The result is that relationships within multidisciplinary healthcare teams perpetuate the hierarchical approach to decision making (Carter et al 2003), and as such are dominated by those with legitimated (e.g. managers) or historical/authority-based powers (e.g. doctors) (Potter & Palmer 2003).

From the discussion presented so far, it would seem obvious that this situation is at odds with the concept of multidisciplinary teams, which implies seamless care, equal recognition of skills of members, and equal recognition of members' contribution.

HEALTHCARE CULTURE AND THE MULTI-DISCIPLINARY HEALTHCARE TEAM

One association that has attracted attention in the literature is the nurse–doctor relationship. This association is not generally discussed within the aegis of multidisciplinary teams, but is more commonly situated within the literature on power and how it is exercised over others (Warelow 1996, Speedy & Jackson 2004). However, medical dominance has been identified as a feature of healthcare systems (Gair & Hartery 2001); therefore, the origins of 'traditional' nurse–doctor interactions and the nature of their association is relevant to the discussion.

It has been argued that, regardless of the expected roles of team members, the more powerful team members direct the contribution of others (Adamson et al 1995, Braithwaite & Westbrook 2005). In that scenario the medical profession invariably dominates, and nurses are generally submissive. This situation is maintained through an effective socialisation (social and professional) based on gender and role differences (Warelow 1996, Gair & Hartery 2001), which are discussed elsewhere in this text, particularly in the chapter on gender issues for Australian nursing (see Ch 12). Meanwhile Speedy and Jackson (2004) present a range of suggestions for nurses and nursing to free itself from domination by (particularly) the medical profession, within an excellent discussion of oppressed group behaviour and its implications for nursing.

While medical dominance of multidisciplinary teams largely remains unchallenged (Gair & Hartery 2001), there are examples of teams lead successfully by nurses (Cameron et al 2000), which does provide some optimism that in future we may see equity among team members.

Senior managers in the organisation also need to recognise that, intentionally or unintentionally, they are instrumental in establishing the values and norms, which set the tone of the organisation (Braithwaite & Westbrook 2004). The culture is based on, and reflects, the policies, procedures and practices that are supported and reinforced at all levels. Individuals and groups then internalise the values and act out their scenes accordingly. Therefore, any organisation that claims to be committed to an integrated and multidisciplinary approach to healthcare needs to identify clear goals for its teams, as well as putting the communication and organisational structures discussed earlier into place. If this is not the case, then the subcultures based on departments, disciplines and charismatic individuals will continue to direct the team, the consequence of which will be that the advantages of the multidisciplinary approach will be lost to the organisation, team members and of course clients.

FACTORS IMPACTING UPON THE EFFECTIVENESS OF MULTIDISCIPLINARY HEALTHCARE TEAMS

A multidisciplinary team brings together individuals from diverse disciplinary and functional backgrounds. The experiences and skills that members bring to the team can be a significant asset when used to advantage for problem solving, decision making, conflict resolution and other activities that enable the team to achieve its goals (Liberman et al 2001). The outcomes will depend largely on how effectively the group of individuals is transformed into a team with common goals. To ensure these teams do function effectively, complex communication procedures must be established and maintained.

The literature on multidisciplinary teams indicates clearly that functional groups must have elements in common (Dion 2004). The most frequently identified attribute is the presence of effective communication; other factors include clear goals (including leadership) and conflict resolution strategies (Arthur et al 2003, Brown et al 2003, Atwell 2004, Jefferies & Chan 2004). Inherent in these attributes is the importance of a sense of common purpose for the team, demonstrated by a mission statement and agreed goals (Crowell 2000, Davis & Thurecht 2001, Brown et al 2003).

Effective communications

Organisations require elaborate channels of communication, both formal and informal, to ensure that everyone in the team shares a sense of common purpose, in this case the provision of high-quality healthcare. This may seem relatively straightforward;

however, in reality the various members of multidisciplinary healthcare teams may have very different views.

Potter and Palmer (2003) presented an interesting illustration of interactions and communications between members of a multidisciplinary team when they reported the outcome from a 360-degree assessment of a multidisciplinary team in a teaching hospital. Some members of the team expressed reservations about the process, and sought exemption from participating, citing lack of time as their reason. During the feedback sessions, individuals in the team were more likely to predict areas of strength identified by their colleagues, but less aware of characteristics colleagues consider to be weaknesses. When negative comments from colleagues were received, the effect of these was not countered by other positive comments. These authors concluded that the 360-degree assessment was a useful tool to identify characteristics of team members and appraise a multidisciplinary team, although the process for feedback and opportunities for professional development need to be considered prior to undertaking the assessment.

Other subsets of 'effective communication' and their importance to the functioning of multidisciplinary healthcare teams can be identified in the literature. It is important, for example, that team members have a clear idea of what colleagues in other disciplines do (Crowell 2000), and the professional language they use (Jenkins et al 2001), to avoid the problems of care being fragmented by the absence of a coordinated plan (Joy et al 2003). Communication between team members from different disciplines offers the opportunity to observe and acknowledge the unique contributions of the roles and expertise of colleagues, and this should then enable team members to work together to achieve the (preferably) clearly stated goals of the team (Jenkins et al 2001). This synergy is only achieved when all members of the team are willing to cooperate (Crowell 2000).

The importance of peers within teams supporting and valuing each other, rather than being critically destructive of each other, was demonstrated by Potter and Palmer (2003). They found that while feedback was generally interpreted as constructive to further development of the team, individuals focused on negative feedback despite the fact that the majority of comments were positive. Encouraging open and constructive discussions among team members encourages trust, leading eventually to everyone feeling that they can put forward ideas and suggestions for improvement. Brown et al (2003) reinforce the significance of peer support, and add the view that managers should reward innovation and encourage personal accountability. This could possibly be achieved through the use of a participative management style, in effect encouraging collaboration in decision making about care, as well as actually providing that care.

Members of multidisciplinary healthcare teams potentially benefit greatly from the sharing of expertise and insight, not least because decisions reached and action agreed tend to be well planned, informed by relevant experience, and owned by the parties concerned, thus enhancing the chances of effecting successful change (Brown et al 2003, Dion 2004).

Clear roles

In effective teams the formal role of each member is generally well established and understood, albeit tacitly at times. While people fulfil these roles (norms of behaviour), the team is likely to be functional. However, conflict can arise when a team member assumes a role that is different from that expected of his or her position in the team, or when the notion of 'equal recognition' is overlooked.

The roles of nurses (who are numerically dominant in health) and doctors (who are undisputedly the dominant power group in health) have been described and analysed within the context of multidisciplinary teams (Warelow 1996, West et al 2002, Braithwaite & Westbrook 2005). In the main, the assumed roles maintain the status quo, with the nursing literature tending to nominate the doctor as team leader. This situation could change, albeit slowly, as increasing numbers of midwives gain admitting rights to hospitals, and nurse practitioners take up their roles.

Braithwaite and Westbrook (2004) have described the 'shared governance' approach to leadership of a multidisciplinary team that is emerging as clinical directorates (CDs), which are replacing traditional structures in hospitals. Shared governance is a dynamic process, which requires team members at every level to play key roles in the decision making that affects the team and the people it serves. As it gains momentum, shared governance is encouraging changes in the structure and functioning of multidisciplinary healthcare teams.

Leadership

The style of leader influences significantly the performance and morale of a team (Kelly-Thomas 1998), although, as Barum (1998) notes, the best leaders may not always be the manager. While traditionally the leader does have responsibilities for the day-to-day activities of the team, contemporary leadership models focus on the need for a leader to have, and to be able to articulate, a vision of what is intended and expected of the team, and to create the 'social environment' in which this can happen. This shift in emphasis from manager as supervisor to one of visionary is, according to Brown et al (2003), reflective of changing professional and community expectations. Leaders with vision are vital in healthcare environments where the system is changing at such a rate that health professionals require an environment that enables them to interpret, create and grow with change.

In recent years, it has been increasingly recognised that nurses can, and indeed should, take a more active role in the management of health services, and that they should do so as nurses, not necessarily as nurses-turned-managers. To this end, leadership development among clinically based nurses is not now taken very seriously; hence, the significant investment by governments in both Australia and the United Kingdom using the Royal College of Nursing's (UK) Leadership Program. This program was developed by Gernalide Cunningham and is based on the work of Kouzes and Posner, who have produced an empirically based model of leadership behaviour(s). Over time, this will inevitably lead to nurses more commonly being seen as leaders of health services, rather than merely participants, which is how they are often viewed today (Buresh & Gordon 2003).

For a variety of reasons doctors are often cast in the role of leaders of healthcare teams. One reason for this is that when medical care is sought, the initial contact is usually with a medical practitioner (particularly general practitioners), and in those cases where onward referral is required, it is often to other doctors. Given that many people only seek to access health services when they are sick or injured, it is not unreasonable for doctors to be considered necessary and important. However, there are issues related to the conventions of this assumption of power, which nurses and those in professions allied to medicine (PAMs) may find problematic. It is also the case that medical practitioners may not always be the best people to take the lead in multidisciplinary healthcare, particularly when outcomes are not 'curative' (e.g. in rehabilitation and developmental disability services). It must, however, be acknowledged that doctors occupy a key role in the care of people requiring health services, not least because the public sees doctors in this light (convention again), but also because modern Western health services are orientated such that they are essentially 'sick services' (Crookes 1992).

This discussion of roles and leadership and their impact upon the effectiveness of the multidisciplinary team leads us to the final issue related to effective teams which we intend to cover—conflict.

The nature of conflict

The traditional healthcare facility has been described as 'a collection of professional fiefdoms', the uniting of which requires attention to organisational, professional and technical barriers (Lenkman & Gibbins 1994). Conflict between and within groups is common, and not necessarily destructive. Functional conflict actually enhances and benefits the organisation's performance. For example, two community health teams may agree that community-based aged care is a priority; however, there may be a conflict regarding how that can best be achieved. Each team applies a different model, both of which result in improved access to services for the elderly—there is not always only one 'answer'.

However, the potential for dysfunctional conflict to interfere with the harmony and outcomes of the group is considerable, and must be addressed effectively. Umiker (1998) identifies six common causes of conflict: unclear expectations; poor communication; lack of clear jurisdiction; incompatibilities or disagreements based on difference; conflict of interest; and operational or staffing changes. Team members may be unclear about their role in the team, policies and procedures, or how outcomes will be measured (West et al 2002).

As we have discussed previously, effective communication between members of teams, and between the team and organisation, is arguably the most significant contributing factor to the team's success. Jurisdiction refers to accountability, authority and responsibility within the team.

Conflict can arise when members do not comply with established expectations— either failure to assume expected roles, or failure to recognise positions with legitimate authority. Conflicts arising from incompatibilities or differences of opinion are complex situations, which can arise from factors as diverse as politics, ethics, values or gender. Conflicts of interest may arise between departments, shifts and individuals, and may be precipitated by operational or staff changes.

Ivancevich and Matteson (1993) describe four factors that predispose to the development of conflict within groups: work interdependence; differences in goals; differences in perceptions; and the increased demand for specialists. Work interdependence occurs when two or more groups must depend on one another to complete their tasks (e.g. conflict may arise between staff working day shift and those working night shift). Differences in goals may arise as groups become increasingly specialised, particularly when limited resources and reward structures within organisations are at stake. Differences in perceptions of reality and disagreements over what constitutes reality can lead to conflict. For example, in a hospital, administrative staff may view a problem differently from the clinical staff. Increased demand for specialisation can also cause conflict between specialists and generalists.

Conflict resolution

Resolution of conflict requires clear procedures for communication (discussed earlier in this chapter) and decision making, commitment to team building, and consideration of factors such as the number of team members and their personalities. The association between the size of the team and job satisfaction is significant in the discussion about health teams. Fargason and Haddock (1992) proposed that the optimum number of members in a team is five; more than that predisposes to conflict, which manifests as increased absenteeism and reduced job satisfaction. However, multidisciplinary teams working in clinical areas usually have more than five members, some significantly more. Team size is therefore potentially a major cause of conflict within multidisciplinary healthcare teams.

A variety of techniques to manage conflict have been identified. Umiker (1998) described strategies such as avoidance or denial of the problem, surrender, compromise and collaboration. Ivancevich and Matteson (1993) include expansion of resources and altering the structure of the organisation as potential strategies. Shell (2001) used the Thomas-Kilman conflict mode instrument in negotiating training. This model speaks of five styles of handling conflict: competing; collaborating; compromising; avoiding; and accommodating. The model described by Tuckman and Jensen (1993) for group formation (forming, storming, norming, performing and adjourning) continues to be used as a framework for conflict resolution. Groups engaged in this process agree on aims, structure, leadership (forming), and then go through a stage of discussion and debate, which may include conflict (storming) to achieve cooperation and collaboration, and to establish team norms. The group is then functional (performing). Depending on the purpose of the group, it may then adjourn.

A common theme in all techniques is the requirement for constructive negotiation via effective communication between the parties. This tends to be the most useful when the conflicts are relatively simple and of a low intensity, and when both parties are relatively equal in power (Eunson 2005). Problem solving and compromise by the parties is frequently required to resolve conflict. Fargason and Haddock (1992) are of the opinion that conflict develops in multidisciplinary teams when individuals approach a problem in a manner that detracts from the quality of decisions made by the team. Problem solving requires meetings between the groups to debate differences and negotiate agreement. Problem solving also requires conflicting groups to display a willingness to work together to incorporate concerns into a consensus decision. Compromise can be used effectively when the goals can be divided equitably, and therefore is most useful when the conflicting parties have relatively equal power and are strongly committed to mutually exclusive goals.

Group decision making is common in organisations, with committees, working parties or teams formed to review a situation and make recommendations. However, that approach does not guarantee quality decisions or consultation with stakeholders (Arthur et al 2003). The traditional, department-based, hierarchical decision-making model is not new to those who have worked in health.

While crucial and ultimately highly profitable decisions have been based on a feeling or hunch, organisations generally adopt a more scientific approach to decision making. A decision-making framework presented by Ivancevich and Matteson

(1993) describes five stages, which takes the team through the process of establishing objectives and identifying alternatives. The alternatives are evaluated, and a course of action is determined and implemented. Research methods frequently used to assist decision making and problem solving in nursing include the Delphi technique and the nominal group technique (Jamieson et al 1998). The Delphi technique is based on structured questionnaires, with responses validated by regular feedback to participants. The nominal group technique also uses structured questions, but differs from the Delphi technique in that the results are available immediately.

Failure to attend to the 'health' of the team and/or absent organisational commitment imposes considerable risks to outcomes. Lenkman and Gibbins (1994) refer to the 'human perspective', which seeks to achieve a balance between organisational and team needs. Failure to achieve that balance results in job dissatisfaction, which manifests as the inability to retain valued employees and attract new team members. These authors have identified six general areas, which if addressed effectively, will significantly enhance the success of multidisciplinary teams and reduce conflict. First, people in the organisation must be committed to change, and opportunities and strategies for effective change determined. Potential barriers to success must be identified, and a framework for implementation (e.g. case management, shared care) agreed upon. The organisation must provide educational opportunities for staff, and opportunities for team building. Managers within the organisation must also recognise that some health professionals find working in teams more difficult than others, and provide support to those individuals.

CONCLUSION

Multidisciplinary teams are formed to achieve objectives; the most obvious (but certainly not the only) reason is to achieve measurable outcomes that are beyond the capacity of individuals or groups from the same discipline. The complexity of new therapies, increasing specialisation (and emergence of new specialities), and the increasing diversity of services that consumers expect, points to the team approach as an efficient and effective model of care. The professions represented in a multidisciplinary team will reflect local needs, priorities and resources.

Health services have traditionally been structured around functional areas of professional expertise; therefore, multidisciplinary teams are unlikely to be successful until the organisation is committed to change, and group processes are in place to support communication within the group, and between the group and the organisation. The culture within the organisation will largely determine the productivity or teams and the degree of satisfaction experienced by the members.

There are potential barriers to the success of multidisciplinary teams, and these must be dealt with at both the group and organisational level. We have discussed precipitating factors for group conflict and, very briefly, presented strategies to prevent, or at least minimise, the effect of conflict on the team. Opportunities for professional development of members, which includes team-building activities, must be provided and supported by the organisation, and evidence of successful problem solving, negotiation and compromise rewarded.

REFLECTIVE QUESTIONS

1 What do you believe to be the strengths and weaknesses of multidisciplinary teams?

2 How do you believe multidisciplinary teams could benefit nurses and the nursing profession?

3 What do you think might be the impact of initiatives such as 'shared governance' and nurse practitioners on the structure and functions of healthcare in the future?

4 Consider ways in which nurses in general, and you personally, could positively impact on the efficacy of multidisciplinary teams.

RECOMMENDED READINGS

Braithwaite J, Westbrook M 2005 Rethinking clinical organisational structures: an attitude survey of doctors, nurses and allied health staff in clinical directorates. *Journal of Health Services Research Policy* 10(1):10–17.

Buresh B, Gordon S 2003 *From silence to voice: what nurses know and must communicate to the public*. Cornell University Press, New York (first published in 2000 by the Canadian Nurses' Association).

Crookes P A, Davies S eds 2004 *Essential skills for reading and applying research in nursing and health care: research into practice*. Bailliere Tindall, Sydney.

Eunson B 2005 *Conflict management: communicating in the 21st century*. John Wiley & Sons, Brisbane.

Speedy S, Jackson D 2004 Power, politics and gender: issues for nurse leaders and managers, pp 55–68. In J Daly, S Speedy & D Jackson (eds) *Nursing leadership*. Elsevier Australia, Sydney.

West M A, Borill C S, Dawson J F, Brodbeck F, Shapiro D A, Haward B 2002 *Leadership clarity and team innovation in health care*. Available from: http://www/modern.nhs.uk/115/23713/25415/Leadership%20Clarity.pdf.

CHAPTER FIFTEEN

Technology, skill development and empowerment in nursing

Alan Barnard

When you have read this chapter, you should be able to:

▲ highlight the importance of technology for nursing practice and skills development;

▲ describe characteristics associated with technology that are important for fostering interpretation and analysis;

▲ outline implications of technology for nursing care with specific reference to empowerment; and

▲ describe key principles and values important for fostering excellence in nursing practice.

KEY WORDS
Technology, empowerment, skill, nursing, technique, clinical practice, healthcare

NURSING AND TECHNOLOGY

This chapter considers the role and importance of technology for nursing practice, with specific reference to skill development and empowerment. Principles important to understanding technology are outlined and the implications of technology for nursing and healthcare are discussed, along with guiding principles and values important to appropriate integration of technology into clinical practice. It is argued that technology is a phenomenon that must be understood adequately to address the many challenges it presents for current and future nurses.

Technology influences the practice of nursing both from the perspective of what we do and how we understand ourselves as practitioners. Nurses talk about technology, develop skills and knowledge to apply technology, interpret technology, praise the qualities of the latest computer applications, worry about loss of human contact and work in a changing workplace. Technology is used, for example, to deliver accurate treatment, to hold water, to cover patients and to observe the internal workings of the human body. Technology advancement is linked to a range of experiences, including shorter length of admission to hospital, greater efficiency, changing skills and knowledge, alteration to employment patterns, specialisation and standardisation of care (Locsin 2001, Rinard 1996, Sandelowski 2000). These outcomes of technological development combined with the interests of dominant social groups, increasing legal liability and the maintenance of technology have produced healthcare practices that are focused sometimes on functionality, sameness, conformity, automation, safety, predictability and logical order.

Technology is significant to the history, contemporary practice and future of nursing. It has always been a part of nursing and in order to understand nursing as a discipline we need insight into its social, theoretical and practical implications. Prior to the twentieth century, technical knowledge and skills developed by trial and error, and were passed down through generations via a practical and oral culture. Nurses relied on experience and faith. Technical skills included magical and aesthetic components that equated with moral and psychic life. Nursing practice relied less on scientific knowledge and explanation than on a personal and intuitive understanding developed and refined through practice (Barnard & Cushing 2001).

The rapid growth of scientific and technological knowledge has bought about enormous changes for nursing and healthcare over the past hundred years, and technology has figured prominently as both a protagonist for development and an influential partner in our practice. Technology remains integral to healthcare and has significantly influenced our workplace, not only in terms of the artefacts and resources we use, but also how we do things, how we organise ourselves as nurses and what we value. In fact, Cooper (1993) went so far as to claim that the process of technological change has advanced to such an extent that many areas of nursing practice are defined by technology. For example, the haemodialysis machine is associated with renal nursing and the ventilator is associated with intensive care practice.

These claims are confirmed further by the increasing importance of competency-based education and practice, which is linked directly to the use of technology(ies). But regardless of whether the claim of Cooper is entirely accurate, it is acknowledged widely that nurses in all specialties are required to not only manipulate machinery and interpret the world around them, but accept increasingly varied and complex roles and responsibilities associated with the emergence of technology (Allan & Hall 1988, Barnard 1998, 2000b, Harding 1980, Reiser 1978, Reverby 1987, Sandelowski 1997a, Walters 1995b, Wichowski 1994).

INTERPRETING TECHNOLOGY

The word technology (tech.nol.ogy) refers to the practical arts, specific implements and the knowledge and/or activity of a group (i.e. technologist). The phenomenon is subject to varied and sometimes inadequate explanation in nursing and is influenced by social status, culture, gender and politics (Barnard 2002, Harding 1980, Pelletier 1989, Rinard 1996). Technology is more than the sum of things we use in healthcare. It has characteristic features that include the development of skills, knowledge and the incorporation of social arrangements and values (Feenberg 1999, Pacey 1999, Winner 1977).

One way to interpret and portray technology is as three concentric circles (see Fig 15.1). Concentric circles highlight the characteristics of technology, and together they therefore emphasise a character-ological interpretation of the phenomenon. The interpretation is useful because it focuses our attention on not only the 'things we use in nursing and society' (at the centre), but also their relations with other characteristics that are integral to meaning.

Artefacts and resources

The smallest and central concentric circle depicted in Figure 15.1, *artefacts and resources*, is technology at its most obvious and refers to the integration, use and application of the 'things' of nursing. Rinard (1996) noted that in modern nursing there have been three key periods of change that have been significantly influenced by technology. The first period was 1950–65 and was characterised by new medical techniques and a significant introduction of pharmaceuticals to care. The second

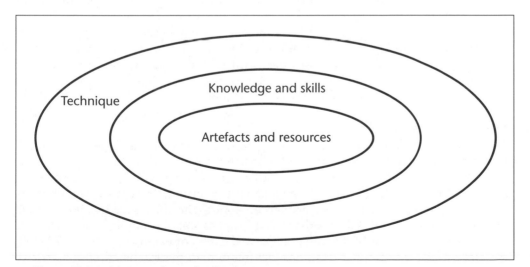

Figure 15.1 A character-ology of technology

period was 1965–80 and was associated with increasing machinery and specialisation. The third period was from 1980–90 and was associated with increasing technical control, streamlining and prediction of care. A more recent period has not been identified by Rinard, but it could be argued that current nursing is within a period of informational retrieval and computerisation.

We are required to use and maintain increasing amounts of technology in daily practice, and it is useful to clarify the various types of technology that are often found in our practice. We use simple, sophisticated, old, new, unique and commonplace technologies that continue to evolve in design and application. It can be observed that there are at least 12 different types of technologies that are artefacts and resources of nursing. These include *clothes* (e.g. shroud, pyjamas), utensils (e.g. bedpan, kidney dish), structures (e.g. hospital ward, isolation room), apparatus (e.g. Jordan frame, wheelchair, trolley), utilities (e.g. electricity, gas), tools (e.g. urinary catheter, syringe), resources (e.g. pharmaceuticals, sterile dressing), machines (e.g. intravenous infusion pump), automata (e.g. computer, refrigerator), tools of doing used to enact clinical practice (e.g. nurse's watch, stethoscope), objects of art or religion (e.g. nurse's uniform), and toys/games used for diversion (e.g. chessboard).

Although some machinery, apparatus, tools and so on are new, increasingly accurate and powered by utilities such as electricity, it is worth noting that there is also a lot of *simple* technology that remains fundamental to daily care (e.g. a shower chair, a stethoscope and a bedpan). Artefacts and resources assist to enact complex assessment and treatment, while supporting us to meet the daily needs of each patient. They can manifest as things to be held in our hand, pharmaceuticals we dispense to patients, volumetric pumps we use to assist enteral feeding, and occasionally as various noises and visual stimuli that we observe, such as colour screens and digital displays.

While an extended debate could be undertaken to examine what constitutes technology that is specific to nursing, for the purposes of this chapter nursing technologies include any technology that we use and/or claim to be fundamental to our daily practice. However, in stating this, it must be recognised that a lot of commonplace and simple nursing technology is not acknowledged as significant (e.g. bedpan) (Barnard 1996, 1998). That is, it lacks recognition as technology by nurses both in clinical practice and in nursing literature. The reasons for the lack of acknowledgment are speculative, but include our emphasis on the application of sophisticated technology, our inclination to uncritically embrace new technologies, a de-emphasis on technology associated with the 'dirty work' of nurses, limited investigation into the historical development of nursing technologies and a lack of substantive scholarship examining the phenomenon.

Knowledge and skills

The second or middle concentric circle in Figure 15.1 portrays technology as *knowledge and skills*. Artefacts and resources have associated meaning(s) and these are in many ways determined by the knowledge and skills associated with the way we use, repair, design and interpret them. Knowledge and skills contribute to the successful use of artefacts and resources, and are as much technology as the objects themselves. Without required knowledge and skills for the use and application of technology, it has limited ability to meet the needs of nursing practice and care. For example, without the skills necessary to use a computer, it is not much more than plastic, metal and electricity, and will not assist daily practice.

Nursing is a practical occupation and our knowledge is expressed most often through the way we perform our work. We focus often on what we do as practitioners and explain technology from perspectives that emphasise daily roles and responsibilities. For example, there has been debate concerning the increasing role of nurses in the use and maintenance of machinery and equipment. It has been argued that nurses have to fulfil the role of technician, and this is significantly distracting us from focusing on the experience of each patient (Brown 1992, Tisdale 1986).

Nurses rely on experience, continuing education, personal development and peer mentors to maintain and develop knowledge and skills. Failure to establish and develop knowledge and skills is inadequate for practice and unhelpful to patient care, colleagues and the requirements of the healthcare sector. Knowledge takes many forms and relates to not only competencies related to nursing intervention, but also organisational policies, current research and changing evidence. As such, technological competence is central to technology–nurse–patient relations and is vitally important for care (Locsin 1995, 1998, Walters 1995a).

Knowledge and skills alter regularly, and thus an active interest in maintaining and advancing competence is a sign of a caring and responsible practitioner who is accountable for the quality of their practice. Attitudes that reflect an offhand and neglectful interest in updating knowledge and skills are inadequate, and reflect a failure to value the importance of the person. It is a denial of the many possible contrary indicated outcomes that might arise from inadequate technology integration and is unprofessional.

One of the most important behaviours that patients look for from nurses is their competence in using technology. Competence reduces anxiety and fear, and increases the likelihood of successful care. Advances in organ transplantation, genetics, designer drugs, gene replacement therapy, microsurgery, virtual reality, e-health, tele-health, and so on, will place unprecedented demand upon each practitioner, and the updating of knowledge and maintenance of competence are now essential elements of quality care.

Technology introduces options for care and can make clinical practice more efficient, quicker and more accurate. Skills alter as a result of technology, and this fact should encourage personal reflection on the nature, relevance and impact of change on individual and collective practice (Barnard 1998, Hill & Summers 1994, McConnell 1990, Reiser 1993, Sandelowski 1996). For example, an automatic blood pressure monitor de-emphasises manual skills related to assessing a person's blood pressure, but demands new skills in terms of integrating electronic data. Many skills that were required previously for nursing are no longer necessary for contemporary practice and new skills emerge regularly to become part of daily care (e.g. boiling urine in a test tube has been replaced by the use of the coloured test strip). Thus we are engaged regularly in a process of reskilling. Skills and knowledge change continually in healthcare and alteration to skill requirements and skills mix is a reality.

The outcomes of technological change are associated with changing technical complexity that very often suit managerial perceptions and decisions related to how technology should be integrated into the organisation of work. Technological sophistication is always about achieving greater efficiency, and technological change is associated with better use of time and resources. For example, the intravenous infusion pump permits nurses to undertake 'other duties' while intravenous therapy is being delivered to their patient at a determined rate. However, the intravenous infusion pump de-emphasises skills associated with visually counting infusion drops per minute and manually determining flow rate. An infusion pump is often a good thing for time saving and control in daily practice, but at a higher level we are reminded that an often unasked question in relation to technology and nursing is 'what skills need to be retained' and 'what skills can fall away' as a result of specific technological change(s).

These are important questions and are fundamentally necessary for current and future professional development. For example, although we have been proactive in acquiring new skills and knowledge for care, we are required sometimes to revisit older, less common ways of undertaking certain assessment(s) and treatment(s), especially in less resourced clinical areas.

But amidst all this change some nurses interpret the process as skills loss, especially when skills associated with caring and human relationships are devalued or ignored. Rinard (1996) postulated that the evolution of technology and nursing is a story of deskilling in which nurses have purposefully gendered nursing knowledge in line with vocational and societal expectations of what is(was) valued culturally as 'feminine', at the cost of serious analysis of skills.

Deskilling and reskilling are issues worthy of analysis, but little has been undertaken within the profession. In fact over the past 60 years nursing has refused to adequately analyse technological change within the contexts of skills alteration, societal trends and the changing nature of nursing work (Barnard 2002, Barnard & Cushing 2001, Fairman 1998, Rinard 1996, Sandelowski 1999b, 2000). Although new clinical activities have been added to the professional role of the nurse, these additions are secondary to a more generalised growth in a sophistication of nursing work.

Most technological development in nursing has arisen as a result of technology replacing older procedures with newer more efficient and reliable technology, and among this there are significant changes occurring to nursing labour. We do things more quickly, more efficiently, with more automation and at times with more accuracy, yet there is a clear disjunction between the social–scientific nature of nursing work, analysis of changing healthcare, theoretical interpretation of nursing and the realities of nursing work. The effects of technological change on the skill of each nurse have been analysed poorly by nurses, but at a practical level changes are linked to increasing technical complexity and alteration to practitioner discretion/autonomy.

Technique

The influence of technology on practitioner discretion/autonomy is most obviously illustrated in the third and most inclusive concentric circle in Figure 15.1, which highlights the concept of *technique*. The third circle extends our character-ology of technology to include the way systems, policy, politics, economics, ethics, organisational management and human behaviour are organised for the benefit of technology. The way nursing practice is organised for, as well as by, artefacts and resources is as much technology as the first and second levels of meaning. Technique is not an entity or a specific thing. It is a way of thinking, and is an attitude that has an enormous influence upon us and society.

A transformation is occurring in which many aspects of our practice that were once instinctive, reflexive, natural and particular to individuals and cultures are being transformed into rational method and instruction. In craft-based technology the worker is able to express themselves with a sense of creativity, pride in personal agency and autonomy in determining action and expression. In automated technology environments these values and experiences have a tendency to be replaced by a sense of dependency on predetermined actions and protocols, a partial exercise of personal ability and preference, and knowledge that personal input can be replaced by another (Ferre 1995).

Technique is a mentality, a discourse and an objectification of naturally occurring phenomena such as reflective thinking, communication and human behaviour. An example to illustrate technique might be the difference between a caring moment with a patient motivated by nothing more than a nurse's compassion for another, versus the preplanned use of efficient communication strategies for the fulfilment of predefined goals and outcomes. The latter has all the hallmarks of technique because there is emphasis, for example, on a 'one best way' to efficiently undertake the activity. According to Lovekin (1991), technique is the consciousness that gives machines force, that sees everything else as machine-like or as needing to serve the machine-like, the ideal toward which technique strives.

Technique reduces the means of production, whether they be machines or nurses, to that which is most technological (i.e. efficient and rational), in order to create a unified activity. Examples of technique in the management of healthcare services are economic rationalism, protocols, risk assessment, action planning, communication strategies, benchmarking, patient dependency models, systems theory, clinical pathways management and standardised care plans.

Technique is a complex phenomenon that is constituted by three subtle yet important characteristics. First, technique adheres to a *primacy of reason* to govern practice. It is a way of thinking, acting and living by which people attempt to control the internal, passionate and emotional world of everyday life via protocols, rules, evidence and general observance to a logical order. Second, it requires a *desire for efficiency* in order to assist its goal and to justify its activity. The desire for efficiency is akin to the inventor or factory owner who seeks to streamline methods and actions in order to obtain certain outcomes. Efficiency seeks practical utility and a guaranteeing of results. There is a striving to reduce waste and the construction of systems that simplify and systematise previously uncontrolled or random activity. We nurses are free to engage in clinical practice, but this freedom is limited much like that of a clock. There is freedom for the hands to move around the clock face as long as nothing 'gets in the way'. The gears and springs move freely within the mechanism, yet there is a clear expectation that behaviour is determined and replicable.

It must be stressed that there is nothing wrong or dangerous per se with a desire for reasoned activity or efficiency. In fact, there is nothing new about rationality or efficiency as reasonable and worthwhile goals. They have both guided invention and activity throughout human history and, after all, who wants to be exposed to ineffective care?

However, the third characteristic of technique brings about new and different activity because it stresses primacy of efficiency in *every realm of human activity and thinking*. Technique has become so prevalent in society, organisations and nursing that people are increasingly incapable of thinking outside its boundaries in their search for meaning. A world has been created that has a tendency to override or minimise the importance of subjectivity and human experience. There is emphasis on control, efficiency and order within a climate of litigation (Harvey 1997, Neuhaus et al 2002, Sinclair & Gardner 2001, Wagner 1992, 1994).

Technique reduces thinking and human-centred activities such as nursing to measurable and predictable outcomes. It has potential to change previously natural worlds of human experience to *other*. That is, technique brings about qualitative transformation(s) in care. Under these conditions nursing practice risks becoming a robotic-like activity that does not require its practitioners to be particularly caring, compassionate or necessarily understanding of the experiences of people (except if it is preplanned as an efficient activity). As a result of technique, a new struggle has emerged for nursing and we need to find ways to authentically respond to individual need(s), cultural difference(s) and personal choice.

TECHNOLOGY, NURSING AND PROFESSIONAL EMPOWERMENT

Empowerment can be measured at an individual, organisational and community level, and is associated with the ability to make independent decisions in our professional and personal life (Masi et al 2003). It is characterised by a sense of control, goal attainment and competence. Professional empowerment is linked to ownership of knowledge, especially knowledge that is attributed to a specialist group or professional elite. Unfortunately, power for nursing has arisen less often in association with our ownership of knowledge because nursing knowledge is associated often with gendered skills of caring that are valued less by society and healthcare (Henderson 2003, Rinard 1996). Notwithstanding we continue to seek recognition as a discipline and seek to produce competent practitioners for clinical environments where technical performance is prized highly (Barnard 1998).

We have accepted new roles and responsibilities that have originated from the introduction of technology and the reassignment of duties from medicine (e.g. diagnostics and assessment). As a result, there is consistent reliance within healthcare sectors on our knowledge and skills, and this fact has been interpreted as a demonstration of our success (Abbey 1978, Boss 1989, Cooper 1993, McClure 1991, Orem 1991, Simpson 2001, Simpson & Brown 1990). Nurses are often the only healthcare workers who possess the knowledge and skills required to operate particular machinery and tools in clinical environments. Technology cultivates for nurses enhanced respect, importance and uniqueness and, when it is used well, these qualities transfer to nursing as a profession (Fairman 1992, Sandelowski 1997a, 1997b).

However, it must be noted that despite the growth of knowledge and skills in nursing and the expansion of roles and responsibilities, the legal, clinical and political responsibility for technology continues to remain predominantly in the control of medicine (Briggs 1991, Brown 1992, Harding 1980, Reiser 1978, Walters 1995b). It is noted by Patel (2002) that even though physicians make up less than 10% of the workforce in the United States, they determine why, how, when, and the frequency with which biomedical technologies will be used, not only in the diagnosis of patients, but also in their treatment. Nurses and other healthcare workers provide well-defined and restricted services that are reflective of the physician's orders. Doctors admit patients to hospital, order most diagnostic procedures and, by and large, have been the decision makers and gatekeepers who determine treatment(s) that patients will receive.

With this continuing reality and the growth of technique in many realms of human activity, empowerment is significantly challenged, both because we lack clear avenues for franchisement and our autonomy is limited by the continual search for efficient order to which we nurses must best fit.

From where then might empowerment arise?

It is commonplace for nurses to judge the effects of technology from perspectives that award it either a positive or negative influence upon clinical practice (known commonly as the optimism versus pessimism debate) (Harding 1980, Sandelowski 1997a). Debates between nurses have been reliant upon whether, for example, technology is believed to reduce menial work, increase comfort, emphasise a harmony between technology and caring, and expand knowledge (optimism) (Abbey 1978, Ray 1987, Simpson & Brown 1990), or undermine patient care, cause fragmentation of health services, foster a lack of caring behaviour and deskill nurses (pessimism) (Calne 1994, Cooper 1993, Henderson 1985, Wilson 1991).

Either perspective (optimism or pessimism) is to some degree an expression of specialist and class interests and value judgments concerning technological development. In reality, both perspectives contain elements of truth. For example, problems related to enhancing a person-focused approach in high-technology areas reflect individual nursing experience(s), assumptions about the role of technology in clinical practice and the organisation of healthcare, rather than any essential conflict between technology and nurses (Barnard 2000b, Sandelowski 1999a, Rudge 1999). In a critical essay on the semiotics of the nursing–technology relationship, Sandelowski (Sandelowski 1999a, 2000) highlighted the way(s) that language/depiction/sign within nursing has served to create a presumed problem between nurses and technology. It was argued that there is growing evidence that current representation of the relationship between nursing and technology does not support the development of nursing, nor does it foster strategies for the appropriate use of technology.

Future professional advancement will demand deeper insight into technology, and this growth will empower nurses because it will equip us to better engage in debate and decision making (Fairman 1998, Fairman & D'Antonio 1999, Locsin 1995, 1998, Walters 1995b). Expertise in clinical practice will be enhanced through our ability to: assess the suitability of technology for healthcare provision; advance person-focused care; sustain effective healthcare initiatives; and reinvigorate cultural, spiritual, moral and social values important to healthcare professions. Thus, it was encouraging to note that the United States Institute of Medicine 2001 report, entitled *Crossing the quality chasm: a new health system for the twenty first century*, emphasised the need for patient-centred and performance-based care that is devised around healing relationships and the provision of healthcare founded on needs and values.

The following guiding principles and values related to technology and nursing are important for empowerment in practice, will equip us to engage in healthcare debate(s) and should foster a desire to reinvigorate social and public service.

Good healthcare matters because people matter

Healthcare and nursing practice must be guided fundamentally by principles that promote, establish and protect human dignity. Protection of dignity is central to all that nurses engage in, and is central to the utilisation and integration of technology in care. Each person and their family have intrinsic value. Their uniqueness and importance must be acknowledged in even the most sophisticated technological environments. Episodes of objectification and loss of human dignity have been linked with technology (Locsin 2001, Rinard 1996, Sandelowski 2000), yet so often an emphasis on the experience and uniqueness of the person is possible with foresight and courage. For example, Barnard and Sandelowski (2001) highlight that even during high-intervention experiences such as emergency resuscitation, clinical measures can be adopted in order to place human experience and dignity central to care. Good healthcare matters because people matter, and this moral value must be continually emphasised, especially within healthcare systems dominated increasingly by technique.

Technology is political

The practice environment of a specialist unit, community facility or an institution impacts on the usefulness of technology. For example, a hospital unit that is designed poorly or resourced inappropriately is unsuitable to accommodate modern machinery and automata. Nurses can spend excess time and effort attending to technology and compensating for the inadequacies of poor resources. When resources do not foster adequately the use of technology, when they are defective or deficient, and support is not provided to foster skills and knowledge, the practice of nursing becomes difficult and stressful. Technology under these conditions becomes a burden to our practice. Funding, ward design, appropriate equipment and resources such as power and gas supply are crucial. When the practice environment is inadequate, the experience of integrating technology into care can be one of frustration, compromised health and safety for patients and staff, inadequate patient care and decreased efficiency and effectiveness (Carnevali 1985, Lumley 1987, McConnell 1990, Pillar et al 1990).

Central to nursing practice is the need to create order in busy, demanding and complex clinical environments because practice alters regularly, policies and procedures are governed by external authorities, and patients are very often acutely sick. Nurses can experience a lack of certainty in clinical practice (unpredictability, varying demands on time, numerous roles and responsibilities) due to the demands of busy and complex clinical practice environments, and we rely upon appropriate technology (Fitter 1987, Hepworth & Fitter 1981, Walters 1994). In the following quotation a nurse explains her experience by stating that:

> [T]echnology has so many advantages that if you are without it and you are busy, you do notice the difference. You tend to be more rushed and you don't have as much time to stop and chat . . . to your patients (Barnard 1998:169).

When technology operates effectively and is appropriately resourced, it provides substantial assistance to establishing safe and predictable patient care and coordinates various elements of clinical practice. Therefore, we need to be involved in determining the direction(s) of technological change and influencing decision making (Allan & Hall 1988, Fairman 1996, Harding 1980, Hiraki 1992, McConnell 1990, Reverby 1987, Sandelowski 1988,1997a, 2000, Walters 1995b). Decisions regarding access to particular technology, or the acquisition and use of machinery and equipment, are always political. Decisions related to technology will impact directly on the practice of each nurse, the organisation, and the patients for whom we care.

The right to quality care

Each person has a right to healthcare resources and quality nursing. Even though access to technology is sometimes restricted as a result of factors such as physical location and managed-care initiatives that place limitations on available resources (e.g. types of pharmaceuticals available in Australia), the dignity and worth of each life supports the view that we are responsible to effectively utilise and integrate appropriate technology.

Technology reveals only part of each person's experience and condition

Sophisticated electronic and computerised technology emphasises a reliance on quantitative evidence that is made available for us as digital display, computer screens and printouts. Although technology offers real and worthwhile indicators as to the physical condition of a patient, an excessive reliance on technology can result in a tendency to accept quantitative evidence in preference to, and in spite of, the thoughts, experiences and feelings of the person. The following quotation from a nurse explains a typical scenario:

> [Y]ou've got this patient who is really grey, sinking in the bed, more and more you've got to be saying, what's happening? Is it just because of his oxygen saturation levels? Is there nothing else going wrong? Should I be checking other things? We've got to have faith in ourselves to go and check through and say what is happening with this patient (Barnard 1998:189).

It is unprofessional to replace patient assessment skills with a singular reliance on information from machinery and equipment. Excessive focus on information from technology without adequate consideration of a patient's total physical and emotional condition can result in treatment and intervention that is inappropriate and insensitive.

Technology is not a neutral object and nurses are not its master

Technology assists to achieve care outcomes that are complex and significant. However, technology is *not* neutral to care and sometimes overrides consideration of cultural, spiritual, emotional, physical and psychological needs along its path to bring about efficient outcomes (Barnard 1997, Sandelowski 2000). That is, it always has seen and unseen impact(s) upon activity, goals and outcomes. It does *not* lead always to outcomes acceptable for patients and nurses, but it is *not* a demonic force leading always to uncaring nurses in inhospitable wards. The use of technology will lead to care which ranges across all possibilities from positive to negative, and expertise in practice needs to be based upon a holistic framework that informs awareness and planning. Holism emphasises the centrality of the person and by extension the values, choices and individual lives that come into our care and management. The increasing emphasis within healthcare upon, for example, standardisation, protocols and integrated systems to manage healthcare delivery have to be balanced against the values and expectations of the person for whom we profess to care.

Technology to a greater or lesser extent alters our capacity to determine and accomplish individual goals, professional approaches to care and principles of nursing practice. It influences what Walters (1994) described as the ability of each nurse to *focus* his or her energies on the person and their ability to *balance* technology with the qualities of caring. Technology can positively and negatively shape a nurse's available time to establish a nurse–patient relationship and be involved in personal care. For example, technology in a clinical environment that malfunctions often will not save time nor allow each nurse to concentrate on practice principles that place the person at the point of primary concern. Poorly integrated technology can make the daily practice of nursing more demanding, time consuming and distracted. In addition, when clinical practice is dominated by excessive policies, protocols and limited resources, as well as constant demands to check equipment, administer drugs and respond excessively to inappropriate alarms, technology becomes a compelling and sometimes annoying influence upon a nurse's time, physical commitment and intellectual attention.

The demands of technology can sometimes intervene independent of strategies used to ensure the smooth operation of a clinical area. Choice of technology affects people's lives and requires users to formulate different ways to do things. It is not surprising that when problems arise from technology it can affect available time to, for example, care for a person's body (e.g. mouth care, hygiene, bathing). We are required to manage the effective integration of technology sometimes at the cost of other roles and responsibilities. The demands of telephones, buzzers and equipment checking can draw us away from the other things we need to do. In the following quote from a nurse the experience is explained:

> All those alarms and monitors, they're geared to catch your attention aren't they? I mean, that's why they have alarms. So the first thing you do when you have alarms is go to it. It's like telephones at home. The first thing that you do when the telephone rings, it doesn't matter how busy you are, you drop everything to go and answer the phone, instead of saying, it's just a phone, leave it ring. I mean you put telephone answering machines on telephones these days, because the phone has to be answered doesn't it? We're geared these days to attend to noises and equipment before we attend to people (Barnard 1998:193).

You cannot use technology without also, to some extent, being influenced by its use. Our ability to display many of the caring behaviours associated commonly with nursing (i.e. a focus on personal experience, empathy, compassion) can be challenged, not often by a lack of compassion, empathy or desire to be involved more with people, but by the influence of technology on roles and responsibilities. The amount of technology in nursing practice does not alter our ability to feel compassion for the experience of others (Barnard 2000a, Brunt 1985). It is simply not true to claim that the majority of nurses do not desire to engage in patient-focused practice founded on compassion and concern. It is true, however, to claim that sometimes technology and the way(s) we use it gets in the way of our ability to express the desire.

CONCLUSION

When technology is used appropriately in clinical practice it improves the effectiveness and efficiency of nursing, empowers carers and establishes predictable measures, assessment and behaviour. It assists greatly in our ability to understand the physical condition of the patient, and saves time by making patient assessment increasingly accurate and potentially reliable. These advantages are extended further when we properly integrate technology into personalised care and our practice is one of expertise and competence. Technology–nurse relations are more than just being able to manage equipment. Nursing practice is changing as a result of technology. It influences the practice of nursing, both from the perspective of what we do and how we understand ourselves as practitioners. There is nothing secondary about the experience of technology. The act of including it in nursing practice introduces patterns of activity that by their very nature change healthcare (Barger-Lux & Heaney1986, Barnard 2002, DeVries & Barroso 2000, Ray 1987, Sandelowski 2000, Walters 1994, 1995b).

Nurses are responsible increasingly for technology in healthcare systems managed by administrative and bureaucratic structures. Knowledge and skills of nursing practice have altered over time, the ends to which we find ourselves working have changed and clinical practice continues to broaden despite a paucity of understanding and explanation as to ongoing changes to arise from technology. More research is needed into technology from the perspective of how we use artefacts and resources in practice, the relationship of clinical practice to theoretical models, ongoing skills and knowledge development, and a plethora of philosophical and sociological issues associated with power, gender, human experience and discipline development. Technology is a complex phenomenon that places before us an abundance of puzzles and questions. It is influential in every realm of social and professional life. Our profession continues to seek recognition, and technology has implications for nursing practice, education, theory and research.

Finally, the question remains, what do we do about technique in our clinical practice in order that we might begin to empower ourselves and the people for whom we care? The answer to the question lies probably in political action, individual activism, making informed choices in care and being willing to create a certain detachment from the imperatives that technique engenders. Being willing to question the use of technology when it does not meet the needs of people and quality care is paramount, but we should not underestimate the challenge that is before us.

Technique is integrated within the sociocultural context of society and nursing, and person-focused practice(s) is a freedom to be won. Being determined by specific technology(ies) is not the issue. In fact the idea is nonsense because the act of freedom lies in victory over necessity, rather than over individual machines and automata. That is, empowerment is most likely to arise through individual and collective acts of resistance to the use of every possible means available in care and the technological order that is increasingly part of us. Healthcare practice that is not wholly determined by technique is a prize to be won in the first instance by our awakening to what is before each of us. Our duty is to occupy ourselves with the dangers, errors, difficulties and temptations of technology.

REFLECTIVE QUESTIONS

1 What does this chapter tell us about the relations between nursing, technology and empowerment?

2 What important issues need to be addressed in order to further our skills in the appropriate use of technology in clinical practice?

3 Based on this chapter, what future research and practice development could be initiated in a clinical practice environment that you have experienced?

RECOMMENDED READINGS

Barnard A 2002 Philosophy of technology and nursing. *Nursing Philosophy* 3:15–26.

Barnard A, Sandelowski M 2001 Technology and humane nursing care: (ir)reconcilable or invented difference? *Journal of Advanced Nursing* 34:367–75.

DeVries R G, Barroso R 2000 *Midwives among the machines: recreating midwifery in the late 20th century*. Accessed 14 September 2000. Available from: http://www.stolaf.edu/people/devries/docs/midwifery.html.

Locsin R 2001 *Advancing technology, nursing and caring*. Auburn House, Westport.

Sinclair M, Gardner J 2001 Midwives' perceptions of the use of technology in assisting childbirth in Northern Ireland. *Journal of Advanced Nursing* 36(2): 229–36.

CHAPTER SIXTEEN

Dealing with distance: rural and remote area nursing

Desley Hegney

LEARNING OBJECTIVES

On completion of this chapter, the reader will be able to:

▲ demonstrate an understanding of the impact of rural life on the health of rural Australians;

▲ explain how the Australian rural and remote environment impacts upon the scope of practice of the nurse;

▲ demonstrate an understanding of the differences between rural, remote area and metropolitan nursing;

▲ describe the role and function of the rural and remote area nurse in Australia; and

▲ explain the issues currently impacting upon the practice role of the rural and remote area nurse.

KEY WORDS
Rural, remote nursing, diversity, health status, service delivery, recruitment and retention, professional development

RURAL AND REMOTE NURSING

This chapter provides an overview of the nature and the different health status of rural and remote communities. In this chapter, the words 'regional', 'rural' and 'remote' refer to the 34% of Australians who live outside a major city (population equal to or greater than 250,000). There is no 'one' rural or remote community; rather, each community in Australia has a different economic base and different demographics that impact upon the health and health needs of rural and remote residents. The Australian myth that rural areas are healthy places to live and that the lifestyle of rural residents is superior to that of those living in provincial and metropolitan cities will be dispelled.

A description of the role of both rural and remote area nurses will be provided, as well as an examination of the similarities and differences in their scope of practice. It will be demonstrated that the role of the rural and remote area nurse is different from that of the nurse employed in health facilities in major cities, and that the core difference is the generalist advanced practice role. This generalist role has resulted in the devaluing of the role of these nurses by other nurses working in more specialised fields.

Identified issues which impact on the scope of practice of rural and remote area nurses will be discussed—issues such as inadequate preparation for the role, lack of access to education and training, personal and professional isolation, and the lack of anonymity associated with working in small rural and remote towns. While some aspects of the role are highly valued by these nurses (e.g. the higher level of professional autonomy), the isolation and lack of preparation for the role often results in low retention rates, especially in the more remote communities (Dowd & Johnson 1995).

It will be argued that it is the rural and remote environment itself that impacts upon the health status of rural communities, and therefore determines the scope of rural and remote area nursing practice. Characteristics of this environment are low population densities, ethnic origin (particularly indigenous populations), isolation from other healthcare providers, the diversity of economic base and activities, and distances between settlements.

RURAL COMMUNITIES

Rural Australia is seen by most Australians as 'the bush'. When visualising 'the bush', most Australians have images of wide-open spaces, clean air, a healthy lifestyle and primary production (agriculture, mining, forestry, fishing). They do not have images of poverty and of indigenous populations with Third World health status. Despite this reality, the myths of 'mateship', 'hardiness', and people surviving through hard times caused by environmental factors (such as drought and flood) and/or economic factors (such as the value of the Australian dollar) still dominate the descriptions of rural Australia. To understand rural life today, however, requires the inclusion of images such as poverty, economic problems and underserviced healthcare needs.

The dominant image of rural Australia is one of being reliant on agriculture. Yet the 768 million hectares, which is the land area of Australia, have a great diversity of resources, opportunities and alternatives for future development (Lovett 1993). The key consideration in modern rural Australia is diversity. That is, no two rural areas are alike and some areas are more advantaged than others. For example, settlements that are in close proximity to capital cities, those on the coastal fringe, those with tourist potential, and the regional centres, are more likely to sustain growth and survive. In contrast, the more remote areas face a more tenuous and difficult future (Lovett 1993).

RURAL POPULATIONS

In 2001, two-thirds (66%) of Australia's population lived in a major city (classified as having a population equal to or more than 250,000). Of the remaining one-third of the population, 21% resided in settlements of 48,000 to 249,999 (known as inner regional areas), 10% resided in settlements of 18,000 to 47,999 (known as outer regional areas), 2% resided in settlements of 5000 to 17,999 (known as remote areas) and 1% resided in settlements of 1000 to 4999 (known as very remote areas) (Australian Institute of Health and Welfare 2004b, 2004c). These settlements do not have an homogenous economic base. Rather, their economic base ranges from mining, indigenous settlements, coastal resorts, retirement communities, regional service centres, and towns which could be considered to be commuter suburbs (as they are located on the periphery of a major city), to those dependent on agriculture, forestry and fishing (Fragar et al 1997).

The composition of the population residing in rural areas of Australia has changed enormously over time. For example, since 1976, there has been a 60% decline in the number of farmers in their 20s. Instead of young people, those entering farming were more likely to choose farming as a mid-career option and therefore be aged 40 years or older. Additionally, younger people's disinterest in farming has meant that many farmers stay longer into their later years, as their children are not interested in continuing the family tradition of farming. All of these changes have meant that the median age of a farmer has increased from 44 in 1981 to 50 in 2001 (Land and Water Australia 2004).

Farms have been subject to severe cost/price pressures, resulting in many farmers being asset rich and income poor (Rolley & Humphreys 1993). In the early twenty-first century, farm incomes have become diverse, with on-farm income comprising only a small proportion of earnings. The economic pressure on farmers has meant that farms have become larger. Thus, as smaller farms are merged to make larger economic units, the farming population has declined (Land and Water Australia 2004). Additionally, many family-owned farms have been replaced by corporate farming. In the late twentieth century the rural landscape had changed considerably with only one in ten people in the non-metropolitan workforce employed in agriculture, and with many people living in retirement in rural coastal areas (Australian Institute of Health and Welfare 2004c).

Rural and remote Australians have some characteristics that are quite different from Australians living in major cities. For example, they:

▲ have larger families;

- ▲ are less likely to be aged between 15 and 34 years;

- ▲ are less likely to be one-parent families;

- ▲ are more likely to live in a house (rather than an apartment) and less likely to pay rent;

- ▲ are more likely to own a car;

- ▲ are more likely to have both partners of the marriage in employment; and

- ▲ are more likely to be employers rather than employees (Australian Institute of Health and Welfare 2004c).

It must be remembered that rural Australia is composed of much more activity than agricultural pursuits and that the income generated by rural women is a vital part of the rural landscape. In a recent report on *Women in business in rural and remote Australia*, it was found that the income derived by regional businesswomen around Australia was diverse and generated income in the order of $1.2 billion per annum (Houghton & Strong 2004). The authors noted that regional women ran businesses which ranged from 'bed and breakfasts and traditional "country craft" business to business in professional and health services, education, manufacturing, and personal and business services' (Houghton & Strong 2004:2). In some cases the income provided much-needed off-farm income, while in other cases, the women lived in town and had no link with agriculture (Houghton & Strong 2004).

While much is made about the isolation of rural communities (and isolation from services will be the focus later in this chapter), some argue that communities are far less isolated than they were in the past. Epps and Sorensen (1993) stated that in the 1970s a typical rural life was one where incomes were largely dependent on seasonal conditions and fluctuations of commodity prices, housing was cheap and functional, and food prices were high. In addition, less emphasis was placed on educational attainment than today, services were fewer and of poorer quality than those of larger cities because of low population density and insufficient demand to make delivery of services worthwhile, and many rural communities experienced outmigration of the young and energetic. People were concerned about the weather, isolation and road conditions, had a strong work ethic and viewed impersonal city life with suspicion (Bessant 1980).

It is argued that rural Australia has been transformed since the 1970s in that technology has reduced the sense of isolation, deregulation of transport has facilitated overnight parcel deliveries to many rural areas, people can travel further by road to obtain goods and services, and larger regional centres often have cultural visits by national and international artists (Epps & Sorensen 1993, Rolley & Humphreys 1993).

Recognising that the face of rural Australia is constantly changing, and that there is no one standard rural town or area, it is time now to examine the myth that the 'bush' is a healthy place to live.

RURAL AUSTRALIA: A HEALTHY PLACE TO LIVE?

The myth of rural Australia as a healthy place to live seems to have dated from the nineteenth century and it appears that, in comparison to industrialised and urbanised Europe, it may have been so (Walmsley & Sorensen 1988). Rural people have been reported to have a more self-reliant attitude to health (Lovett 1993). They are renowned for their independence, resourcefulness, capacity for hard work, stoicism in the face of adversity, generosity and community-mindedness (Rolley & Humphreys 1993).

Two major reports have been published by the Australian Institute of Health and Welfare (Strong et al 1998, Australian Institute of Health and Welfare 2004c) on the health of regional, rural and remote people in Australia. The findings of these reports indicate that rural and remote Australians have considerable differences in morbidity and mortality rates to those Australians living in major cities. These data do indicate that regional, rural and remote Australia is not a healthy place to live. For example:

▲ death rates are about 1.1 times higher in inner and outer metropolitan regional and remote areas than in major cities, but 1.5 times higher in very remote areas (Australian Institute of Health and Welfare 2004c);

▲ the death rate for indigenous Australians is three times higher than for non-indigenous Australians (Australian Institute of Health and Welfare 2004c);

▲ the life expectancy of rural populations is less than that of people living in major cities (Strong et al 1998); and

▲ rural populations have higher hospitalisation rates, especially for falls and burns (Strong et al 1998) and lower life expectancy (Humphreys 1999).

It is not possible in a chapter of this size to cover the findings of these two reports—I will leave it to the reader interested in rural health to do so. However, some important points need to be made about what impacts upon the health status of rural people in Australia.

If one was to take a whole-of-health view, as does the national rural health policy *Healthy Horizons*, then one would need to examine various issues, such as the differences in access to education (primary, secondary and tertiary), the physical environment within rural areas and its impact on health, the socioeconomics of rural areas, the impact of distances between towns, and the supply of goods and services (such as fresh fruit and vegetables) (Australian Government 2004a). One would also need to consider the access of rural Australians to healthcare services. Some of these factors will now be considered.

Socioeconomics

A number of studies have found links between low socioeconomic status and the health of the individual in rural areas (Fragar et al 1997, Strong et al 1998). Poverty is now higher in rural districts than in major cities and is a significant variable in terms of rural health. This poverty is compounded by high unemployment rates in rural and remote areas, a higher proportion of unskilled labour in the workforce and, with the exception of some remote mining communities, a lower family income (Fragar et al 1997). The socioeconomic indexes for areas (SEIFA) applied to the 1991 census data indicates that socioeconomic disadvantage increases as population density declines (Strong et al 1998). Thus the more 'remote' the population, the greater is the socioeconomic disadvantage.

Problems posed by distance

Rural Australia is characterised by low population densities and varying distances between towns (Strong et al 1998). These low population densities are of 'critical importance in understanding problems of service provision' (Humphreys & Rolley 1991:23). Rural people 'in need' are more dispersed and isolated in their distribution than city residents in major cities, and this makes the provision of even basic services extremely expensive (Rolley & Humphreys 1993).

It is well documented that accessibility is the main issue for rural residents (Australian Institute of Health and Welfare 2004b, Humphreys & Rolley 1991, Macklin 1991). This lack of accessibility is caused by remoteness. Remoteness has been defined as:

> . . . access to a range of services, some of which are available in smaller and others in larger centres: the remoteness of a location can thus be measured in terms of how far one has to travel to centres of various sizes (Department of Health and Aged Care and Geographical Information Systems Classification of Australia 2001, cited in Australian Institute of Health and Welfare 2004b:2).

Populations in Australia (and thus the health status of these populations) are now reported on according to one of three 'remoteness classifications'. However, all of these classifications have limitations, and the readers of this chapter are referred to the discussion about these strengths and weakness as outlined in *Rural, regional and remote health: a guide to remoteness classifications* (Australian Institute of Health and Welfare 2004b).

Accepting that rural and remote Australians are affected by remoteness, and despite Macklin's (1991) statement that 'universal coverage and equity of access to the healthcare system are two important principles which are widely accepted' (p 5), in rural and remote areas of Australia the reality is that the majority of residents do not have access to the range of services available in major cities. The barriers of access to health services by the rural and remote population have been identified as: lack of healthcare professionals; cost and limited access to specific services; and lack of culturally acceptable services.

Lack of healthcare professionals

There is wide agreement that rural and remote Australian communities are underserved by appropriately trained health professionals. Additionally, there is evidence that urban-background medical practitioners are less likely to remain in rural practice for more than 3–5 years. This contrasts with medical practitioners with a rural background, who are more likely to choose a rural career and remain in practice for longer (Hays et al 1997). Further, in many of the more remote areas of Australia, communities are unable to attract a medical practitioner and are dependent upon rural and remote area nurses to provide their healthcare (Macklin 1992). The shortage of rural registered nurses is also now impacting on healthcare delivery in rural and remote areas (Australian Institute of Health and Welfare 2004c).

The problem of recruitment and retention of medical practitioners to rural areas has been the subject of several discussion papers (e.g. *The future of general practice*, Macklin 1992). Schemes focusing primarily on medical practitioner recruitment and retention such as the Rural Incentive Program (Hays et al 1997), the Rural Clinical Schools (Australian Government 2004b) and the university departments of rural health (Humphreys et al 2000) have been introduced to address this problem.

The same level of attention has not, to date, been given to the issues of the recruitment and retention of other health professionals such as nurses and allied health, mainly because medical practitioners are seen as 'employees' of the Australian

Government (through Medicare reimbursement), whereas nurses and allied health professionals are normally employees of state or territory governments (Hegney 1996). However, as the shortage of nurses has increased, both the state/territory governments and the Australian Government have begun to offer incentive programs for nurses. For example, the Australian Government now offers the aged care nursing scholarship scheme, as well as the rural and remote nurse scholarship program, which provides support for undergraduate, reentry, upskilling, postgraduate and conference scholarships (Australian Government 2004c). Examples of state and territory government scholarships include:

▲ the NSW Nursing and Midwifery Scholarships (New South Wales Health 2004);

▲ the Victorian government's postgraduate scholarships (State Government of Victoria 2004);

▲ the Queensland Health Rural Scholarship Scheme (Queensland Health 2004); and

▲ the studies assistance grants scheme of the Northern Territory (Northern Territory Government 2004).

Since 1991, when the first national rural health conference was held in Toowoomba, Queensland, there has been a plethora of rural health organisations. For example, the National Rural Health Alliance (NRHA), which is an organisation comprised of key professional and consumer rural organisations, is now responsible for most of the rural health policy. Professional organisations, such as the Rural Doctors' Association of Australia (RDAA), the Association for Australian Rural Nurses Inc (AARN), the Services for Australian Rural and Remote Allied Health (SARRAH), the Council of Remote Area Nurses of Australia (CRANA), the Isolated Children's Parents Association (ICPA), the Country Women's Association of Australia (CWA), are all member bodies of the NRHA. Despite the work of these organisations, in 2004 there is still a shortage of Australian-born medical practitioners, nurses and allied health professionals in rural and remote Australia. This lack of a 'stable, efficient and well-educated workforce' directly impacts upon the viability of rural health services (Kenny & Duckett 2003).

Cost and limited access to specific services

Strong et al (1998) in their examination of the health resources available to rural and remote residents noted that:

▲ nurses provide a higher proportion of healthcare in rural and remote Australia than in metropolitan Australia;

▲ nursing home beds are less likely to be available as remoteness increases;

▲ Medicare data indicate that people living in rural and remote zones use less services than those living in major cities; and

▲ the number of doctors (including medical specialists) and pharmacists declines as an area becomes more remote.

People in rural areas therefore, while experiencing increasing levels of poverty, have to face increased costs of travel and accommodation should they require anything other than basic primary care services. While schemes such as the Isolated Patients' Travel

Assistance Scheme have been available for some time, patients usually have to pay the costs up-front and seek reimbursement later. This can be problematic if the rural person was unaware of their entitlement or wishes to claim after they have sought treatment (McGrath et al 1999). The financial and personal cost of travel for treatment in a major centre does mean that some rural people will either choose more radical initial surgery options (e.g. women will choose to have a mastectomy for breast cancer rather than radiotherapy and chemotherapy) or they will delay treatment until it can no longer be avoided (Hegney et al 2005a, Humphreys & Rolley 1993, McGrath et al 1999).

Lack of culturally acceptable services

This has been one of the reasons for the 'Fourth World' health status of the Aboriginal and Torres Strait Islander people (Peach et al 1998, Strong et al 1998).

The economic activity of the area

Lawrence (1987) stated that there are high levels of stress-related illnesses such as hypertension and psychiatric disorders among farming families due to the close connection of business and personal life on the farm. In addition, suicides among the male rural and remote populations are higher than those in metropolitan areas (Fragar et al 1997).

These earlier studies' findings have been confirmed with data from the Australian Institute of Health and Welfare. For example, death rates from coronary heart disease are higher in rural and remote areas than in major cities, with the male death rate twice that of the female death rate (Strong et al 1998). Similarly, the rates for hospital separations for both male and females for coronary heart disease are higher than for people living in major cities. A similar pattern is found in male suicide rates, with males living in rural and remote areas more likely to commit suicide than males in major cities. In contrast, female suicide rates are higher in major cities than in rural and remote areas (Strong et al 1998).

Additionally, rural and remote Australians exhibit a greater incidence of unhealthy behaviors such as:

▲ rural women are more likely to be overweight in comparison to women in major cities;

▲ rural men have significantly higher alcohol consumption than men residing in major cities;

▲ rural women have higher self-reported high blood pressure than women living in major cities; and

▲ both men and women living in remote areas represent the highest proportion of people who smoke tobacco (Fragar et al 1997, Lawrence & Williams 1990, Strong et al 1998).

However, with regard to breast cancer screening and pap smear tests, there is little difference in the participation rates between women from different geographical locations (Strong et al 1998).

There is evidence, however, that rural living has its positive advantages. Sorensen and Epps (1993) suggest that there are lower levels of crime in rural areas. In addition, housing costs are lower than in major cities and rural residents, in the main, have the advantages of a pollution-free environment (Walmsley 1993).

It is quite clear that the health status of rural and remote area people is lower than that of urban dwellers; it is also apparent that rural people have access to a reduced range of health and community services. Rural and remote area nurses, therefore, provide essential healthcare facilities to these communities, sometimes being the sole provider. Before proceeding to a discussion on the health services provided by these nurses, let us first define what is meant by the terms 'rural' and 'remote area' nursing.

RURAL AND REMOTE AREA NURSING

A remote area nurse is:

> . . . a registered nurse whose day-to-day practice encompasses all or most aspects of primary healthcare. This practice most often occurs in an isolated or geographically remote location. The nurse is responsible, either solely or as a member of a small team, for the continuous, coordinated and comprehensive healthcare in that location (CRANA 1993, cited in Dowd & Johnson 1995:36).

In contrast, 'rural nursing' has no one agreed definition. The most cited definition defines rural nursing as the practice of nurses in the rural environment and where no medical practitioners are employed full time in a hospital, but are 'located within the town' (Hegney 1997a). This definition has its limitations, as it defines rural nursing 'by default'. That is, it does not define rural nursing by what rural nurses do; rather, it states that rural nursing practice is defined by the absence of other health professionals. However, the definition does recognise that it is the rural environment that determines the context of rural nursing practice and, therefore, the advanced generalist practice nature of the rural nurse's role.

Both definitions highlight the similarities and differences between rural and remote area nursing. Remote area nurses are isolated from medical and allied health support staff, and therefore their practice is more autonomous than that of the rural nurse, who has medical and allied health staff located within the town. For remote area nurses, medical support is usually provided by a medical practitioner located in a distant location (e.g. the Royal Flying Doctor Service). Remote area nurses are often the only health professional providing healthcare to the community—with or without the support of indigenous health workers. In contrast, rural nurses are more likely to work in an interprofessional team, with at least one medical practitioner practising in the town and experiencing varying levels of support from allied health professionals, depending on the size of the town and its surrounding area.

Another difference between rural and remote area nurses is the model of healthcare delivery on which their practice is based. Remote area nurses provide, on the whole, a primary healthcare service, whereas rural nurses predominantly work from a medical model health service (Cramer 1994, Hegney 1996, Wakerman & Field 1998). The similarities and differences of the practice of rural and remote area nurses are also reflected in their workforce profile.

Demographic characteristics of the rural and remote area nursing workforce

In 2001, while the number of registered nurses and enrolled nurses working in rural and remote areas aligned with the percentage of the Australian population residing in these areas (approximately 66%), there were more enrolled nurses than registered nurses employed in rural and remote areas (Australian Institute of Health and Welfare 2003). For example, approximately 55% of enrolled nurses were employed in major cities in contrast to approximately 69% of registered nurses.

With regard to hours worked, nurses employed in very remote locations worked 33.8 hours per week compared to the 30.9 hours per week worked by nurses employed in a major city (Australian Institute of Health and Welfare 2003). The longer hours worked by remote area nurses reflects their working environment, where they are likely to be the only nurse employed in the health service and on-call 24 hours a day, 7 days a week.

The scope of practice of the rural and remote area nurse

Nursing roles in rural and remote Australia are different not only from the role of nurses employed in major cities, but also from each other. The role differences are caused by many factors including:

▲ geographical location (e.g. a nurse working closer to a regional or major city will usually have easier access to medical and allied health services and be more likely to work in an interprofessional team);

▲ the population density of the area (as the population increases the more cost-effective are generalist and specialist medical and allied health services; this means that either on-site or visiting services are available);

▲ the type of employing institution (e.g. community compared with hospital facility);

▲ the type of community, its economic base and health needs (e.g. remote area nurses working in indigenous communities have a different role from remote area nurses working in mining communities); and

▲ the number and type of services available within the community, which also impact on health (e.g. generalist and specialist healthcare services, access to transport, educational facilities, levels of public sanitation).

It is the context of practice, it has been argued, that determines the role and function of the nurse (Hegney 1996). The increased level of responsibility and autonomy within the practice role accepted by rural and remote area nurses is described as high compared with nurses employed in major cities (Dowd & Johnson 1995). The level of responsibility has been linked to the high job satisfaction level of rural and remote area nurses (Cramer 1994, Hegney et al 1997).

Research in Australia on the role and function of rural and remote area nurses has revealed that the majority of the community believe these nurses are competent in a vast array of nursing skills, acquired by education and experience, and possess skills that are highly valued by the community in which they work (Burley & Harvey 1993, Kreger 1991).

This advanced practice role, which has been described as 'Jack-of-all-trades', or 'extended', 'expanded' and 'multiskilled', is not new to these nurses; rather, it has been the norm for rural and remote area nursing practice since white settlement (Hegney 1997c, Offredy 2000). In small rural and remote health facilities, the broad scope of the role means that nurses are providing care, as well as dealing with situations external to the health environment, including the wellbeing, development and safety

222

of the local community in which they work (New South Wales Health 1998). Rural and remote area nurses, therefore, must have skills and knowledge:

> . . . beyond that acquired in basic nursing education, as well as the advanced knowledge and skills to meet the needs of the population unserved, or underserved by the medical services normally available in urban communities (McMurray et al 1998:9–10).

Until relatively recently, with the introduction of the nurse practitioner program in Australia, the advanced practice role of rural and remote area nurses was not recognised or legitimised in law (Dowd & Johnson 1995, Hegney 1997c, McMurray et al 1998). In 2004, the introduction of the advanced practice role for rural and remote area nurses was not uniform in Australia. For example, while New South Wales, South Australia and Victoria either had in place rural and remote area nurse practitioners (Offredy 2000), or were in the process of introducing this role, Queensland was still undertaking trials to ascertain the effectiveness of such a role. Rather than a nurse practitioner role, Queensland has introduced a rural and isolated practice nurse endorsement where existing rural and remote area nurses, following an education program and using health management protocols, can administer and supply restricted and controlled drugs without a medical officer order (as long as it is listed on a drug therapy protocol). The changes to Queensland's Health (Drugs and Poison) Regulations have ensured that registered rural and remote area nurses endorsed for rural and isolated practice now have legislation which legitimises their medication practice (Hegney et al 2005b).

Factors impacting upon rural and remote area nursing practice

Before an advanced nurse practitioner in Australia becomes a national reality, there are other aspects of rural and remote area nursing practice that need to be addressed. These include educational preparation, access to continuing professional education, recruitment and retention issues, dealing with personal and professional isolation, lack of anonymity, promoting rural and remote area nursing as a desirable career, and strengthening communication between rural and urban health authorities, and professional groups. This chapter will now address some of these issues.

Anonymity

In small towns people know each other and are often related. For the rural and remote area nurse, this knowing and being known by the community has advantages and disadvantages (New South Wales Health 1998). Several authors have described the lack of anonymity of remote area nurses and the need for those in small communities to have 'time out' because of their high visibility within the small community (Cramer 1992, Kreger 1991, Siegloff & Hegney 1996). Additionally, remote area nurses who are employed in indigenous communities experience a level of visibility within the community for which they often have not been prepared (Cramer 1992).

The rural nurse employed in a small rural community, and the remote area nurse, are often well known by the rural community, as the majority of nurses remain in one health service for long periods of time (Hegney et al 1997). In contrast to remote area nurses, it is not uncommon for rural nurses to have grown up in the area in which they are employed, and to have kinship ties with other members of the community (Hegney et al 1997). This means that the nurse often has to provide care to relatives and friends. Thus, in adverse advents, the nurse has to cope with personal feelings of loss, as well as those of the patient and/or family (Siegloff & Hegney 1996).

As well as being a member of a small community, rural and remote area nurses can provide healthcare to several generations of the same family. This aspect of their role has been described as 'womb to tomb care' (Hegney 1996). Studies have suggested that rural nurses have a 'unique insight' into their community and its needs because of the length of time that most rural nurses work in rural communities (Burley & Harvey 1993). In contrast, the majority of remote area nurses do not have the same work history within one community as do rural nurses.

Rural communities have the expectation that the nurse will be an integral member of the community. Thus it is suggested that nurses lose their anonymity by virtue of their rural and remote area practice—they are never off-duty (Hegney 1996). Leaving the community or 'getting out' is, for some nurses, an important coping mechanism. To do this, however, nurses must have access to relief staff locums (New South Wales Health 1998). The lack of locum relief is a barrier that has been identified as impacting not only on the nurse's ability to leave the community for 'time out', but also for continuing professional education.

Education and training

Education and training levels have a significant impact upon rural and remote area nursing practice.

Lack of preparation for the role

A feature of the literature with regard to the role of the nurse employed in remote area and small rural communities is the lack of preparation for their role (Cramer 1992, 1994, Dowd & Johnson 1995, Hegney et al 1997, Kenny & Duckett 2003). A study of 57 remote area nurses (Cramer 1992) found that the majority believed they were totally unprepared for their role. A major contributing factor to their lack of preparation for the role is the lack of orientation to practice (Cramer 1992, Hanna 2001, Hegney et al 1997). For remote area nurses the lack of preparation for working in indigenous communities has resulted in 'reality shock' (Cramer 1994, Hanna 2001). Additionally, the lack of preparation for remote area practice has been linked to the higher turnover rate (as much as 300% per annum in some locations), as well as burn-out (Cramer 1992, Dowd & Johnson 1995).

Attempts have been made to address this lack of preparation, with orientation courses for remote area nurses now conducted in some states (e.g. Queensland and Western Australia). As the majority of the remote area nursing workforce is employed in indigenous communities, cultural awareness programs are considered an essential part of this orientation (Dowd & Johnson 1995). Similar programs, however, are not routinely provided for rural nurses. Several recent studies indicate that there remain inadequacies in access to education (and career-enhancing opportunities) between nurses who are employed in major cities and nurses who work in rural and remote areas (Courtney et al 2002b, Hegney et al 2003a).

Undergraduate, postgraduate and continuing education and training

Since 1991, there has been recognition that rural and remote area nurses require adequate preparation for their role in the form of formal higher education programs and orientation courses (Wakerman & Field 1998). Postgraduate programs have been provided by several universities (e.g. Monash University, La Trobe University, James Cook University and the University of Southern Queensland). These programs are at the graduate diploma and masters' levels and may be nursing-specific or interprofessional. An audit of these programs in 1998 suggested that none prepared the nurse for an advanced practice clinical role (McMurray et al 1998). However, since this time several universities have introduced either an undergraduate double degree (e.g. Monash University) or a postgraduate program (e.g. the Masters of Advanced Nursing Practice (Rural and Remote) at the University of Southern Queensland). The masters' programs are usually very clinically focused and many are accredited as nurse practitioner preparation programs.

For those nurses who are unable to enrol in formal programs, continuing professional education and training courses are available through other sources such as rural health training units, university departments of rural health, universities and hospitals. However, studies of rural and remote area nurses suggest that remote area nurses in particular still have problems accessing education and training programs (Hegney et al 2003a). There are many reasons for this, many of which have been reported for considerable periods of time and remain unaddressed. For example, reasons for problems of access include the cost of the programs to the student and the shortage of clinical practice placements for students in rural areas.

Because of changes to Australian Government funding, the majority of university postgraduate courses are now fee-paying. The cost varies between universities, but it affects the ability of rural and remote area nurses to enrol in a course. There have been some attempts to address this barrier. For example, in 1998 the Australian Government provided funding in the form of rural and remote scholarships (through the Royal College of Nursing Australia) for rural and remote area nurses to attend formal and informal education and training courses (Australian Government 2004c). These funds were competitive and therefore not all rural and remote area nurses were able to take advantage of the scholarships. In 2004, while not particularly targeting rural and remote area nurses, postgraduate students are able to access the Postgraduate Education Loan Scheme (PELS). PELS is a loan that is repaid through the taxation system once the person's income reaches a certain threshold (Australian Government 2004d).

The shortage of clinical practice placements for students in rural areas, as well as a lack of preceptor/mentors who can supervise students during the program, is another barrier to access (Hegney 1996). While some states provide some funding for clinical placements (New South Wales Health 2004), the majority of undergraduate students are required to self-fund clinical placements in the rural or remote area health facility. This is an added cost, which often means that a rural clinical placement is limited for many nurses (Neill & Taylor 2002).

The lack of graduate programs in rural and remote areas limits employment in a supervised capacity for the newly graduated registered nurse seeking employment in these areas (Hegney et al 1997, New South Wales Health 1998).

The Australian literature contains a wealth of information on the lack of access to education and training of rural and remote area nurses. It particularly focuses on the need for appropriate, accessible and flexible programs delivered within the rural clinical environment (Dowd & Johnson 1995, McMurray et al 1998, Lampshire & Rolfe 1996). Barriers to education and training that have been identified include family commitments, inability to afford unpaid leave, lack of locum relief staff, lack of finance, lack of information on what courses are available, lack of employer support, and the unsuitability of many courses for rural nursing practice (Hegney et al 1997, Hanna 2001, Hegney et al 2003a, McMurray et al 1998).

The extensive literature on education and training for rural and remote area nurses recommends that they be educationally prepared for their role prior to employment, have access to suitable education and training after their employment, and be able to enrol in programs which give articulation between higher education providers (Hegney 1997c, 1997d, Kenny & Duckett 2003). It was also recommended that the clinical environment be an equal partner in the preparation and continuing education of rural nurses (Hegney et al 1997).

Professional isolation

Related to the need for an adequately prepared nurse is the ability of the nurse to provide a health service in relative isolation from the nursing profession and other healthcare providers. Distance does not necessarily mean isolation. Nurses can feel isolated in metropolitan settings, especially if they are working as a sole practitioner (such as midwife or occupational health nurse). The literature suggests that rural and remote area nurses do feel isolated in their practice, and the major cause of this isolation is the distance between health services and, therefore, nursing, medical and allied health support (Dowd & Johnson 1995, Hegney et al 1997, Neill & Taylor 2002). Distance, in these cases, limits the ability of nurses to form peer networks with other nurses and healthcare professionals (New South Wales Health 1998).

To address the isolation of remote area nurses, the Council of Remote Area Nurses in Australia (CRANA) received federal government funding for the provision of a 'Bush Crisis Line'. This crisis line, which has a toll-free number, can be used by rural and remote area nurses 24 hours a day.

Relationships with other healthcare professionals

A factor that often influences the level of responsibility of rural and remote area nurses is the number of medical and allied health professionals employed by or appointed to the health service. This varies between health facilities, ranging from remote area nurses often working alone and relying on off-site medical services (such as the Royal Flying Doctor Service) to rural nurses who have resident medical officers, medical specialists and a wide range of allied health professionals working in the town.

In small rural hospitals and remote communities where there are no resident medical officers, the first patient contact in an emergency is the nurse. General practitioner contact can be unavailable for periods ranging from 30 minutes to 4 hours depending on locale and travelling time for the doctor. Additionally, in many of these facilities there may be no allied health staff, such as pharmacist, radiographer, physiotherapist or occupational therapist. In these facilities, nurses dispense medications on a telephone order from an off-site practitioner (or an endorsed rural and isolated practice nurse or nurse practitioner may work from a protocol), take X-rays and provide allied health services. For those nurses who rely on the orders of part-time or distant medical and allied health professionals, role relationships are vitally important, not only to the nurse but also to the quality of healthcare which is delivered to rural and remote residents (Blue & Fitzgerald 2002).

Despite the rhetoric of interdisciplinary teams in rural areas, there is often role conflict between the nurse and the medical officer (Blue & Fitzgerald 2002, Hegney

1998). A major cause of the conflict between rural nurses and medical officers occurs when the off-site medical officer is required to attend a patient in the hospital. During the day, it may be that the medical officer is conducting a consulting session with private patients. During the evening and night it is often the case that the nurse, having assessed the patient, must discuss the patient with the off-site medical officer. These telephone conversations are reported to be a source of stress for many rural nurses, as often the medical practitioner does not wish to attend the patient in the hospital (unless it is an emergency) (Hegney 1998, Hegney et al 2003b).

Additionally, many medical practitioners undervalue the skills of rural nurses by not recognising their experience and expertise. This may lead to a situation where medical practitioners limit the nurse's ability to deliver holistic care and only allow them to deliver fragmented care (e.g. requesting that a community nurse check on a client's blood pressure without giving a concise picture of the client's condition or any prescribed medication, or a referral to the nurse for care) (Lampshire & Rolfe 1993). The pressure that medical practitioners place on rural and remote area nurses to work outside their role is associated with a higher rate of medication violations (McKeon et al 2003).

Recruitment and retention

While much has been written about the shortage of medical practitioners in rural and remote areas, until recently very little attention has been paid to the increasing shortage of rural and remote area nurses and midwives in Australia (New South Wales Health 1998, Senate Community Affairs References Committee 2002). A report by New South Wales Health in 1998 stated that the top specialties for which positions were being actively recruited for the rural nursing workforce were 'generalist, mental health, intensive care, midwifery, operating theatre, emergency department, orthopaedic, community health and paediatrics' (p 4). Similarly, the shortage of experienced remote area nurses has been well documented (Dowd & Johnson 1995).

Factors that have been linked to poor retention include lack of understanding of the role, poor accommodation, the lack of a career pathway, little to no child-minding facilities, the lack of access to affordable and relevant education and training, lack of employer support, the level of work-related stress, legal aspects of the role (particularly with regard to the administration and supply of medications), relationships with medical officers, inadequate locum relief, and the violence often experienced by remote area nurses (Cramer 1992, Dowd & Johnson 1995, Hegney et al 1997, 2003a, 2003b, 2003c).

As with the shortages of remote area nurses, the recruitment of rural nurses is becoming problematic in Australia. The factors that have a negative impact on the decision of nurses to work in rural areas include the lack of promotion of rural nursing as a desirable career option, the low number of clinical placements that are available for pre-registration undergraduate nursing students, and the lack of graduate year placements in rural health facilities (Courtney et al 2002a, Hegney et al 1997, McMurray et al 1998, New South Wales Health 1998).

CONCLUDING REMARKS

The majority of nurses who practise in rural and remote areas find their practice rewarding, despite the demands of autonomous practice and the hardships associated with isolation. However, the provision of healthcare to rural and remote communities would not occur without this nursing workforce. The introduction of a legitimised advanced nurse practitioner role is, therefore, a positive step and will lead to improvements in the quality of healthcare provision in rural and remote areas. This is particularly important in remote areas of Australia where population densities make the employment of a medical officer uneconomical. This is not to say that the rural or remote advanced practice nurse is a medical officer replacement—rather, with their focus on the delivery of primary healthcare, these nurses provide a different health service. In the twenty-first century, as in the nineteenth and twentieth centuries, it is nurses who provide the majority of healthcare services to rural and remote Australians.

REFLECTIVE QUESTIONS

1 Working in relative isolation from other healthcare professionals, how can the rural and remote area nurse implement primary healthcare with a focus on prevention in the community in which they are employed?

2 What programs could be introduced to attract and retain rural and remote area nurses?

3 What is the level of educational preparation that would best suit the beginning rural and/or remote area nurse? Note that this may involve several different programs—before commencement of employment and during employment.

RECOMMENDED READINGS

Australian Institute of Health and Welfare 2004 *Rural, regional and remote health: a guide to remoteness classifications*. AIHW, Canberra.
Australian Institute of Health and Welfare 2004 *Rural, regional and remote health: a study on mortality*. AIHW, Canberra.
Bushy A 1998 Rural nursing in the US: Where do we stand as we enter a new millenium? *Australian Journal of Rural Health* 6:65–71.
Strong K, Trickett P, Titulaer I, Bhatia K 1998 *Health in rural and remote Australia: the first report of the Australian Institute of Health and Welfare on rural health*. AIHW, Canberra.

Online resources

Australian Government, Department of Health and Ageing: http://www.health.gov.au. This site gives you access to various information on rural health policy.
Australian Institute of Health and Welfare: http://www.aihw.gov.au. This site contains the statistical reports on rural health and the labour force.
National Rural Health Alliance: http://www.ruralhealth.org.au. This site gives you access to all the member bodies of the alliance. It is the most useful site for rural health.

CHAPTER SEVENTEEN

Professional organisations: why do we need them?

Judy Lumby & Tracey Osmond

After reading and reflecting on this chapter, readers will be able to:

▲ recognise the need for continuing professional development throughout one's career;

▲ list three major trends influencing society today;

▲ explicate the difference between an industrial and professional organisation;

▲ list five characteristics of a modern professional; and

▲ rationalise the responsibility for continuing professional development from both an individual and societal perspective.

KEY WORDS

Professionalism, continuing professional development

WHERE HAVE TODAY'S PROFESSIONAL ORGANISATIONS DEVELOPED FROM?

According to Black (2003) it could be argued that today's professional organisations have their earliest roots based in the ancient Greek and Roman civilisations where such groups were formed as 'artificial families', differentiating themselves from the rest of society based on common beliefs, values and ethos. In ancient Greece the most important of these were male drinking clubs, while the Roman *collegia* included 'social clubs, burial societies and cultic groups' (Black 2003:3). So some may wonder . . . has much changed?

It is, however, more commonly acknowledged that contemporary professional organisations have their strongest links to the medieval guilds, in particular the craft guilds that emerged in Europe in the Middle Ages. These guilds were strengthened in the move from the feudal organisation of labour to the emergence (and importance of) skilled artisans, journeymen and master tradesmen. Medieval guilds took their place between 'family and state' as a distinctive type of social entity (Black 2003:12). They imposed moral standards upon members, which often combined both their *rights* and *duties*, and created for the membership a *legal entity*.

Guilds were viewed as an 'occupational milieu', in which professional ethics could develop without state coercion (Black 2003:13). Black argues that guild membership was important both 'psychologically and practically', as it incurred serious and enduring obligations and benefits affecting one's self-perception and moral entity (p 14). It gave one a position in society and enabled one to ply a trade, thereby crucially affecting one's economic status. The guild, therefore, gave skilled tradespeople and the emerging professions societal status, which hitherto could only be achieved through birthright.

An additional role of the guilds was to provide for the social security of its members. Kieser (1989:551) notes that guilds provided 'reciprocal obligations in assisting sickness and death cases. Some guilds even had money chests to support the unemployed. Social security also applied to widows and orphans.'

During this time other types of guilds were established, remnants of which survive to this day. Krause (1996:9) describes today's universities as 'guild survivor(s) and profession maker(s)'. The scholars' guild emerged in Europe at the time of the craft guilds (1100–1200 AD) when scholars attached to cathedral and church schools organised themselves as a *universitas magistribus et pupillorium* or 'guild of masters and students' (Krause 1996:9). It was at this time that the 'traditional professions' became firmly entrenched in the academy as 'the university was primarily a producer of arts graduates, of physicians, of lawyers both civil and canon' (Krause 1996:11), while practical professions remained the domain of the guilds (e.g. surgeons, pharmacists and grocers in Florence comprised the medical guild) (Krause 1996:12).

The evolutionary changes that have occurred between the Middle Ages and the last century become apparent from the preceding overview when we consider the organisations that represent the profession of nursing today. The role of universities in the undergraduate preparation of professionals has certainly evolved from this time, with the more practice-based professions having to strive harder for recognition than those of the more traditional established professions. The work of the guilds in relation to working conditions and social security has evolved into the domain of the unions, who seek improved salary, benefits and job security for their respective workforces. The role of the guilds in seeking standards of workmanship and quality has evolved into the regulatory bodies that govern the professions, namely the professional registration boards of the states and territories of Australia. The establishment of the professional colleges in the mid-twentieth century in Australia was to stem the need for health professionals to travel to the United Kingdom to gain postregistration qualifications.

NURSE TRAINING AND REGISTRATION

The first recognised training program for nurses was established in Australia by Lucy Osburn at Sydney Hospital in 1868 (Bowd 1968:5) under the Nightingale system. From that time, those trained nurses, in the absence of any other regulatory authority, established the Australian Trained Nurses Association (ANTA) in 1899. This body's major aims were to improve and standardise the training of nurses, thereby ensuring consistency and quality in nursing care in Australia through a system of registration for trained nurses. By the early twentieth century most states of Australia had established branches of the ATNA (Queensland, 1904; South Australia, 1905; Western Australia, 1907; Tasmania, 1908), while in Victoria the Victorian Trained Nurses Association (VTNA) was established in 1901.

Through the work of the ATNA and the VTNA, nurse regulatory authorities were established across Australia by the mid-1930s (South Australia, 1920; Western Australia, 1922; New South Wales, 1924; Victoria, 1924; Tasmania, 1927; Queensland, 1928; Australian Capital Territory, 1933) (Russell 2000:14). While nurse training schools were becoming well established in hospitals across Australia by the early twentieth century, Pratt and Russell (2002:1) state that 'as far back as 1912, the establishment of a Faculty of Nursing at the University of Sydney was being urged'.

NURSING COLLEGES

In the absence of postregistration courses being available in Australia for registered nurses prior to 1949, the ANTA provided 'lectures subsidiary to general nursing' to its members during winter months (*Australasian Nurses' Journal* 1903:2). Formal moves towards the establishment of a College of Nursing for Australian nurses are attributed to the appointment of Miss Muriel Knox Doherty as the pioneer Sister Tutor at Royal Prince Alfred Hospital, Sydney, in 1933 (Pratt & Russell 2002:2). Miss Doherty had begun corresponding with Miss Grace Wilson, Matron of the Alfred Hospital in Melbourne, during 1933 in relation to postregistration plans for their respective states. It was always Miss Doherty's vision that an Australian College of Nursing be developed under a federated model, as evidenced by the following:

> All along the stress has been on a national College of Nursing acting in an advisory capacity to the Federal Government and the State Bodies in a similar capacity for their states . . . [t]he latter (autonomous bodies) to be established first followed by a Federal Council elected by the state Colleges (Doherty, cited in Pratt & Russell 2002:6).

The establishment of the colleges progressed somewhat along the lines envisaged by Miss Doherty; however, there were divergences from this vision. Between 1933 and 1949 there was much correspondence, meetings and conferences between the key nursing organisations and nursing leaders of the day, remembering that World War II (1939–45) also delayed progress. Seen as paramount to the cause, Miss Doherty believed state unity was the first step towards federal unity: 'if we have state unity . . . we could immediately present a united front and bargain with our present state government' (Doherty 1947, cited in Pratt & Russell 2002:8).

The barrier to the state unity to which Miss Doherty refers is the number of nursing organisations that had developed in each state, representing nurses' interests, which at times overlapped. In 1947 these consisted of: in New South Wales, ATNA (NSW Branch), the NSW Nurses Association (NSWNA, registered as an industrial union in NSW), and the Institute of Hospital Matrons of NSW and ACT (IHM). In Victoria, there was the Royal Victorian College of Nursing (this organisation was the Victorian branch of the ANF) and the Trained Nurses Guild (TNG), which was an organisation registered with the Federal Court of Conciliation and Arbitration with branches in other states. There were also nurses' unions (similar to the NSWNA) in Western Australia and Tasmania.

Federally, the organisations consisted of the Australian Nurses Federation (ANF), with six state branches, including ATNA (NSW) and the RVCN, and the National Florence Nightingale Memorial Committee of Australia (FNMCA), which was established in 1947 (Pratt & Russell 2002:5).

It is as a result of the combined efforts of key members of each of the above organisations, amalgamations of some of these groups and the political context of the day that finally saw the establishment of two colleges of nursing in Australia (for a detailed account of these events, see Pratt & Russell 2002), the New South Wales College of Nursing (established 10 January 1949) and the College of Nursing, Australia (based in Melbourne, established 2 April 1949). Today these two national professional nursing organisations continue to represent all registered nurses and enrolled nurses across Australia: the College of Nursing (incorporating the NSW College of Nursing) and the Royal College of Nursing, Australia.

Since their establishment over five decades ago they have evolved into quite diverse organisations. The College of Nursing is a membership organisation, which lobbies and undertakes research, but is also one of the largest faculties of nursing in Australia in that it conducts a major educational program at graduate level, nationally and internationally. The Royal College of Nursing, Australia, which is situated in Canberra, does not conduct a formal educational program, but is involved mainly in lobbying and managing scholarships for the federal government as well as representing Australian nurses at the International Council of Nurses (ICN).

Today, there are several colleges across Australia representing specialty branches of nursing and midwifery.

UNIONS

The evolution of nursing unions and industrial organisations representing nursing interests is inextricably linked to the evolution of the colleges, as previously discussed. Today's nurses' unions have developed as a federated model—namely, the Australian Nurses Federation (ANF)—with state-based groups structured in various ways. The

ANF represents nurses in terms of awards and work-related cases involving equity, safe and supportive work environments, and legal cases against individual nurses who are union members. The ANF has state entities in each of the Australian states and territories. In New South Wales and Queensland, these state branches are the New South Wales Nurses Association (NSWNA) and the Queensland Nurses Council (QNC) respectively, with the remaining states known as the ANF (Vic), and so on.

SOCIAL AND CULTURAL CHANGES IMPACTING ON PROFESSIONAL ORGANISATIONS

In our contemporary society, a professional organisation does not have the same boundaries as in the past when few roles were identified as 'professional' and few groups were therefore in 'professional organisations'. In Australia in particular, because of the way in which most of our nation was colonised, the majority of workers were unionised and certainly not 'professionalised'. Professions were few and far between apart from doctors and lawyers who in the early days of colonisation were not really professionalised either, if we consider their past practices against today's standards.

Over the last three decades our society has undergone greater changes socially, economically, demographically and industrially than in the three decades prior. Some of this can be put down to the change of women's place in society, as they gained first sexual and then economic freedom. We no longer live in a world where women do all the caring and men establish the culture, although this has not changed as much as many would desire. We no longer live in a world where we can assume a family describes a group including a man, a woman and three or four children. Indeed the *2005 Year Book Australia* (compiled by the Australian Bureau of Statistics) states that the so-called 'nuclear family' now only represents 47% of all households, and in 20 years this is predicted to reduce to one-third of all households. There is an increasing trend towards single households, couples who will remain childless 'by choice or circumstance' and parenting by same-sex couples.

In terms of nursing and its environment, the healthcare system of the 1960s clearly delineated general practitioners as the priests of society. They were the father confessors, they birthed the babies, looked after the children and the parents, and even the next generation. Specialisation was just emerging. In terms of the patient population, life expectancy was less for men and women, although more men in their middle age died due to heart disease; women died in childbirth; small neonates did not survive; and intensive care, ventilators, hyperalimentation and advanced pharmacology as we know it today were only being introduced. Nurses were clearly the blue-collar workers in the healthcare system, and for this reason they were joiners, not leaders. Because marriage and children excluded women from the workforce, those women who were in the workforce were single women or women without children. Men in nursing were rare because many hospitals did not allow them into training programs.

The changes in terms of gendered roles and responsibilities have likewise been considerable, meaning that no longer is there a woman left at home caring for the family and the community. We can no longer identify the male as the main breadwinner, or in some cases as the one who does the breadwinning. Women are consistently achieving academically on a par and even above their male counterparts in some previously male-dominated professions such as medicine, and in the corporate world women are slowly emerging as highly competent leaders of commerce.

While the above trends may not appear to link directly to the topic at hand—that is, the changes in professional organisations—indirectly they do. Just as changes to the social structure of the Middle Ages forced the emergence of the guilds, contemporary societal trends continue to shape professional organisations. This is because the changes in family and social groupings reflect lifestyle changes, which impact on how individuals choose to live their lives. This choice may be quite deliberate or one brought about by opposing options, such as a relatively comfortable life economically with a balance of work and play or a more stressful life, which is less balanced but involves having children and a mortgage. The ability to have such choices reflects a level of economic wellbeing above that of the majority of our parents or grandparents—a level that has increased the number of material goods acquired in any one lifetime, leading to higher expectations in terms of acquisitions. After all, real choice is a 'middle class' prerogative.

Peter Singer (1993) explores this 'world of self-interest' as he calls it in his text *How are we to live? Ethics in an age of self-interest*. He claims that it has changed the way in which we think in the world. We are self-absorbed and have lost our sense of community. But individual society cannot be solely to blame for this change. Globally, Westernised societies have voted in conservative governments, which have changed our structures through political interference—socially, culturally and economically. There has been a shift towards deregulation of markets and removal of government funding for the three pillars of a civilised society. These pillars are education, health and social welfare, and in Australia all three have been eroded over the last decade.

We now have increasingly privatised, 'user pays' health and education systems, meaning fewer individuals from 'poor' families will be able to afford higher education or optimal healthcare. In terms of social welfare, there are subtler changes regarding changing eligibility criteria and greater levels of bureaucracy, which are daunting to those who are illiterate or intellectually or mentally disabled. Compounding this is the increase in technology, which has destroyed many jobs for manual workers.

Our world is so different from the one in which most of us were born as to be like another planet. It has changed across all of its cultural structures and is governed by very different ideologies. It is a world of difference and diversity, which has caused John Ralston Saul (2001) to ask the question:

> [W]hat drives a successful society or a successful life, by which I mean a good life? Is it our talents and characteristics? Is it our virtues? If that were so civilization would be little more than competing certainties. One talent against another. Talents allied against others. Even virtues opposed to each other. Benevolence against selfishness. Generosity against ambition. Tolerance against intolerance (Ralston Saul 2001:7).

In his book *On equilibrium*, Ralston Saul challenges us to question how we can balance our competing interests—namely, how do we live our lives fully as individuals while also being responsible citizens? After all, it is our context that will enable us to fully develop individually, so if we neglect the society around us it will be at our individual peril.

This brings us to the question of joining groups and in this way contributing to society at large and inadvertently to your individual world. Membership organisations such as unions were once an essential part of the scene culturally, not only for nursing but for other poorly paid groups in the Australia of yesteryear who needed a strong lobbying power within industry. They were identified as essential for representing individuals, such as women and the poorly educated, who in the main did not question or speak out for their rights.

The pervasive ideology in nursing of commitment, dedication and even subservience, of getting together and supporting each other, reinforced the need of nurses to join groups. Thus it is that nursing has had an historical commitment to groups, to social bonding and commitment.

But change has also affected nursing. The move to shift nursing to the higher education sector has meant that all newly registered nurses in Australia now have an undergraduate degree and already many of our senior specialist nurses have higher degrees including masters and doctorates. This has changed the face and the culture of nursing, moving it out of the blue-collar worker milieu into a culture and image of professionalism. Not that this has necessarily been validated in many quarters, but it has definitely been reflected in increased salaries and more informed and assertive registered nurses.

The downside for the profession is that the graduates are well aware of their potential and know they do not need to remain in nursing. This may not necessarily be because they dislike the role, but has more to do with the changing nature of work today where individuals no longer stay in one job or role for their lifetime, but change every five or so years moving across disciplinary boundaries, developing new skills and building on those they already have.

In such an environment, is it any wonder that the obligatory joining up to an organisation, whether it be a union or a professional group, no longer prevails? Pryor (2005) claims that:

> [T]rade unions like traditional churches are struggling to maintain membership and influence particularly among the young. In the decade to 2003, union membership in this country declined by 26%. Bureau of Statistics figures show some of the biggest falls were among the under 24 age group (Pryor 2005:11).

In comparing churches with unions, Pryor (2005:11) goes on to suggest that unions need to use some of the marketing tools such as those used by Evangelical churches, which are attracting an increasing number of young people. As she writes 'these days even young shop assistants tend not to see themselves as "prisoners of want" or members of the "servile masses" who need to rise up against the bosses', which was the rationale behind the early union movement.

For many reasons we can therefore no longer assume that individuals perceive an advantage in joining an organisation, whether it be a union or a professional group. One exception in healthcare is the specialist group, which individuals join in order to stay abreast of clinical trends and research outcomes, and to build networks of professional colleagues. In this way individuals enhance their practice and career. In some cases this has placed the specialist groups in direct competition with their larger and more general professional colleges. A prime example is the struggle between the very traditional and powerful Australian Medical Association (AMA) and the Australian College of Rural General Practitioners (ACRGP) who, in 2005, are claiming separate status as a specialist group within medicine similar to the Royal Australian College of Surgeons (RACS). Their claim is even being disputed by the

Royal Australian College of General Practitioners (RACGP), which claims to represent the general practitioners who are working in rural practice.

In nursing we have not set up the same college structure as medicine, in which practitioners are credentialled for their roles. Instead we have parallel structures. Academic structures work through the university sector, preparing graduates who are then credentialled through the registration boards, against nationally recognised standards, namely the Australian Nursing and Midwifery Council (ANMC, formerly the Australian Nursing Council Inc or ANCI) Competencies for the Beginning Nurse. National nursing organisations have established themselves as those groups that provide advanced practice standards and guidelines for those nurses moving into specialist or advanced generalist practice domains. Nurse practitioners (the expert nurses within our profession) are regulated by the state and territory registering authorities and are authorised on the basis of their ability to demonstrate expert practice against established criteria, including academic preparation at masters' level in most jurisdictions.

At last count there were 53 specialist nursing groups nationally. In heeding lessons of the past, both in Australia and from our international colleagues, these national nursing organisations (NNOs) began to meet biennially under the auspices of the ANF. The NNOs have formed a coalition to discuss and progress issues impacting on advanced nursing practice in general, while each specialty group represents the specific needs of their members from a specialist or context-specific perspective. A national nursing organisation in Australia is defined as one that has members in four or more states/territories. Members are:

▲ all enrolled nurses and/or registered nurses;

▲ the nursing section of a multidisciplinary group; or

▲ a clear network of registered nurses within such groups who can ensure a nurse representative and feedback to nurses in the practice area.

As we have fragmented due to the specialisation of the profession, membership numbers have reduced in most groups, making it a major issue for strategic planning. The question of how to attract young members in today's world is a continuing topic of debate and discussion (Pryor 2005).

But just as our new world requires that we change our personal ways of living, it also insists that we adopt new ways of thinking, which can be unsettling. After all, we gradually build a construction of concepts over time about our world, which makes it very difficult to move beyond. In healthcare this is increasingly problematic because it is a system that assumes so much. Assumptions include that there is an ultimate truth, that things move along a continuum, that life is linear and that the only way to make sense of the world is through an empirical approach. Even the theories that have challenged this seem to have passed over our system of healthcare, leaving it unchanged. Theories such as Eisenberg's Uncertainty Principle and Chaos Theory are but two. A nurse's world validates these theories, as individual lives demonstrate how uncertain things are and how, in many cases, chaos makes the most sense. But of course nurses work in a world based on the certainty of science.

So what does all this mean for our professional organisations? Somehow we need to rethink the balance of the personal with the professional and construct organisations that allow for this balance. That means rethinking what was appropriate in the past and revisioning the future. After all, professional organisations not only exist for the members; they also rely on members to make them sustainable. Today individuals are too busy, their dollar is too malleable, goods too available and choices too abundant. Individual nurses will quite rightly be very selective in what and who they join. In turn, professional groups need to be accountable to their members and their directors need to ensure corporate governance of the highest standard. Consultation needs to be widespread and consistent. Decisions involving resources need to be transparent.

The future issues that professional and industrial bodies need to address are closer together than ever before in Australia. Just as a blurring of boundaries between disciplines and professions has occurred, so it is that industrial and professional issues have blurred. To be a professional today is not about shoring up an elitist stance, which sets you apart from others, as in the past. Elitism today, except in someone's head or dress, is mainly the food of comedians and cartoonists. To be a professional, one needs to have a balanced life. Professional environments are those that ensure the workplace is suitable; the salary commensurate with work done; continuing professional development is in place; safe and flexible work practices are working; family friendly policies are on offer; and staff are consulted, reviewed, oriented, mentored and not discriminated against.

More importantly in today's world of self-regulation is the need for individuals to take responsibility for their own professional learning and life. Rapid changes in technological advances demand almost constant changes in professional knowledge and practice. Lundgren and Houseman (2002:237) state that 'the rate of turnover of knowledge is now estimated to be 4 to 7 years'. In this context, completion of an undergraduate degree is merely the starting point to a lifelong commitment to improving and building upon professional knowledge and practice. This is the reality of professional practice in the twenty-first century. What is yet to become widely accepted is how individual professionals plan for, undertake and demonstrate their continuing professional development.

Current issues related to the regulation of healthcare practitioners and their continuing professional development (CPD) include:

▲ the need to differentiate between recency of practice and continuing competence;

▲ the need to differentiate between continuing education and continuing professional development;

▲ the need to explore the roles and responsibilities of key stakeholders in promoting CPD—namely professional colleges, regulatory authorities and health service employers—and how their involvement can influence the individual professional's commitment to CPD; and

▲ the need for cultural change in nursing, other health professions and healthcare systems to support and promote a commitment to continuing professional development and lifelong learning.

KEY STAKEHOLDERS FOR CONTINUING PROFESSIONAL DEVELOPMENT

The importance of the workplace or professional context is recognised as a key catalyst for learning. However, distinctions are made about the importance of the roles of key stakeholders in influencing involvement in CPD. Three broad groups of key stakeholders are described as:

1. the individual professional, in particular how they explore motivations for a commitment to CPD, such as seeking peer evaluation, seeking mentors (informal relationships), developing personal education plans/identifying professional learning needs, commitment to lifelong learning, self-awareness and self-evaluation (Evans et al 2002, Touger-Decker 2002, DiMauro 2000, Vuorinen et al 2000, Friedman & Phillips 2002);

2. professional organisations, such as colleges and regulating authorities (Brockett & Bauer 1998); and

3. the employer/organisation, including organisational culture, management support for CPD, job satisfaction and CPD integrated into human resource systems.

In the context of demonstrating continuing competence as a component of CPD, the literature strongly suggests that it is *ultimately the responsibility of the individual nurse* (Evans et al 2002, Touger-Decker 2002, DiMauro 2000, Vuorinen et al 2000, Friedman & Phillips 2002). However, these authors clearly state that the individual nurse cannot do this in isolation.

The professional association has a responsibility in providing assistance and guidance for the individual nurse in planning for, undertaking, communicating and evaluating professional development. Brockett and Bauer (1998) also suggest that the professional association has a strong role to play in providing networks and services that support the individual nurse's endeavours in seeking mentors, career guidance and advice.

The role of the board of nursing (or regulatory authority) is ultimately to protect the public. A number of authors (Gibson 1998, Whittaker et al 2000, Radcliffe 2001) argue that an accountable profession, routinely demonstrating CPD and competence, is the best assurance for public safety and quality healthcare. In this context, and at a time when healthcare consumers are more informed than ever before, nursing boards/regulatory authorities cannot ignore the need for mandatory evidence of CPD and competence for renewing authorisation to practise for much longer.

The role of the employer is to provide an environment that values and demonstrates a commitment to employees who actively undertake to maintain their clinical competence. This may be through the provision of educational opportunities, study leave, multidisciplinary learning opportunities, human resource policies that support workplace learning, peer support and review systems (mentoring, preceptorship), organisational structures that engender the characteristics of a learning organisation, or a variety of other organisational practices that support workplace learning.

The purpose of the *National review of nursing education: our duty of care 2002* (commissioned by the Australian Government) was 'addressing nursing education in relation to patient and client health outcomes' (Heath 2002:1). After wide consultation, review of submissions and the commissioning of a number of research projects, the Review Committee had the following to say about CPD for Australian nurses:

> The comments received showed universal support for nurses to undertake professional development activities and continuing education. These activities are seen to be an integral part of a profession. If nurses are to further their professional standing and

facilitate improved quality of care for their patients, professional development and continuing education must be strongly promoted. Although there was some debate, the general view was that professional development was the responsibility of both the individual and the profession. It was noted, however, that employers also have a responsibility to ensure the currency of skills and knowledge of their employees (Australian Government 2002:205–6).

If we consider all these things, it is clear what our colleges and organisations have to do. We have to work closely together across all these issues to ensure nurses are placed in the very best environment possible, to do their work safely and skilfully. The days of discriminating between whether something is the responsibility of an industrial or a professional body are over. Nursing organisations need to work together in lobbying, education, research and policy formation, embracing diversity and difference.

We need to all work towards one agenda—one that is centred on a new health workforce to meet the needs of healthcare in the future. And we need to demonstrate why our organisations are dynamic and worthwhile joining.

Let's set the agenda!

REFLECTIVE QUESTIONS

1 What advantages do you think membership of professional organisations have for undergraduate nursing students?

2 How do you think specialist nursing organisations differ from industrial organisations?

3 How do you think membership of a professional organisation will enhance your future nursing career?

RECOMMENDED READINGS

Australian Government 2002 *National review of nursing education 2002: our duty of care*. Commonwealth of Australia, Canberra.

DiMauro N M 2000 Continuous professional development. *Journal of Continuing Education in Nursing* 31(2):59–62.

Pratt R, Russell R L 2002 *A voice to be heard: the first fifty years of the New South Wales College of Nursing*. Allen & Unwin, Sydney.

CHAPTER EIGHTEEN

Meeting the needs of individuals

Mary FitzGerald

LEARNING OBJECTIVES

After reading this chapter, students will be able to:

▲ appreciate the ideal of meeting the needs of individuals;

▲ understand the ways that nurses can assess the needs of individuals;

▲ identify the systems in nursing that are conducive to individualised nursing;

▲ acknowledge the problems of providing an individualistic service; and

▲ develop creative means to provide an individualistic nursing service to clients in the contemporary healthcare climate.

KEY WORDS

Individualised care, continuum, dependency, nursing assessment, nursing process, care planning

WHY INDIVIDUALISE CARE?

Individualised care, or care that is specifically designed to meet the distinctive needs of each and every client nursed, is much applauded as a central and valued tenet of good nursing practice. It is supported in nursing literature, educational establishments and, to a large extent, practice. Value Statement 1 of the *Code of ethics for nurses in Australia* reads: 'Nurses respect persons' individual needs, values, culture and vulnerability in the provision of nursing care' (ANCI 1993; note that the ANCI is now known as the Australian Nursing and Midwifery Council (ANMC)).

It seems reasonable to assume that it is in the client's best interest to offer a nursing service that caters to each specific person, and nursing in Western countries such as Australia, the United States and the United Kingdom has certainly adopted the provision of individualised nursing as a core value. There is an assumption that an understanding of the biopsychosocial needs of each person, and a service that accommodates as many of these needs as possible, is more likely to foster improvements in patients' health status, comfort and satisfaction with service than one that delivers a standard service to people according to their medical diagnosis.

In its purest form, individualised nursing constitutes one end of a continuum; at the other end lies a routine service in which all people are treated the same according to their grouping (e.g. age or diagnosis) and where nurses are required to follow protocol rather than make decisions. The reality of practice probably falls somewhere between these two extremes. It is arguably one of the profession's greatest challenges to maintain the delivery of individualised care in spite of institutional and policy pressures that militate against core nursing values such as this. Hence, the real challenge confronting nursing has less to do with the maintenance of current practice than with the generation of creative solutions and strategies that preserve and develop those core values that nursing has treasured.

Manthey claims that American nurses practised individualised nursing in the 1920s:

> The nurse took care of the sick person from the time the need for care was identified until it no longer existed; care was personally administered by the nurse according to the assessment she [sic] made of the individual needs of the patient. There were no rules or regulations, no routine procedures, no hospital policies, time schedules, or supervisors. She practiced nursing with a degree of independence unheard of in modern hospital nursing (Manthey 1980:2).

It is notable that the service described above was provided in the community, away from the complex and medically dominated hospital system where there is a tendency for people to gain a medical diagnosis and perhaps lose some of their personal identity. Later we will consider whether rising levels of dependency among patients in the community might lead to the increasingly medical aspects of care detracting from personal identity, as it has done in hospitals in the past. A strong resurgence of interest in the individual patient returned to nursing in the 1970s against a social backdrop of rising individualism, consumerism and the escalation of the professional classes. The driving philosophies were existentialism and humanism. The focus of philosophers

241

was on the individual as an intelligent human being capable of autonomous decision making, and upon the quality of individual existence. Bevis (1978), a leading American academic, described 'humanistic existentialism' as a modern phase in nursing, with rising value placed upon human life, uniqueness of individuals, quality of life, and freedom of human beings to choose.

The nursing theorists of the late 1970s embraced these ideals and incorporated them, relatively uncritically, into their conceptual models of nursing (Meleis 1997, Pearson et al 2005). In turn, conceptual models of nursing and their authors have been extremely influential in the academic and educational development of nursing (Field & FitzGerald 1989). While they have not been used everywhere as frameworks or guides for nursing practice, they have been used to guide nursing curricula and research. My point is that throughout their education nurses are taught in theory to value the concept of individualised care, but this is taught without a great deal of theoretical consideration for the difficulties of delivering this ideal of nursing in practice. Nursing students frequently experience a degree of disillusionment and stress in practice when they believe that patients do not receive the kind of individual attention they are taught and believe to be necessary.

The practice development movement described by Garbett and McCormack (2002) focuses strongly on person-centred care. This movement is practice rather than theory driven and in the United Kingdom has made headway in the provision of individualised care to patients in contemporary settings. It should be noted that they tend to use the term person-centred care to denote care that is personalised. McCormack in 2004 (p 33) reviewed the literature regarding person-centred care in relation to the care of elderly people and, drawing particularly on the work of Kitwood (1997), identified four core concepts of person centredness: being in relationships with others; being in a social world; being in the place or the context in which the person expresses his or her personhood; and being with self or self-concept.

While essentially supporting individualised nursing, I would like to present in this chapter some perspectives that portray it as problematic. By looking at individualised nursing in a critical way it is more likely that the forces that support or obstruct it in practice may be understood. This should contribute to a healthily realistic approach to its implementation and development in nursing practice. Before dealing with the problems of individualised *nursing* there will be a section dealing with the assessment of individual *needs*, for this is the starting point in any nurse–patient relationship and it is an area where a nurse's time and skill are required to reveal the patient. The systems that are conducive to the delivery of individualised care will also be discussed, along with the evidence there is for their implementation. Lastly, there will be a few suggestions for improving the level of individualised care and the means of evaluating it.

ASSESSMENT OF INDIVIDUAL NEEDS

Assessment of the person who requires nursing is the crucial factor in identifying the individual needs of any client. Although assessment is usually associated with the first encounter of nurse and patient, when a history is taken on admission, the process of assessment can and should continue throughout the nurse–patient relationship. In all encounters with a patient an astute nurse is able to recognise and collect useful information that will help him or her know both the patient and the specific nursing he or she requires. Data can be collected both objectively and subjectively, but before detailing the type of data that are required some time should be spent considering the conditions that affect the collection of information.

The type of relationship that a nurse establishes with a patient affects the quality and amount of information that he or she can gather about that person. Although this may sound obvious, it is of such significance that it is worth dwelling upon. Usually relationships are built up over a period, but time to build relationships with patients is becoming scarcer for the nurse. There are some places where there is time and this should always be appreciated and capitalised upon. Consider the difference between a typical surgical ward and a nursing home that provides residential accommodation for the older person. It is far more likely in the latter institution that the nurses will know the patient and be able to cater to him or her as an individual. This is more a function of the patient's length of stay than of the amount of time available to the nurse in this setting, but it does facilitate the development of the relationship.

Nurses who only come into contact with people for a short period of time require a particular skill to be able to establish a working rapport with their patients quickly. This is not necessarily a skill that can be taught, because different people will respond in their own way to particular circumstances; the astute nurse will gauge the best way to communicate with new patients in order to reassure them and encourage them to talk. New nurses should watch the skills of nurses in long-stay and short-stay situations, and reflect upon the ways that the more experienced nurses establish, or fail to establish, relationships with patients. All nurses—new and experienced—need to reflect on the impact of the changing context of practice on the nurse–patient relationship, for it may well be that this important connection is becoming harder and harder to achieve.

In most areas of nursing, either in hospital or in the community, there are structured systems for assessing patients when they are first encountered. In selecting the form of assessment, it is preferable for the team of nurses to establish a degree of consensus on the nature of nursing and what it is that they are offering patients. Without this consensus the questions may result in the collection of routine data that are unhelpful in assisting nurses who are endeavouring to offer a holistic individualised service to patients (Pearson et al 2005).

In its simplest form, an assessment structure may be merely a checklist of questions required to establish the individual's bare biographical and physical benchmarks. These forms are not conducive to individualised nursing in its broadest sense, for they are not intended to extract detailed information about the person's feelings or lifestyle. However, they may be highly efficient for the service being offered (e.g. in areas where the encounter between nurse and patient is very short and the patient's main purpose is to receive treatment for a medical condition). It should also be acknowledged that not all patients require or even want a 'therapeutic relationship' with a nurse. Other frameworks for assessment are more complex and conducive to the nurse making much deeper inquiry. These assessments are commonly based on one of the theoretical nursing models, and adapted by nurses to their locale. By way of examples, I would point to the assessment frameworks given by two nursing models (Neuman 1995, Roper et al 1990).

Roper et al (1990) state that, at assessment, the nurse aims to establish what the patient is able or unable to do for each of the activities of living with regard to physical, sociocultural, psychological, environmental and politico–economic factors that affect the person. These well-known activities of living are:

- maintaining a safe environment;

- communicating;

- breathing;

- eating and drinking;

- eliminating;

- personal cleansing and dressing;

- controlling body temperature;

- mobilising;

- working and playing;

- expressing sexuality;

- sleeping; and

- dying.

Objective information is gathered by *observation and measurement*. For example, it is possible to observe how restlessly or peacefully a person sleeps, and to measure the length of time they sleep at night. There will inevitably be an element of subjectivity in the nurse's judgment, but this should be contained in order to generate an accurate and reliable profile of the person. *Subjective information* is gathered from the person and it represents their *perception of reality*. Remember that perceptions are real in their consequences, and to that extent they are as important as objective measurement. It is this information that truly reveals the individual and enables the nurse to know how the person can be nursed most beneficially.

Remember, too, that often the nurse's own subjective judgments and perceptions, coupled with all of the demands placed upon them, serve to filter and in some cases impede the reception of information from the person. Here are some examples from a patient obtained during a phenomenological research study (FitzGerald 1995) who has asthma and who consequently has extensive experience of hospital and health services:

> . . . and the senior sisters would come down on their shifts and say, 'Hello, youse back again?' and I am in bed there—'Oh those are lovely flowers, isn't that a pretty nightie?' They wouldn't stop and say, 'How are you coping, do you need any help?' And I used to think, 'Silly bloody bitches, why don't you stop and sit down and ask—just talk to me?'
>
> . . . and her job is to dismiss, err, discharge people and she comes around—it's a stupid job she has got—and she said to me 'Ah Peggy now you're,' [as] she just rubbed my toes, 'Now you just look after yourself won't you, now you're right, aren't you, you don't need any help when you get out?'
>
> When I was on the [ward] the asthma clinical sister came around—'Ah Peggy do you want any magazines or anything?' . . . [pause] . . . I was half dead and on a drip.

You could characterise Peggy as 'difficult', but she is a classic example of someone who was nursed often and whose many individual needs, beyond the purely physical, were neither recognised nor met. Peggy was not just difficult. Her needs were complex and longstanding, she had a lifetime of illness and all that goes with it, and it is undoubtedly the case that had the nurses involved discussed these needs with her they would have found themselves out of their depth. That would have been perfectly reasonable, and she could have been referred to the appropriate services. However, the point is that these needs were never even identified. A thorough nursing assessment may have afforded Peggy the opportunity to express these needs.

In contrast to the relatively structured assessment offered by Roper et al (1990), Neuman (1995) advocates the use of just six questions to elicit information from the patient. The questions are:

1   What do you consider to be your major problem, difficulty or area of concern?

2   How has this affected your usual pattern of living or lifestyle?

3   Have you ever experienced a similar problem before? If so, what was that problem and how did you handle it? Was your handling of the problem successful?

4   What do you anticipate for yourself in the future as a consequence of your present situation?

5   What are you doing and what can you do to help yourself?

6   What do you expect caregivers, family, friends and others to do for you?

The information, once obtained, is then inserted into a more conventional assessment format. This approach seems more likely to engage the person and thus to produce a more personal profile than a checklist of questions such as Peggy was subjected to over and again during her long hospital career. In a study to examine the practice of individualised nursing, Brown (1992) concluded that open-ended questions were by far the most likely to elicit information that was significant to the individual.

Individualised nursing cannot really get off the ground without an assessment, for little is known about the characteristics of the patient. There are many ways of obtaining information for assessment, and formal frameworks should not impede nurses from making the most of any encounter with a patient. However, if nurses are to work in teams that offer some reliable and consistent standard of service across the team, assessment information needs to be written so that all nurses have information about clients readily to hand. Commonsense would dictate that the nurse who initially spends time with the patient and writes the assessment is the best person to be assigned to the patient, but of course this depends upon the system of work allocation in an area. The next section of this chapter will deal with this aspect of individual nursing.

SYSTEMS FOR INDIVIDUALISING NURSING

Individualised care can mean a number of things in nursing, but it is integral to such contemporary professional developments as total patient care, the nursing process, nursing models for practice, patient-centred nursing, primary nursing, information giving and patient autonomy.

In recent years the primary vehicles used to enhance individualised nursing have been the nursing process (a written systematic process of assessment, goal setting, planning and evaluation) and total patient care (the assignment of patients to nurses for their entire nursing during a shift). The nursing process was an initiative that appeared to flounder in practice, although it was hailed in theory as the most appropriate means of professional decision making geared to the individual's requirements for nursing. Total patient care has persisted, and it is now uncommon to find nursing work allocated by tasks.

However, the degree to which nurses are able to meet individual needs without provision in the system for continuity of care is questionable. Primary nursing (Manthey 1980) is a system of work organisation wherein one nurse is assigned responsibility for the prescription and delivery of care to a patient, from the time they first require nursing to the time they are discharged. Primary nursing in reality incorporates both total patient care and the nursing process, because the primary nurse is responsible for the delivery of care and the written prescription of care (Ersser & Tutton 1991, Long et al 1999, Pearson 1989). The primary nurse has to write an assessment and plan in order to ensure that any other nurse caring for the patient gives the same treatment and knows the person's individual needs. The most reliable way to do this is to write the nursing notes tailored to the individual's needs.

From my experience of providing individualised nursing through using the nursing process and primary nursing, I would claim associated benefits for individuals in terms of continuity of care, quality of service and accountability for nursing delivery (FitzGerald 1991, 1994). However, the amount of scientific evidence regarding the efficacy of individualised nursing is disappointing (Black 1992). Predominantly this is because the variables in clinical practice are impossible to control and it is difficult to state with certainty the cause of any improvements.

While there is no conclusive empirical evidence that demonstrates the efficacy of individualised nursing, it is an integral part of the movement named by Salvage (1990) 'new nursing'. The vanguard of 'new nursing' in the United Kingdom was found in the Nursing Development Units at Burford and Oxford. On these units the primary therapy was nursing and attention was focused on the needs of individual clients. A study to compare patient outcomes and quality of care for patients who had been admitted to the nursing unit (treatment group, $n = 84$) and patients who were left to follow a normal hospital pathway (control group, $n = 74$) demonstrated the following for the treatment group:

- ▲ higher quality of care;

- ▲ higher levels of independence on discharge;

- ▲ slightly longer hospital stay; and

- ▲ lower cost per day.

While the majority of studies reported higher ratings of quality after the implementation of primary nursing, it is not always apparent exactly what is the cause of the improvement. Indeed MacGuire (1991) found, in a study of the introduction of primary nursing, that both the control and the experimental wards had improved quality scores. She concluded that this was a result of increased attention to quality measures rather than primary nursing, because primary nursing was only introduced to the experimental ward.

When a team of nurses in an Australian hospital introduced and researched the effectiveness of primary nursing, they too found it difficult to prove its effectiveness, even though they have adopted it and continue to use it (Long et al 1999). In Victoria, Pearson and Baker in 1992 reported consistently higher quality scores in a nursing-led ward that practised primary nursing in a 'contemporary nursing' environment, than a ward from the acute sector. The nursing-led unit nurses had a philosophy (adapted from Henderson 1964) that encouraged these nursing approaches:

▲ the adoption of systematic problem-solving;

▲ the use of scientifically derived knowledge;

▲ the development of transforming relationships with patients;

▲ a holistic approach; and

▲ active participation of the patient in his or her own care (Pearson & Baker 1992:4).

This Victorian project was a small descriptive study that compared data from the nursing records by using the Phaneuf (1976) Nursing Audit to measure quality of care in the following functions:

1   Application and execution of the physician's legal orders.

2   Observations of symptoms and reactions.

3   Supervision of the patient.

4   Supervision of those participating in care (except the physician).

5   Reporting and recording.

6   Application and execution of nursing procedures and techniques.

7   Promotion of physical and emotional health by direction and teaching.

The functions where there were the biggest differences between the two wards (the nursing unit scores were consistently higher) were 2, 3, 4 and 7.

As individualised nursing is predicated on the assumption that the consumers of our services are competent and autonomous human beings, their autonomy should be respected and encouraged. Above all else, the person who knows the individual best is the individual himself or herself, and nurses are technically capable of encouraging patient autonomy by a system of nursing where the patient is encouraged to identify, voice and ensure provision for his or her own needs.

In brief, the required systems for the provision of nursing that meet individuals' needs are those that provide for continuity of care, a system of record keeping that maintains a record of needs and outcomes, and one that helps to maintain and develop the patient's sense of personal autonomy within a healthcare setting.

THE PROBLEMS WITH INDIVIDUALISED NURSING

The first problem with individualised nursing is that on the whole it is not problematised—that is to say, individualised nursing is accepted as the ideal towards which nurses should strive. Uncritically accepting individualised nursing negates the possibility that there may be other competing ideas that have merit, and closes off any prospect of exploring those other ideas. In critiquing individualised nursing I want to traverse some of these ideas and their implications because it strikes me that there must be some middle ground that reconciles the best of individualised nursing with the needs of cost containment and the general wellbeing of society as a whole. For individualised nursing to survive the current reality of practice, it must first be perceived as achievable in practice amid the current realities of practice, and for this the middle ground is essential.

Nurses recognise very early in their careers that the ideals they learn in their schools often bear little resemblance to the realities of practice (Department of Human Services and Health 1994, Kramer 1974). The disillusionment experienced by newcomers to nursing stems from a conflict between the ideals and personal expectations of individualised care on the one hand and the realities of practice on the other. The response of nurses to this discrepancy is important. Faced with a less than ideal situation, they may either see themselves as professional failures (in which case they may leave nursing or avoid promotion) or accept the status quo as unalterable (in which case they may steadily draw the conclusion that the ideal is unachievable and therefore not worth pursuing). Either way, individualised nursing is not advanced, and this may well be a reason why people such as Peggy (remember Peggy?) can regularly attend a hospital for more than 20 years and still perceive that they have not received individualised care from nurses. Individualised nursing should not necessarily be taught as a theoretical imperative but discussed in what Brown (1992:39) describes as its 'empirical adequacy'—that is, how it is brought about in everyday practice.

Taking a broad view, individualised nursing can be regarded as being grounded in humanism, which is a philosophy that is not universally accepted. It is firmly anchored in Western moral philosophy, but many cultures preserve an emphasis on community rather than individual needs. In these cultures—which we often, and somewhat arrogantly, like to characterise as undeveloped—nursing as we know it hardly exists. Instead, care is provided not according to need but according to the community capacity, with a far greater emphasis on public health than treatment and cure of sick individuals. When we refer to individualised nursing we are usually firmly fixed in the illness paradigm. The change of focus to public health and preventive care tends to look to the health of groups rather than individuals per se.

Lest we fall into the error of assuming that the influence of humanism is universally seen to be beneficial, we should look carefully at the individualism advocated by some right-wing governments as an excuse to increase individual responsibility and reduce welfare (Bowers 1989). There are social commentators (Saul 1997, Turner 1991) who are concerned about the rising individualism in Western civilisation, which has resulted in an inwardly focused culture of the self to the detriment of the collective good.

At a local level an example is the patient who has absolutely no regard for the other patients in the ward, while vigorously pursuing his or her own ends. A warning has been sounded by McMahon (1996) that nurses who have responsibility for only a small group of patients are at some stage likely to make these people their priority at the expense of other patients. There is the frequently told story of the patient making a desperate request of a passing nurse being told 'I'm not your nurse'. Although that is an overused example, these are difficulties that the ward team needs to discuss in order to arrive at a collective solution—which may well be to temper any such examples of rigid insistence upon individualised nursing.

The last problem I will mention is with regard to the operationalisation of individualised nursing. There is some resistance among nurses to the introduction of systems that change their practice and increase either their workload or responsibilities. Nurses are adept at blaming rising workloads and reduced staffing levels for most ills in the health service. They are successful in doing this because, to a large extent, it is true. However, there is an attitude among a proportion of nurses that resists added responsibility because it requires additional education and/or a higher commitment to work.

Individualised nursing and some of the associated systems bring the patient and his or her problems closer to the nurse. As we saw from Peggy, often these problems are not easily solved and are likely to increase stress levels in a profession that is already highly stressed. I hear all sorts of explanations for resisting continuity of care, writing assessments or evaluations, or continuing education. These nurses are important because they are able to resist change, not merely by virtue of their numbers and established positions in the system, but because almost all of us are weary of change and perceive nursing development as change for the sake of change. However, the bottom line is that nurses are responsible for and accountable to patients, who enjoy an array of rights that includes the right to high-quality care. Nursing as a profession has declared that high-quality care is individual care.

MEETING THE NEEDS OF INDIVIDUALS

Rather than teach specifics, the intention of this chapter is to introduce a range of issues associated with meeting the needs of individual patients. There is an array of textbooks on the subject that will give details of how to learn skills of assessment, care planning, systems of work organisation and critical reflection. The nurse who wishes to provide an individualised nursing service to his or her patients must become skilled at establishing relationships with a broad range of people. To do this requires refining skills of personal insight, observation, measurement and listening, learning to analyse and interpret this information and, in the light of their disciplinary knowledge, using it to help the person towards health goals. This nurse also has to be able to communicate these plans to the rest of the nursing team and stand accountable for decisions.

However, it is almost impossible for a nurse with these skills to work alone to provide an individual service to patients. It must be confusing and frustrating for patients to receive care on one shift from someone who knows them, and then to meet a nurse on the next shift who not only doesn't know them, but who wants to stick to a routine of his or her own. The team needs to value individualism and work together to ensure that the patients in their area are known personally and treated in the light of this knowledge. Newcomers to an area should not, however, be too hasty in assuming—merely because the hallmarks of individualised nursing (primary nursing) are not apparent—that there is no consideration for the individual patient. Rather, they should look for alternative indicators.

One way to influence practitioners to change is to look carefully and positively at what is being done. We have already established that individualised care is a central tenet of nursing and, if this is true, forget for a while about the theory because it should be evident in nursing practice. In a very small study, Brown (1992) tape-recorded the conversations between an experienced midwife and three expectant mothers. Having searched the data for examples of nursing actions that fitted the unique characteristics of the client, Brown analysed the individualised nurse–client interactions as: specific affective support; health information; decisional control; and professional/technical competencies (Brown 1992:40).

In a similar vein, nurses may look for examples of nursing that are tailored to the individual needs of patients in their practice. How is it, even though work is very busy, that some individuals' needs are catered for? The positive things need to be examined, and ways to encourage this type of care considered, reinforced and developed further. Perhaps a ward has a particularly well-thought-out discharge plan that is specifically tailored to the individual and their home situation; or maybe the nursing team takes particular care to deal sensitively with relatives, knowing something about their relationship with the patient and when and how to give them information.

It may be that there are not many examples of individualised nursing and the team needs to consider introducing some changes. An example might be a commitment to improving written assessments, with a proviso that others in the team will read them if it is the first time they have looked after a particular patient. Another idea may be to reconsider the patient allocation system to try to reduce the number of different nurses each patient has to deal with during any treatment phase. This type of exercise brings alive the values and beliefs of the team. If they espouse a belief in individualised care, they should be able to give examples from their practice that represent reality.

If a team decides that individualised care is not a priority in their area (and this could be quite legitimate), they should be able to justify this decision and articulate their priorities. It could be that the nurses on a day-surgery unit believe that their main aim is to ensure the physical safety of each patient and that the number of patients treated each day is high enough to keep the waiting time for surgery down to the minimum. Their focus would be upon the identification of potential complications, information giving and efficiency.

The evaluation of individualised nursing should be considered from a process and an outcome perspective. In terms of the process, it is relatively easy to evaluate, for there are many indicators of individualised nursing. For instance: Are assessments holistic? Are they written within a certain time of admission? Do other nurses read them when first assigned to a patient? Does the plan reflect the individuality of the person? How many different nurses does a patient have looking after him or her in the space of three days? Outcomes, on the other hand, are far more difficult to establish because, as already mentioned, there is little empirical evidence that individualised nursing affects patient health outcomes. Apart from being more satisfied with their nursing as indicated in quality assurance measures, it is difficult to identify specifics. Commonsense would dictate that rather than measuring specific outcomes over a range of patients, outcomes must relate to individuals' health goals; however, it is extremely difficult to demonstrate that individualised nursing was the cause of improvement.

Future trends in nursing will impact upon the delivery of individualised nursing because they shorten the patient–nurse contact time and the context in which nursing takes place. There has been a dramatic downward shift in hospital admission rates and, importantly, length of stay. The logical next step is hospital-in-the-home. Nurses are beginning to experiment with this development and we need to establish exactly what nursing is required in these circumstances, and how it will be possible to capitalise on the new context to preserve and develop the patient's sense of identity and autonomy.

CONCLUDING REMARKS

On the face of it this chapter has focused on the provision of individual nursing, but surreptitiously it is about the interface of theory and practice. It is about the ways in which theory can and should inform practice and, in its turn, about the ways in which practice should give expression to its theoretical underpinnings. It is also about the concurrent development of theory and practice. At its heart, though, lies the assumption that nursing has a collective professional aspiration to deliver the most beneficial nursing it can. This is only possible when open but critical minds are brought to bear on the whole picture—and this includes the aims and aspirations of both the profession of nursing and the discipline of nursing, the needs and expectations of the consumers of nursing, and the various contexts of the delivery of nursing.

Whatever its source, there does appear to be a human imperative to do good and, in particular, to do good for one's fellow human beings. Nursing as a whole reflects this imperative and it clearly articulates this in its professional codes and charters. In this chapter it has been shown that expressions of the imperative to do good can, by that mere fact, escape critical evaluation, and to uncritically classify individual nursing as good is a case in point. While long experience as a nurse tells me that meeting the needs of the patient in an individualised way is the optimal way in which to deliver nursing, a critical perspective reveals that this is not without its problems. Besides advocating individualised nursing, there should be openness to other ways of delivering quality nursing.

REFLECTIVE QUESTIONS

1   Consider the following after your next clinical practicum. How many patients did you nurse? In what ways did you attend to their individual needs? What systems or people in the area helped you to attend to each patient?

2   Consider the reporting mechanisms, both written and verbal, in the area and ask yourself how reports made by the registered nurses help to ensure that individual needs of patients are recognised by the nursing team.

3   With no further resources, either in terms of time or money, how can a team of nurses in any area improve their ability to offer an individualised service to their patients?

RECOMMENDED READINGS

Madjar I, Walton J eds 1999 *Nursing and the experience of illness: phenomenology in practice*. Allen & Unwin, Sydney.

McCormack B 2001 *Negotiating partnerships with older people: a person centred approach*. Aldershot, Ashgate.

McMahon R, Pearson A 1998 *Nursing as therapy*. Stanley Thornes, Cheltenham.

Pearson A, Vaughan B, Fitzgerald M 2005 *Nursing models for practice*, 3rd edn, Chs 1–4. Butterworth Heinemann, London.

Sacks O 1995 *An anthropologist on Mars*. Picador, London.

CHAPTER NINETEEN

Healthy communities: is there a role for nurses/nursing?

Gay Edgecombe

LEARNING OBJECTIVES

When you have completed this chapter, you will be able to:

▲ describe the role of nurses involved in healthy community programs;

▲ recognise the importance of regular community assessments;

▲ understand the 'new' public health;

▲ understand the importance of early intervention; and

▲ play an active role in policy development and implementation.

KEY WORDS
Community assessment, early intervention, healthy communities, health promotion, social support, public health

TOWARDS STRONGER COMMUNITIES

The majority of nurses and midwives employed today spend limited time in the community. For many, their only experience is their clinical placement as a student. But for those who do decide on a career as a community nurse, they are rewarded by the expanded scope of practice. For example, this can involve delivering services to populations of school children and families with infants and young children. These universal public health services are designed to facilitate and support healthy communities.

A key strategy used by such services is a strength-based approach. Strengths-based approaches focus on identifying and building on the existing strengths of individuals, families and communities. Deficit-based approaches of the past focused on single issues, people's gaps and inadequacies, and community problems. Such approaches can reinforce perceptions of loss, low self-esteem and failure. This change signalled a shift in thinking from the 'old' public health to a 'new' public health. In the former, public health agencies usually decided what was best for communities. In the latter, communities are actively engaged to decide on priorities and preferences for health (Baum 2002, Keleher & Murphy 2004, McMurray 1999). The five action strategies from the Ottawa Charter (World Health Organization 1986:i–v) illustrate this change:

1 The development of healthy public policy.

2 The creation of supportive environments.

3 Strengthening community action.

4 The development of personal skills.

5 Reorientation of health services.

Marshall (2004:175) has taken the five action areas of the Ottawa Charter and developed a useful table (Table 19.1) to illustrate examples under each action. Table 19.1 provides an example from a local government's maternal and child health service initiative that was begun by two local maternal and child health nurses (Higgins & Jones 2004).

The public health movement began in the nineteenth century with the goal to keep nations well across the life-span through providing direct public health services to populations (universal maternal and child health services), enacting government legislation (e.g. to provide safe water, milk, food; set standards for housing) and nationwide programs (e.g. immunisation, chest X-ray screening for tuberculosis) (Duckett 2004, Baum 2002). Early public health service providers included public health nurses, school health nurses, maternal and child health nurses, health visitors and occupational health nurses. Each of these nursing specialties focused on a section of the population and provided a universal service to that population. The generalist public health nurse provided a range of services to local communities and worked with the specialist nurses and other members of the public health team to provide school and maternal and child health services.

Table 19.1: Ottawa Charter action areas: an example

Build healthy public policy	Create supportive environments	Strengthen community action	Develop personal skills	Reorient health services
Infant nutrition. Support for breastfeeding in public places	Pram walking groups. Stops at supportive coffee shops	Pram walking groups established by mothers	Education sessions about breastfeeding and exercise	Multidisciplinary teams in health services, local government planning team and parents

Sources: Adapted from B Marshall 2004 Health promotion in action: case studies from Australia, in H Keleher & B Murphy (eds) *Understanding health: a determinants approach*, p 175, Oxford University Press, Melbourne; and Y Higgins & C Jones 2004 *Baby take a walk in the park*, City of Darebin, Melbourne.

Public health nursing has been developing along with the public health movement for the last 100 years under the auspices of national, regional and/or local government public health departments. Although the range and scope of this development varies greatly between countries, the main reasons worldwide for the development of public health nursing have been crushing poverty, inequity, and lack of basic health services, environmental pollution and infectious disease. The strong, informed leadership capacity of public health nurses has been vital in ensuring that innovative programs are implemented, evaluated and receive ongoing funding.

HEALTHY COMMUNITIES

Terms such as 'healthy settings', 'community health' and 'community wellness' have evolved through public health initiatives over the last century. The Healthy Cities projects were developed in response to the Ottawa Charter (World Health Organization 1986). The Charter called for the 'creation of supportive environments'. Most work by the World Health Organization (WHO) to date has related to WHO Healthy Cities projects initiated by the WHO Regional Office for Europe (Baum 2002, World Health Organization 2003). Many countries in other WHO regions, including Australia, have initiated a range of healthy community projects (Baum 2002:474–508). The WHO Healthy Cities project has four overarching actions:

1 Action to address the determinants of health and the principles of health for all.

2 Action to integrate and promote European and global public health priorities.

3 Action to put health on the social and political agendas of cities.

4 Action to promote good governance and partnership-based planning for health (World Health Organization 2003:1).

If you are just beginning to work as a community nurse in any setting, it is very useful to find out exactly what other community nurses in the different specialties are doing to support healthy communities.

UNIVERSAL HEALTH SERVICES

It is important that nurses understand the importance and meaning of universal service provision. Such services are usually free at the point of access to all families. Examples in Australia are Victoria's Maternal and Child Health Service; the QUIT Program; and drug and alcohol services (Duckett 2004:167, Keleher 2004:102). In the past, many more services were provided in this manner to people on the basis of their need, but a growing number now have a fee or co-payment requirement.

'OLD' AND 'NEW' PUBLIC HEALTH

Table 19.2, adapted from Baum (2002:36), is very useful when trying to compare the changes that are still taking place in public health. Many of the strategies of the 'old' public health are still very important in the 'new' public health. This can be very confusing for new community nurses to unravel and understand.

Table 19.2: 'Old' and 'new' public health

'Old' public health	'New' public health
Focus on improving physical infrastructure, especially in order to provide adequate housing, clean water and sanitation	Focus on physical infrastructure, but also on social support, social capital, behaviour and lifestyles
Legislation and key policy mechanisms, especially in the nineteenth century	Legislation and policy rediscovered as critical tools for public health
Medical profession has central place. Public health nursing has developed with close links to the public health team	Recognition of intersectoral action as crucial. Medicine only one of many professions contributing
In the nineteenth century, public health was one of a series of social movements that worked to improve living conditions. Primarily expert-driven but community action was evident	Philosophy places strong emphasis on community participation, but in some practice this is not achieved, despite increasing success
Epidemiology legitimate research method	Many methodologies recognised as legitimate
Focus on disease prevention and health is seen as absence of illness	Focus on disease prevention, health promotion and a positive definition of health
Primary concern with the prevention of infectious and contagious threats to human health	Concern with all threats to health (including chronic disease, mental and ageing), but also concern with sustainability and viability of the physical environment
Concern with improving the conditions of the poor and special needs groups	Equity an explicit aim of new public health philosophy

Source: Adapted from F Baum 2002 *The new public health,* 2nd edn, p 36. Oxford University Press, Melbourne.

POPULATION-CENTRED MODEL VERSUS INDIVIDUAL-CENTRED MODEL

Community health nurses need to be very familiar with the population-centred and individual-centred models of practice. This is because they work with both models simultaneously if they are providing direct services to a population such as mothers with young infants. The population-centred model relates to objectives for the whole population, and the need to link as many individuals as possible into services that help to achieve population objectives (Duckett 2004, Keleher 2004).

The individual-centred model relates to objectives for an individual client and the need to link the client into as many resources as possible, which will help achieve the client's personal objectives.

Government-supported public health services will give priority to the population-centred model and expect the community health nurse to manage the conflict between the two models. Table 19.3 has been adapted from Holman (1991:54) and sets out some of the differences in the two models.

EARLY INTERVENTION

A key strategy for nurses working in the community is early intervention. Early intervention can mean intervening early through working with parent(s) during pregnancy and infancy, or it can mean intervening early during a key transition point or pathway in an individual's life. Through early intervention and referral, issues can be dealt with before they become entrenched problems. Such problems/issues have causal pathways (Keating & Hertzman 1999) that require careful planning because:

▲ they are complex;

▲ they start early in life;

▲ they arise in social and environmental adversity;

▲ they are inadequately researched; and

▲ available research is fragmented and undertaken in silos and does not inform solutions (Stanley 2002).

How do causal pathways assist us? Adolescents, for example, may be experiencing all or some of the following elements:

▲ no sense of belonging/connectedness;

▲ no sense of control/chronic stress;

▲ no social support/social skills/social networks;

▲ limited participation with family/school/community;

▲ no significant adults about; and

▲ no experience of success (Stanley 2002).

This information is very useful for secondary school nurses to consider when working with troubled students.

256

Table 19.3: Population-centred model versus individual-centred model

Elements	Population-centred model	Individual-centred model
Goal:	The public good	The individual
Market forces:	Supply driven	Demand driven
Scope of programs:	Universal and/or targeted	The individual and family
Short-term utility:	None or negative*	Good for individual
Long-term utility:	Good for individual and population	May be good for individual
Discretionary component:	Low	High
Resource allocation and control:	By policy	By budget
	Undesirable	Desirable
Pricing effect:	Centralised control with strong motivational systems	Peripheral control with a system of checks and balances
Management:	May be linked into a state government regionalised structure and/or local government structure	Healthcare provider
Staff development:	Standardised	Individualised
Information systems:	Population-based	Client-based
Model of evaluation:#	Allocative efficiency	X-efficiency

Notes:
*Examples of short-term negative utility are the pain of an immunisation injection or the withdrawal symptoms of smoking.
#Allocative efficiency is concerned with the comparative benefits of investing funds in pursuit of different objectives. X-efficiency is concerned with the comparative cost of servicing a given objective using different strategies.

Source: Adapted from C D J Holman 1991 *Building the future of community and child health services*, p 54. Health Department of Western Australia, Perth.

According to Stanley (2002), the best way to intervene was at:

▲ key developmental transition points; and

▲ early and later intervention points.

There has been a renewed interest in intervention early in life as a result of new research on brain development, particularly during the first three years of life (Keating & Hertzman 1999) that has:

> . . . clearly shown that a child's brain development is intimately linked to, and influenced by, the child's environment—a complex interaction between genetic inheritance and experience (Department of Human Services 2001:1).

Early intervention has always been a feature of public health programs. But the success of early intervention is dependent on the communication skills of front-line health workers such as community health nurses.

COMMUNITY ASSESSMENT

A key aspect of community health nursing practice is to understand the local community. It is very useful to undertake a community assessment when working in a community setting for the first time. Then, in order to keep up-to-date with changes, an annual community assessment needs to be carried out. Stanhope and Lancaster describe community assessment as a:

> . . . process of critically thinking about the community and getting to know and understand the community as a client. Assessments help identify community needs, clarify problems, and identify strengths and resources (Stanhope & Lancaster 2002:183).

There are a number of excellent databases to assist with community assessment evidence. For example, the Australian Institute of Health and Welfare is an excellent portal for all sorts of data on community health and population statistics. The Australian Institute of Health and Welfare produces a biennial report *Australia's health*, which is downloadable from their website. This is a good summary of workforce data, health status of communities, hospital data and many other variables. Community health nurses can obtain data from this source for most communities where they are employed. *Evidence-based healthcare* (Muir Gray 2001) is a very useful background text for community assessment. It contains lists of key websites. Other useful websites are listed in the box below.

Useful websites

- Australian Bureau of Statistics at http://www.abs.gov.au/
- Australian Institute of Health and Welfare at www.aihw.gov.au/knowledgebase/index.html
- Communicable Disease Network of Australia and New Zealand at www.cda.gov.au/cdna/index.htm
- Evidence-based nursing at http://www.nmj.com/data/ebn.htm
- Joanna Briggs Institute at www.joannabriggs.edu.au/pubs/approach.php

---

Bronfenbrenner's (1979) ecological model of human development is being revisited by leaders in child health (Australian Institute of Family Studies 2002:xi, Keating & Hertzman 1999, Scott 1992) because of the growing interest in how families relate to their local communities and larger social systems (Scott 1992:204). Therefore, revisiting this model is timely for community-based nurses undertaking a community assessment.

Another useful document to have on hand is *Social determinants of health: the solid facts* (Wilkinson & Marmot 2003:1–32). This publication provides evidence supporting the impact of the 10 main social determinants on our health:

1 **The social gradient.** Life expectancy is shorter and most diseases are more common further down the social ladder in each society. Health policy must tackle the social and economic determinants of health.

2 **Stress.** Stressful circumstances, making people feel worried, anxious and unable to cope, are damaging to health and may lead to premature death.

3 **Early life.** A good start on life means supporting mothers and young children: the health impact of early development and education lasts a lifetime.

4 **Social exclusion.** Life is short where its quality is poor. By causing hardship and resentment, poverty, social exclusion and discrimination cost lives.

5 **Work.** Stress in the workplace increases the risk of disease. People who have more control over their work have a better health.

6 **Unemployment.** Job security increases health, wellbeing and job satisfaction. Higher rates of unemployment cause more illness and premature death.

7 **Social support.** Friendship, good social relations and strong supportive networks improve health at home, at work and in the community.

8 **Addiction.** Individuals turn to alcohol, drugs and tobacco, and suffer from their use, but use is influenced by the wider social setting.

9 **Food.** Because global market forces control the food supply, healthy food is a political issue.

10 **Transport.** Healthy transport means less driving and more walking.

Cultural diversity is a feature of Australian communities. The Department of Human Services (2004b:7) in Victoria has published a useful *Cultural diversity guide*. The policy statement's core principles are valuing diversity, reducing inequity, encouraging participation, and promoting the social, cultural and economic benefits of cultural diversity. McMurray (2004:16–17) points out the need for evidence-based nursing practice that is culturally sensitive. She notes that with the 'increasing trend towards home and community care', there is an urgent need for 'culturally appropriate information that can foster empowerment'.

HEALTHY COMMUNITIES: NURSING INITIATIVES

There are numerous examples of initiatives being designed and implemented by nurses and midwives in the community that support healthy community development. Three such projects are briefly described to illustrate how nurses and midwives are embracing the 'new' public health.

Initiative 1: maternal and child health nursing

In 1996–97, the Department of Human Services funded 39 New Initiatives Projects over three years to enhance the existing Maternal and Child Health Service for families with high needs. The projects aimed to improve the health and wellbeing for families who fell broadly into two groups—those who had underutilised or who did not utilise the universal Maternal and Child Health Service, and those who had high needs requiring additional services. These families were perceived to include families from culturally and linguistically diverse backgrounds, young unsupported parents, families from low socioeconomic groups, Aboriginal families and rurally isolated families.

Many of the New Initiatives Projects incorporated a range of service types that included centre-based, home visiting and group activities. As well, models included outreach services, day-stay projects, and mentor and volunteer projects. In most projects, maternal and child health nurses delivered the service; however, a number also employed family support, ethnic youth and Aboriginal family support workers to work with them.

Evaluation design

A team of researchers (Edgecombe et al 2001) evaluated the 39 projects over three years. The evaluation was implemented in two phases. In the formative phase (phase 1, June 1998–May 1999), preliminary data on projects were collected, the evaluation design was reviewed and revised, data collection instruments were piloted, and project staff were made familiar with the evaluation data requirements. The evaluation team adopted a consultative approach that was critical in establishing and maintaining the cooperation of project staff and managers, and to maximise the quality of the data collected.

In the summative phase (phase 2, May 1999–December 2000), data were collected on projects and families using a range of instruments and with consent from families. Data on project implementation were revised and updated until August 2001. During this phase, site visits were undertaken. Networking between projects teams was encouraged to enable successes, progress and problem-solving strategies to be shared. This was particularly helpful for the Aboriginal project teams and project teams targeting adolescent mothers.

From the outset, several factors impacted upon the evaluation methodology adopted by the evaluation team and its capacity to compare project models, including those targeting specific client groups. These included variations in:

▲ funding levels;

▲ worker qualifications;

▲ models of service delivery;

▲ target groups;

▲ starting dates;

▲ managerial support; and

▲ acceptance and integration with the universal Maternal and Child Health Service.

Other issues that impeded the evaluation team included:

▲ lack of standardisation in service delivery and record keeping;

▲ lack of readily available and incomplete data;

▲ project model/design changes during the evaluation period;

▲ lack of understanding in some projects at different levels of management of the requirements of an evaluation project; and

▲ lack of access by some local, regional management staff and nearly all project staff about the New Initiative Projects and the evaluation process.

Feedback from families

Feedback from participating families was overwhelmingly positive, with almost all who responded to the service-user survey indicating they would recommend the project to others, and would use it again themselves. Many families provided details of the ways in which the projects had had a significant and positive impact for their families. Overall, the projects succeeded in achieving their objectives of:

▲ engaging families who had either underutilised the Maternal and Child Health Service in the past or had additional needs;

▲ improving the health and wellbeing of infants and children;

▲ improving maternal health and wellbeing;

▲ improving parent–child interaction; and

▲ improving links to the universal Maternal and Child Health Service and other relevant services.

The most significant outcome of these projects, as reported by families, was a dramatic improvement in parenting confidence (see Fig 19.1).

Parents stated:

'Helped me to find out how much I understand my baby, so it's easier for me to cope with the baby when she's crying.'

'This service has made us more aware of child health and wellbeing; it has made us feel more confident about raising children and puts us more at ease. They also help explain the stages of child rearing.'

'Has given me the confidence and skills needed to be able to feed properly and establish a sleep pattern.'

Parents found the projects particularly helpful in having someone to talk to, receiving help with handling the child's sleeping and other behaviour, and accessing information on child health, development, feeding and safety. Many mothers showed a significant reduction in stress levels and attributed this to the projects. For example, a mother who experienced postnatal depression and a delay in admission to hospital said:

'It was one of the most useful and helpful programs I was involved with. I couldn't have done without it.'

Parents reported an increase in their knowledge of services and resources. Projects that worked with families who had previously underutilised the Maternal and Child Health Service demonstrated improvements in compliance with ages-and-stages child health and development assessments and immunisation.

Analysis of the feedback from families indicated that the following factors related to staff characteristics, service delivery, and project structure and resourcing were important in achieving these outcomes.

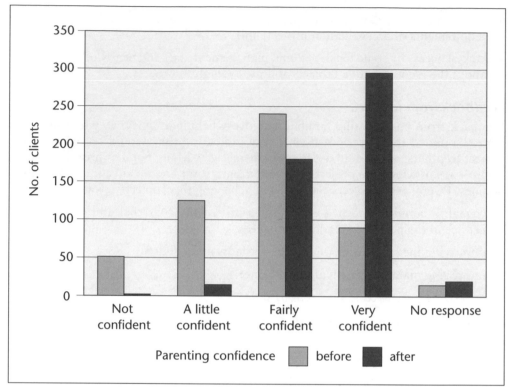

Figure 19.1 Confidence in parenting before and after participation in New Initiatives Projects
Source: Service-user survey, Q9 and Q10. In G Edgecombe, P Rogers, S Kimberley, C Jackson, D Myers, V Mancini, P Needham, S White, G Marsh & M Stewart 2001 *Maternal and child health New Initiatives Projects evaluation (NIPE)*. Department of Human Services, Melbourne.

Staff characteristics

Factors relating to staff characteristics included:

▲ a trusting relationship between staff and clients;

▲ skills and knowledge of staff in terms of advanced family advocacy skills and cultural awareness and competence;

▲ understanding of child health and development, maternal health and parenting, and the capacity to provide anticipatory guidance to parents; and

▲ ability of staff to assist parents to improve the capacity of families to access, mainstream services, including the generic Maternal and Child Health Service through: knowledge of and linkages to relevant local resources; capacity to work as part of a team within the project and with other services involved with the families; and capacity to provide ongoing support after referral to secondary and tertiary services if needed.

Service delivery

Factors relating to service delivery included:

▲ time and timeliness, including: sufficient time available for clients in terms of intensity and duration; and timely and early intervention in response to initial and emerging issues and problems;

▲ confidence of being able to get a quick response to referrals and emerging problems and questions;

▲ availability of home-based services;

▲ opportunities to meet and talk with other similar parents;

▲ assertive outreach to ensure that families are engaged;

▲ comprehensive range of services so that interventions may be tailored to meet individual families' needs; and

▲ culturally acceptable service, including: appropriate venue; and availability of interpreters and printed materials that meet families' linguistic and cultural diversity.

Project structure and resourcing

Factors relating to project resourcing included:

▲ appropriate level of resourcing for project scope and aims;

▲ adequate infrastructure, such as a base office, computers, mobile telephones and cars; and

▲ continuity of project funding.

Factors relating to project management included:

▲ strong supportive management; and

▲ continuity of project managers.

Factors relating to support for staff included:

▲ regular clinical supervision; and

▲ continuing education related to the role and promoting best practice.

Key findings

On the basis of the evidence from this evaluation, the following key findings emerged:

▲ Well-targeted flexible services successfully improved health and wellbeing outcomes for families.

▲ Services were most successful in improving outcomes when they were fully integrated with the universal Maternal and Child Health Service and linked well to other services.

▲ Flexibility in models of service delivery and service activities was critical for families with additional needs.

▲ Families reported that they particularly benefited from social interaction with other parents through groups, community-based services and activities.

▲ Clinical supervision was generally provided in an ad hoc fashion or not at all. Where this was available, maternal and child health nurses and family support workers' confidence, practice and insight into the need for some families for high-duration and high-intensity services was improved and affirmed.

▲ Evaluation data supported existing research that recommends high-duration, high-intensity support (up to three years) for adolescent parents and families with complex problems.

▲ Appropriate management of worker caseloads was critical to ensuring occupational health and safety of the project workers and in some instances the viability of the projects.

▲ Timing of the intervention impacted on outcomes. Early identification through skilled clinical assessment and early referral was essential to prevent problems becoming entrenched. In some instances, due to late referral, unnecessary resources were required to assist families.

Programs, particularly public health programs such as maternal and child health services, must be continually evaluated if they are to survive for another century. Policy makers require evidence to support funding decisions for large universal services.

Initiative 2: secondary school nursing

Victoria's Secondary School Nursing Program is a useful service to examine as it follows the principles of the 'new' public health. The Department of Human Services, Victoria, employed the first 20 secondary school nurses during April 2000. The next 80 nurses were employed and orientated to their new role on 30 May 2001, 15 June 2001 and 19 July 2001.

The goals of the program are as follows:

▲ **Goal 1**: Play a key role in reducing negative health outcomes and risk-taking behaviours among young people, including drug and alcohol abuse, tobacco smoking, eating disorders, obesity, depression, suicide and injuries.

▲ **Goal 2**: Focus on prevention of ill health and problem behaviours by ensuring coordination between the school and community-based health services.

▲ **Goal 3**: Support the school community in addressing contemporary health and social issues facing young people and their families.

▲ **Goal 4**: Place nurses in areas of greatest health needs and socioeconomic disadvantage.

▲ **Goal 5**: Provide appropriate primary healthcare through professional clinical nursing, including assessment, care, referral and support.

▲ **Goal 6**: Establish collaborative working relationships between primary and secondary school nurses to assist young people to deal with any difficulties in their transition from primary to secondary school (Department of Human Services 2000:3).

The role of the secondary school nurse was designed to be in line with government policy and was summarised by the Department of Human Services in July 2000 (Department of Human Services 2000:3):

▲ **Primary care/health education**: Nurses will provide health-related counselling, information, education and advocacy to individuals and groups within the school community.

▲ **Community liaison**: Nurses will help to establish linkages between students, parents, school staff and relevant primary health services in their local community.

▲ **School welfare team participation**: Nurses will work within the school as a professional member of the school welfare team, and this may include liaising with relevant primary school welfare staff to support the transition from primary to secondary school, particularly for vulnerable students.

▲ **School team participation**: Where appropriate, nurses will participate in the broader school community by attending relevant staff and committee meetings, attending in-service programs for school staff, and contributing to the school's planning, evaluation and review processes.

A study by Edgecombe et al (2004) followed the new secondary school nurses from July 2001 until the end of 2002 as they implemented the new policy. One aim of the study was to: 'improve understanding of the issues involved in implementing new nursing programs in Victoria, including an examination of public policy processes'.

Figure 19.2 illustrates the policy processes in which secondary school nurse participants were involved. Key themes to emerge from the findings included the speed at which the program was implemented and the care taken by policy makers and nurses alike to implement the policy on the ground in the way it was intended. Orientation of new school nurses was viewed by all participants as essential to ensure uniform policy implementation across the state. Barriers encountered by nurse participants were many and related to school structure, school policy, school staff, lack of Department of Human Services policy for some issues, and lack of adequate space in some schools.

Due to the majority of the 100 new secondary school nurses being actively engaged in the research that examined their implementation of the new secondary school nursing program (Edgecombe et al 2004), many now have a greater understanding of the policy-making process.

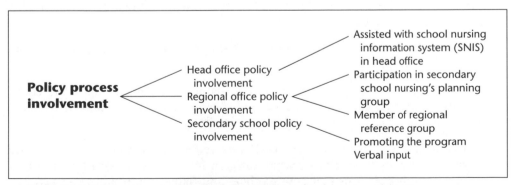

Figure 19.2 Policy process involvement of secondary school nurse participants
Source: Survey Q47. In G Edgecombe, M Hope & M Ward 2004 *Because you're a nurse—I thought I would come and see you: a participatory action research project of Victoria's Secondary School Nursing Program.* RMIT University, Melbourne.

Initiative 3: midwives and maternal and child health nurses continuity of care protocols

Nurses working in the community have many opportunities to become involved in policy development and policy implementation (Hennessy & Spurgeon 2000:ix). Not all take up these opportunities. Hennessy asks, 'Do nurses understand how to use the political and economic processes so that their extensive first-hand knowledge of patients, and their needs, is related in policy developments?' Many community-based nurses get these opportunities in Australia through state/territory health departments, nurses' boards and national professional organisations. There are many examples of nurses' and midwives' involvement in policy development and implementation. A recent example is the 2003–04 team of policy makers, maternal and child health nurses and midwives who worked together to develop protocols for midwives and maternal and child health nurses to follow to ensure women receive continuity of care through pregnancy and childbirth.

The protocols were launched in 2004 (Department of Human Services 2004a:1) and are being used across the state. The aims of the protocol are to:

▲ enhance continuity of care for mothers and their babies from pregnancy through early parenthood by maternity and Maternal and Child Health Services;

▲ promote and strengthen professional partnerships between maternity and Maternal and Child Health Services;

▲ clarify processes to identify and engage families, with emphasis on those who are vulnerable or at risk;

▲ promote mutual understanding of the respective roles and responsibilities of Maternal and Child Health Services and maternity services; and

▲ promote standardised and complementary approaches to the transfer of information between maternity and Maternal and Child Health Services.

The principles underpinning the protocol are:

▲ Effective continuity of care, provided by maternity and Maternal and Child Health Services within the local community, supports mothers and their babies during the first weeks following birth.

▲ Shared philosophical basis and common focus between services supports more effective service provision.

▲ Coordinated service to recent mothers and babies is dependent upon maternity and Maternal and Child Health Services working collaboratively and with a clear understanding of each other's role and responsibilities.

▲ Provision of preventive services or early intervention through collaborative care planning is usually more effective than the later provision of targeted or statutory services. The best interests of new mothers and babies are usually met through family-centred practice.

▲ Information provided to families should be accessible and culturally sensitive, including use of interpreter services.

▲ Information exchange between maternity services and Maternal and Child Health Services should occur with the knowledge and consent of the mother, unless this action would put the baby at significant risk of harm. In this instance, the welfare of the baby takes precedence.

This initiative is very important because midwives and maternal and child health nurses have had ad hoc connections for more than 100 years. Let's hope they begin to coordinate their universal services professionally to ensure parents and their new babies receive integrated care.

Summary

These three examples are focused on facilitating healthy community development across an entire state. Wherever you work in Australia or overseas, there will be programs similar to the ones discussed here.

CONCLUDING REMARKS

The role of nurses and midwives in supporting healthy communities is as important today as it was in the nineteenth century. Their leadership and social support roles are vital for individuals, families and communities. There are many examples of innovative practice that embrace the 'new' public health and which build social capital. Examples of nurses' impact on community health and empowerment are to be found across the life span in places where communities live, work and play.

REFLECTIVE QUESTIONS

1 Describe the role of nurses in establishing and sustaining healthy communities.

2 What are the key aspects of a community assessment? What local, national and international databases will you utilise?

3 What strategies will you utilise in supporting healthy communities?

RECOMMENDED READINGS

Duckett S J 2004 *The Australian health care system*, 2nd edn. Oxford University Press, Melbourne.

Hennessy D, Spurgeon P 2000 *Health policy and nursing*. Macmillan Press, London.

Keleher H, Murphy B 2004 *Understanding health: a determinants approach*. Oxford University Press, Melbourne.

McMurray A 2003 *Community health and wellness,* 2nd edn. Mosby, Sydney.

Muir Gray J A 2001 *Evidenced-based healthcare*. Churchill Livingstone, London.

CHAPTER TWENTY

Diversity challenges in the context of multicultural Australia

Akram Omeri

LEARNING OBJECTIVES

Upon completion of this chapter, the student should be able to:

▲ examine the disparities of cultural diversity that influence health access and outcomes for multicultural Australia;

▲ examine the major multicultural policy directions and their impact on healthcare systems and practice domains in Australia;

▲ critically analyse the relevance of social policy to the provision of healthcare and nursing services;

▲ understand the importance of minimising inequities in the provision of healthcare services in Australia and in contemporary nursing practice; and

▲ examine and discuss the impact of evidenced-based transcultural nursing knowledge in promotion of health and wellbeing of people from culturally and linguistically different backgrounds in Australia.

KEY WORDS

Cultural diversity, poverty, indigenous people, rural-remote, refugees, culturally congruent care

INTRODUCING MULTICULTURAL AUSTRALIA

Australia has been recognised as a culturally diverse society with advanced multicultural policies (Office of Multicultural Affairs 1989, National Multicultural Advisory Council 1999). In Australia, since World War II, cultural diversity has had a focus on ethnicity, which is characterised by differences in views on healthcare and lifeway practices, diversity in languages and religions of the approximately 200 cultures residing in this country, and diversity in the Aboriginal population, the nation's first people.

This diversity is underpinned by the wide range of contexts where nurses practice, often influenced by variation of land, climate and the settings/contexts where healthcare is delivered, such as rural-remote, community health, in the home, and a number of acute settings within or outside hospitals in urban settings. A shift from hospital to home and community care has been the trend in healthcare in the past two decades.

Inequality in health status also distinguishes groups from linguistically and culturally diverse backgrounds, including Aborigines. This chapter will examine issues and aspects relating to healthcare from rural-remote areas and refugees, and reflect on poverty as a growing social issue that impacts on the health and wellbeing of specific and diverse groups.

With the reduction in communicable diseases and death rates from major cancers and cardiovascular disease, the twentieth century saw a marked improvement in the health of Australians and an increase in life expectancy for most (Mathers et al 1999, Australian Institute of Health and Welfare 2000). However, in spite of such improvements, inequalities between socioeconomic groups continue and, for some groups, inequalities are on the increase (Burton 2004, Dobson 1999, Khabir 1999, Marmot 2000, Turrell & Mathers 2000, 2001).

Health is declared as a right not a privilege (International Council of Nurses 1973, Universal Declaration of Human Rights 1948, World Health Organization 1947). Over the past 50 years, inequalities have grown both between and within nations (Cornia 1999, World Bank 1999, 2000, Schrader 2004), with the rate of growth greater in recent decades (United Nations Development Programme 2002–2003). Paradoxically, although global wealth has never been greater, the distribution of wealth is 'extraordinarily unequal' (World Bank 2000, cited in Schrader 2004:17).

The purpose of this chapter is to inform and create a mindset for student nurses in Australia, for inquiry into the challenges of diversity, with the aim of seeing culture care as leading the promotion and provision of culturally meaningful care, and as an essential core of the profession of nursing. The desired outcomes are to:

▲ create an incentive for nurses to pursue transcultural nursing studies in order to further their sense of knowing about diversity beyond the celebration and rhetoric of multiculturalism;

▲ build upon transcultural nursing knowledge through research and to understand the implications of culture-specific knowledge for improving nursing practice; and

▲ develop sensitivity towards cultural diversity that brings unity, respect, tolerance and a fair go for all.

AUSTRALIA'S POPULATION: THE CULTURAL MOSAIC

In December 2004, Australia's projected population was 20,221,215. This projection was based on the estimated resident population as of 30 June 2004, when Australia celebrated having reached a target population of 20 million (Australian Bureau of Statistics 2001). In 2001, the Australian Bureau of Statistics reported that about 23% of Australian residents were born overseas and more than half of these were born in a non-English-speaking country (Singh & de Looper 2002, cited in Australian Institute of Health and Welfare 2002c).

Indigenous Australians (Aborigines and Torres Strait Islanders) comprised 2.2% of the total population. Of this number, the largest proportion (25.1%) resided in the Northern Territory and the smallest in Victoria (0.5%), according to the 2001 Census.

The 2001 Census also revealed changes in immigration patterns. Traditional sources of immigrants—United Kingdom as the majority with 5.5%, New Zealand 1.9% and Italy 1.2%—remained dominant, and the three most common ancestries were Australian (35.9%), English (33.9%) and Irish (10.2%).

However, the three most prominent languages spoken at home, after English, were listed as Chinese languages (2.1%), Italian (1.9%) and Greek (1.4%). In 1996–97, about 31% of Australia's intake was born in 'East Asia', including Southeast and Northeast Asia. These changes in spoken languages reflect changes in the sources of immigrants that have gradually broadened since the 'White Australia Policy' was relaxed three decades ago (Castles et al 1998).

The practice of classifying immigrants into those from English-speaking-backgrounds (ESB) and those from non-English-speaking-backgrounds (NESB) is criticised as being too broad, given the increasing diversity and complexity of the immigrant population (Iredale & Nivison-Smith 1995, cited in Castles et al 1998). The distinction reflects immigrants from ESBs as sharing the British-based culture, institutions and traditions extant in Australian society. It does not serve to reflect the diverse cultural bases of the increasingly large proportion of immigrants from other NESB cultures (Castles et al 1998).

The Australian Bureau of Statistics (2001) identified a number of religious denominations that have implications for health and nursing care. These are Buddhism, Hinduism, Islam and Judaism, with a significant number (1,571,633) recording no religious beliefs. Around 5224 people identified themselves as practising Australian Aboriginal traditional religions. These figures, indicative of cultural diversity by no means unique to Australia, have prompted governments to design policy frameworks to manage diversity.

Martin (1978) argues that multiculturalism was never 'the cause' but a necessary response to cultural diversity. She argues that previous government policies have failed to keep up with the reality of the growing cultural diversification of Australia, as a result of its postwar immigration program (Martin, cited in Hage & Couch 1999).

MULTICULTURAL POLICIES: ASSIMILATION TO INCLUSIVENESS

In the health area, two policy principles have emerged from the numerous multicultural policies developed over the past 30 years to deal with Australia's diversity. The first is 'access and equity' which, in practice, becomes equality of access to health services for all. The second is 'inclusiveness' which, when applied in practice, means the provision of culturally appropriate services to meet the needs of people from culturally and linguistically diverse backgrounds.

Table 20.1 lists the policy principles that have guided policy development from 1945–99. To gain a deeper understanding of the historical perspectives of multicultural policies, students are encouraged to refer to the many references provided (specifically, Commonwealth of Australia 1999a, National Multicultural Advisory Council 1999,

Table 20.1: Periods in immigrant policy development

Years	Policy	Features	Health policy implication
1945–70	Assimilation	Predominantly White Australian Anglo-Saxon policies	Absence of government assistance
1970–80	Integration	White Australia Policy relaxed and gradually abandoned Some cultural characteristics tolerated	Relevant services provided Welfare needs of migrants being addressed
1980–89	Multiculturalism	Pluralistic approach to immigration Policies to limit discrimination on racial and ethnic grounds Cultural and ethnic diversity becoming more accepted in Australian society Cultural identity, social justice and economic efficiency were adopted	Provision of various health services Equality of access to culturally appropriate services
1983	Mainstreaming	Redirecting service delivery from marginal to a central base Concern of government institutions based on social equity and access; economic efficiency and cultural identity	Promotion of culturally sensitive health services Equality of access to health services by immigrants
1999	Inclusiveness	Diversity Multicultural policies built upon civic duty, cultural respect, social equity and productive diversity The term multiculturalism to remain Inclusiveness	

Castles et al 1998, Garrett & Lin 1990, Office of Multicultural Affairs 1989), and also the publication section of the website of the Department of Immigration and Multicultural and Indigenous Affairs (2002, 2003).

Policy in practice

Policy directions have been criticised by many over the years. In highlighting the gaps between policy and practice at a conference designed to reflect upon Australia's multiculturalism, Castles (1999) proposed four objectives to achieve a fairer and more democratic society. These included spreading the rights and obligations of citizenship to permanent residents through multicultural citizenship and transnational belonging. He also advocates social inclusion and institutional change to remove cultural barriers to the full participation of all citizens.

Castles (1999) notes that changes over time to Australia's citizenship rules have yet to achieve a culturally neutral form of belonging based on actual societal membership irrespective of origins. He argues that full participation, in all areas of society, is a crucial part of multicultural citizenship (cited in Hage & Couch 1999).

In the Australian context, policies of inclusiveness have been criticised as monoculturalism in another guise, promoted by policies of integration (Hage & Couch 1999). Inclusiveness can have an homogenising impact upon cultural diversity, reducing its significance in practice. By extension, it can also devalue advanced practice in transcultural nursing by nullifying the worth of culture-specific nursing care that is meaningful and congruent with the cultural care needs of people. Misinterpretations of inclusiveness could lead to stereotyping, discrimination and cultural blindness (Omeri 2003) in the provision of health and welfare services, thus propagating inequalities in care practices.

The obvious diversity of Australia's population is not reflected in the provision of healthcare services, including nursing services. Improved transcultural education for students or a closer connection between education, practice and policy for nursing services is not apparent, despite significant moves on the part of transcultural nursing since the 1990s (as noted by Omeri 1996, 1997, 2000, Omeri et al 2002). In nursing and healthcare, diversity management is limited to ethno-specific services and cultural assessment to country of origin, religion, language spoken and the need for interpreters (Omeri 1997). Omeri concludes that the links between policy and practice and, more specifically, between nursing education and practice are abysmal and merely rhetorical.

Several diverse groups, including those with an ethnic orientation, Aborigines, refugees/asylum seekers and people in rural-remote areas, are chosen to demonstrate disadvantages of cultural diversity. A discussion on *Poverty profile of Australia* (Royal College of Nursing Australia 2004) will set the scene for addressing the reflective questions outlined for discussion at the end of the chapter.

IMPACT OF POVERTY ON HEALTH

Cultural factors in combination with poverty are recognised in Australia and overseas as having a significant impact upon health (Canadian Institute of Health Information 2003, Fuller et al 2004, Royal College of Nursing Australia 2004, Senate Community Affairs References Committee 2004, International Council of Nurses 2004a, 2004b). In 2004 there were about 1.2 billion people living in absolute poverty in developing and transition economies (Rawson 2004). The International Council of Nurses (2004b) states that poverty and health are linked in four ways:

1 ill health leads to poverty;

2 poverty leads to ill health;

3 good health is linked to higher income; and

4 higher income is linked to good health.

Income is a key factor in relation to poverty, but other factors are also significant for good health. In a broader definition of poverty, such things as access to health services, clean water, sanitation, literacy levels and infant mortality (United Nations Development Programme 2002–2003) are included.

Perceptions of poverty are different from country to country. For example, what is perceived as poverty in a country like Australia may be quite different from what is perceived as poverty in a country like Sudan. This widens the factors implicated in poverty to include such things as isolation, powerlessness, vulnerability and physical weakness (World Health Organization 1997).

Poverty and disease are inextricably linked in a direct correlation with wealth: the poorer the person the greater the incidence of ill health; the richer the person the less frequent the incidence of ill health. Disease often further impoverishes the poor (Freudenberg 2000).

Socioeconomic and environmental factors, such as low income, poor housing, overcrowding, job insecurity, unemployment, few community resources, poor education, social exclusion, reduced social approval and self-esteem, are known to have an impact upon health. While government policy can have a significant impact upon health by redistributing wealth and ensuring access to health services, poor social and economic circumstances contribute to disempowerment and hopelessness among the poor and serve to keep the poor in ill health (Schrader 2004).

To attack poverty the World Bank stresses the importance of governments in distributing and channelling resources into public services for healthcare and investing in education (World Bank 2000). Healthcare expenses are redistributed to the community where tax is paid according to the ability to pay. The most effective and efficient health systems are universal health insurance schemes, such as Medicare (Blendon et al 2002, Deeble 1999).

In Australia, changes have been implemented recently which have signalled a move away from tax-based support for health services. The changes, such as reducing bulk billing and the introduction of co-payments, expect more from consumers. This 'user pays' model impacts negatively upon people on lower incomes who are unable to meet the costs and, therefore, have reduced access to services or treatment. People's socioeconomic status affects their health throughout their life. The cumulative experience of social conditions across the life span impacts on health (Schrader 2004).

In Australia, several inquiries have been undertaken in an attempt to discover the extent of poverty in the country. One of the most significant and influential was undertaken by Henderson who led a Commission of Inquiry into Poverty in 1972 and produced the Henderson report. The inquiry focused on the extent of poverty and the groups most at risk, the income needs of people in poverty, and issues relating to housing and welfare services. Its main findings were:

▲ Over 10% of income units in 1972–73 were below the Commission's poverty line. A further 8% were defined as 'rather poor', having an income of less than 20% above that line.

▲ About 7% of income units were below the poverty line after housing costs were taken into account. Those renting from private landlords were the poorest group.

▲ About three-quarters of those below the poverty line before housing were not in the workforce.

▲ Overall, female sole-parent families comprise the largest proportion of very poor people.

▲ The group with the largest percentage gap between its income and the poverty line comprised large families on wages on or just above the minimum wage.

▲ Very few young men were voluntarily unemployed and thus below the poverty line (cited in Senate Community Affairs References Committee 2004).

In 2001, the National Centre for Social and Economic Modeling (NATSEM) reported that 13% of all Australians lived in poverty in the year 2000. The association between socioeconomic disadvantage and poor health has been widely researched in Australia and overseas (Harding et al 2001, Harding & Szukalska 2000, Australian Institute of Health and Welfare 1998). In brief, evidence to the Commission and a range of studies into poverty and deprivation have established that poverty is more likely to occur among particular groups in the population in Australia, including indigenous Australians, the unemployed and people dependent on social security benefits (Senate 2004). In Australia, many groups, including specific cultural groups such as indigenous Australians (Andrews et al 2002, Goold 2001), refugees (Omeri et al 2004, Proctor 2004a, 2004b, 2004c) and those in rural and remote areas (Jamrozik et al 2005, Jong et al 2005) of Australia, remain disadvantaged in accessing health services and in receiving appropriate and equitable care.

RURAL-REMOTE INEQUALITIES

The problem of poverty and disadvantage for people in many rural and regional areas across Australia is evidenced by the generally lower incomes, reduced access to services such as health, education and transport, as well as declining employment opportunities. These factors are compounded by the problems of distance and isolation (Royal College of Nursing Australia 2004).

The provision of services to rural and remote areas is problematic due to distance, low service density and the social and cultural adaptation needed to make them effective (Jong et al 2005). In cancer care, for example, Jong et al (2005) have highlighted the need for improved primary healthcare, and access to expert multidisciplinary services in a coordinated fashion for rural and remote populations. These authors call for cooperation between governments for the successful development of pathways with innovative information systems, to improve interaction between the many services in cancer care to address inequalities in cancer care in rural Australia.

The need to maintain an appropriately educated rural nursing workforce emerged as one of the major issues impacting on rural hospital service delivery in a study conducted by Kenny and Duckett (2003) that explored issues relating to the provision of services in rural hospitals in Victoria. In spite of the established need for postgraduate education for rural nurses, it was suggested that the future rural nursing workforce will need to be recruited from undergraduate courses in regional universities.

Bushy (2002) compared and contrasted nursing practice in rural areas, based on selected publications from Australia, Canada and the United States, to examine the rural phenomenon in greater depth and from an international perspective. The aim was to challenge nurses to collaborate, study, develop and refine the foundation of rural practice across these countries and cultures. Bushy observed that global economic forces are influencing healthcare delivery systems internationally. The health environment is tempered by: declining resources; increasing competition among international markets; and changing consumer demands and their expectations of healthcare providers. The findings from the literature revealed concerted efforts in all three nations to reduce cost, improve access, ensure quality and improve consumer satisfaction with healthcare. This in turn is placing greater demands and stress on healthcare professionals in urban as well as rural-remote areas, leading to burnout and consequent departure from the profession.

Internationally, changes are occurring in how healthcare is financed. In the United States, there is a trend towards less privatisation with an effort to expand and develop a 'seam-free' healthcare system (Bushy 2002:108). In Australia and Canada, the trend seems to be for more privatisation and less government management. In all three nations the trend is towards decentralisation of financial control and management of healthcare resources. In the United States it is decentralised from the federal to the state governments; in Canada, from the national government to provincial governments; and in Australia, from the federal government to state and territory governments. Unfortunately, states and provinces often do not have the financial resources to carry out federally mandated initiatives and that disadvantages rural-remote areas further (Bushy 2002).

Bushy (2002) found similarities in nursing practice in rural environments in the three countries and found that the role of rural nurses is expanding. In all three countries, greater numbers of nurses are being prepared for advanced practice roles, especially nurse practitioners, certified nurse midwives, and certified nurse anaesthetists. Similarly, nurse education programs in the three countries are planning curricula for expanded nursing practice roles (Bushy 2002, Hegney 1997a, 1997b, 2000).

A CASE FOR ABORIGINAL PEOPLE

Although the rural-remote population does not hold a specific cultural group in terms of ethnicity, it is home to many who are disadvantaged. Higher unemployment, distance, isolation, poor housing and lack of access to health and welfare services are some of the disadvantages they face. More than a third of Australians live outside major cities, with 3% living in remote or very remote areas (Australian Bureau of Statistics 2003, cited in Jong et al 2005). Rural and remote areas are home to many indigenous people, who represent a special culture of disadvantage in many ways, which is significant for diversity and nursing care.

Aboriginality: health inequality

The indigenous people of Australia are recognised as the traditional owners or original inhabitants of Australia (Bush & van Holst Pellekaan 1995, Goold 2001).

For indigenous people, spiritual wellbeing is a significant part of health (Winch 1989, Goold 2001, Bush & van Holst Pellekaan 1995, Eckermann et al 1996, Omeri & Ahern 1999).

Along with the welcome support for reconciliation, indigenous people encounter more negative responses from the larger population, such as racism and paternalism, which may influence their lifestyle practices (Eckermann et al 1996). Problem health areas for indigenous populations include: higher infant mortality rates and shorter life expectancy than the non-indigenous population; high suicide rates; poverty; unemployment; and land rights issues.

Health for Aborigines is wellbeing in all aspects of their identity. Identity for Aborigines is inextricably linked to family, community and the land. Ill health, therefore for Aborigines, is not just the presence of physical disease, but also alienation from those factors that comprise identity, culture, land and community, without which wellbeing may not be achieved.

Thus health is constructed as a community concept that includes physical, social, emotional, spiritual and cultural wellbeing (Bush & van Holst Pellekaan 1995, Omeri & Ahern 1999, National Aboriginal Health Strategy 1990, cited in Aboriginal and Torres Strait Islander Commission 2000).

REFUGEES: A CASE FOR CONCERN

Addressing disparities influencing access to health services and minimising inequalities in the provision of healthcare in Australia and in nursing practice have been highlighted in the research literature for refugees (McMurray 2003, Hertzman 2001, Kawachi & Kennedy 1999). Of the 5.7 million immigrants who have arrived and settled in Australia since World War II, 10% have been refugees or other humanitarian entrants (Refugee Council of Australia 2000, 2002).

In the past 50 years, over 600,000 refugees and displaced people have been resettled in Australia, many of whom were reported to have close family ties to Australia. The overall size of the Humanitarian Program quota in 2002–03 was 12,000 new places, the same as the preceding year. Of this number, 4000 places were set aside for use in the 'refugee' category; 7000 places were available for the Special Humanitarian Program; and a further 1000 places were made available to meet possible onshore needs (Department of Immigration and Multicultural and Indigenous Affairs 2002b).

Refugees may have experienced severe deprivation, trauma and torture that can lead to post-traumatic stress disorder (PTSD), a condition that can profoundly affect a person's health and capacity to resettle. There is a body of literature on the medical and psychological responses of people to war and conflict, and on the situation of Afghan refugees in Australia (Harris & Telfer 2001, Procter 2004b, 2004c, Silove et al 1998, Steel & Sil 2001, Sultan & O'Sullivan 2001) and internationally (Halimi 2002, Keyes 2000, Lipson & Omidian 1997). Specific factors that impact on resettlement, not unique to the Afghan people but poorly understood outside of relief agencies, are reviewed by Lipson and her associates as well as others (Khamis 1998, Summerfield 2000). It should be noted that these factors affect the Afghan people's perceptions of the resettlement process and have the ability to create inherent conflicts of understanding between refugees, refugee support agencies and host countries.

AUSTRALIAN GOVERNMENT NATIONAL PRIORITIES IN RESOURCE ALLOCATION

The current national priorities for action within the Integrated Humanitarian Settlement Strategy (IHSS) framework, as described by the Department of Immigration, Multicultural and Indigenous Affairs (2002a, 2002b), include:

▲ English-language training;

▲ access to the labour market;

▲ settlement information;

▲ access to housing;

▲ enhancing support to sponsors of migrants and refugees;

▲ translating and interpreter services;

▲ integrating services for humanitarian entrants; and

▲ enhancing support for the ethnic aged (Department of Immigration and Multicultural and Indigenous Affairs 2002b, Refugee Council of Australia 2002:11).

IMPLICATIONS FOR PROVISION OF CULTURALLY COMPETENT NURSING AND HEALTHCARE

Leininger's theory of Culture Care Diversity and Universality (1991–94) highlights the important role nurses can play in promoting culturally congruent health and nursing care to disadvantaged populations. For example:

▲ Care (caring) is essential for wellbeing, health, healing, growth, survival, and to face handicaps or death.

▲ Care is the essence of nursing and health and a distinct, dominant, central and unifying focus (Leininger 1991a).

▲ The cultural context and care values makes a major difference in how care is expressed and care takes on meanings to clients and especially families or cultures.

▲ Cultural care values, beliefs and practices are influenced by and tend to be embedded and influenced in the worldview, language, religious (or spiritual), kinship (social), political (or legal), educational, economic, technological, ethnohistorical and environmental contexts.

▲ Every human culture has generic (lay, folk, or indigenous or emic) care knowledge and practices, and usually professional (etic) care knowledge and practices which vary transculturally.

▲ Culturally congruent or beneficial nursing care can only occur when the individual, group, family, community or culture care values, expressions or patterns are known and used appropriately and in meaningful ways by the nurse with the people (Leininger 1991b:84–6).

These assumptions can be helpful to nurses seeking to understand, respect and value cultural differences impacting upon care for diverse populations in diverse contexts.

There are countless studies to support the assertion that when care is culturally congruent with the values and beliefs of people, health and healing will improve in quality and cost-effective ways. The *Journal of Transcultural Nursing* (1989–present) represents one example of an international refereed journal, which regularly reports on evidence-based research in transcultural and cross-cultural nursing. Transcultural nursing research also demonstrates that when care meets the cultural lifeways of people, access to health services improves. Application of Leininger's three modes of actions and decisions as portrayed in the Sun-rise Enabler (Leininger & McFarland 2002), based on the theory of culture care diversity and universality, could prove beneficial. These action modes, described briefly here as a guide to the provision of culture-specific nursing care to diverse populations, are:

▲ *Cultural care preservation/maintenance.* Evidenced-based transcultural knowledge will inform practitioners as to what culture care modes could or need to be maintained and preserved without clashing with treatment modalities that need to be applied. For example, for Afghan refugees in New South Wales, understanding of Islam and its code of practice is extremely important. Their religiosity and their practices need to be understood and preserved by nurses and other health service providers to promote culturally meaningful care and respect for their beliefs in order to achieve the best healthcare outcomes (Omeri et al 2004).

▲ *Cultural care accommodation/negotiation.* Accommodating culture in healthcare in culturally meaningful ways is the provision of health-related information in the language of specific cultural groups. Knowledge of cultural and religious festivities relating to significant life events, such as birth and death, is also important transcultural knowledge that needs to be understood and accommodated by nurses and other healthcare professions when appropriate.

▲ *Cultural care repatterning/restructuring.* Repatterning a cultural lifeway is a process of change, which involves giving up the old culturally meaningful ways and adopting new and different care patterns. This process of change is often a three-way process involving the clients as receivers of care, and the nurse or other healthcare professionals as providers of care, as well as the healthcare system. In some aspects this change is very slow and at times may not be possible. It involves a great deal of negotiation and involvement of the clients.

Transcultural nursing allows nurses to think about what may be different or similar among people relating to their special care needs and concerns. As nurses discover the client's particular cultural beliefs and values, they learn ways to provide culturally sensitive, compassionate and competent care that is satisfying and meaningful to the client and congruent with their lifeway practices (Leininger & McFarland 2002). This process of discovery of cultural knowledge, in addition to enabling nurses to develop deep understanding and appreciation for cultures, will allow nurses to develop insights about their own (self-awareness) cultural background and how to use such knowledge appropriately with clients, families, communities and healthcare services.

Transcultural nursing concepts address an essential domain of knowledge to guide transcultural nursing practice. Cultural imposition is one transcultural nursing concept that often leads to cultural clash, dissatisfaction, intolerance, anger, prejudice, discrimination, non-compliance, and a host of other behaviours. Cultural imposition practices, which often stem from cultural ignorance, cultural blindness, ethnocentrism and biases, remain a major and unrecognised problem in nursing. Cultural imposition is defined as: '. . . the tendency of an individual or group to impose their beliefs, values, and patterns of behaviour upon another culture for varied reasons' (Leininger 1995:66, Leininger & McFarland 2002:51). Cultural imposition practices between nurses and clients can be observed in situations in which the nurse believes his or her views are the right, best and most therapeutic professional way and that the client's views are strange, bizarre, and not desirable for their health (Leininger & McFarland 2002:52).

Health and illness are largely culturally defined, constructed and maintained, and so local health systems tend to fit their values and practices (Kleinman 1980, Helman 1994). Additionally, Western scientific theories based on high technologies may be of limited benefit in some cultures because of cultural differences.

Underpinning transcultural nursing are values of equity, justice, fairness, understanding and tolerance of difference. Leininger's theory has been used to identify underserved ethnic populations within a community, and is described as the first step in eliminating inequalities in healthcare among racial and ethnic minorities, and providing culturally congruent healthcare (Zust & Moline 2003).

Transcultural nursing concepts provide ways to identify ethnocentric practices that come about through cultural blindness. Culturally sensitive and aware transcultural nurses, as primary health and nursing care providers, can advocate on behalf of clients, families and communities for healthcare that is equitable because it is culturally congruent, culturally competent and accessible.

CULTURALLY COMPETENT NURSING CARE FOR CULTURALLY DIVERSE POPULATIONS

Culture reflects the values, beliefs, customs, thoughts, actions, communications and belief systems of a racial, ethnic, religious or social group. Competence, on the other hand, implies a capacity to function within the cultural context of an integrated pattern of behaviour, as described by a designated group, community or an institution. Combining these concepts enables a system, community, institutions or group of professionals to develop a congruent set of behaviours and policies to function effectively in a culturally diverse situation. Cultural competence means honouring diversity and respecting differences in interpersonal styles and attitudes. It also reflects those values that underpin policy, administration, education and services provided (Mays et al 2002).

Cultural competence has been defined as: '. . . a set of congruent behaviours, practices, attitudes, and policies related to embracing cultural differences that are integrated into a system or agency or among professionals' (Mays et al 2002:139). It means having the knowledge, awareness and sensitivity of culture sufficient to meet the culture care needs of individuals, families, groups and communities. It involves respect for difference and a desire to learn and accept diversities.

Some view cultural competence as a continuing process of becoming culturally aware, gaining cultural knowledge, and achieving cultural skills (Campinha-Bacote 1999, Leininger & McFarland 2002). It is also described as cultural openness in professional care contexts, achieved through cultural self-awareness and continuing development of transcultural skills (Wenger 1999). Cultural competence refers not only to individual health professionals but also to service agencies, systems and institutions that have the capacity and ability to respond to the unique needs of populations different from the mainstream (Isaacs & Benjamin 1991, cited in Mays et al 2002).

Assuring culturally competent nursing and healthcare is the responsibility of systems, agencies and institutions (Omeri 2003). There is a growing understanding revealed in the literature that organisations providing culturally and linguistically appropriate services (i.e. culturally competent services) have the potential to reduce cultural and ethnic health disparities (Anderson et al 2003).

The nursing profession is responsible for developing cultural competence in its practitioners, not only in its novitiates, but also on a continuing basis as measured by the demonstration of requisite skills, knowledge and attitudes. However, there is no agreement as to how continuing competence should be monitored, nor is there any provision for continuing education in transcultural nursing for faculty and nurse administrators in Australia.

The relationship between continuing education and nursing practice relating to cultural competence remains an area to be evaluated in spite of the development of standards designed to foster excellence in transcultural nursing practice. Leuning et al (2002) proposed a set of standards for transcultural nursing, which are based on Leininger's culture care theory and Campinha-Bacote's model of cultural competence. These standards are intended to provide criteria for the evaluation of nursing care, a tool for teaching and learning, as well as increasing public confidence in the nursing profession (Leuning et al 2002).

CONCLUDING REMARKS

Meeting the healthcare needs of diverse populations in Australia is one of the greatest challenges faced by nurses and healthcare professionals. This chapter has provided an overview of population trends relating to cultural diversity and the ways it impacts on the roles of nurses and healthcare professionals. It has highlighted issues relating to globalisation and the impact of poverty on health and subsequent disadvantage of populations such as those in rural-remote areas, Aboriginal people, and refugees in accessing health and other services. Furthermore, the impact of policy directions on healthcare and education were discussed. Culturally congruent and competent nursing and healthcare were proposed as a way to improve practice in caring for such populations. This chapter also highlighted the importance of transcultural nursing knowledge and its application for practice in an attempt to improve the health and wellbeing of the diverse populations in Australia.

REFLECTIVE QUESTIONS

1   What are some of the factors influencing healthcare of diverse populations in Australia? Reflect upon those discussed in this chapter.

2   How can poverty be defined? How is it linked to health?

3   Take some time to think about your own cultural beliefs in relation to health and healthcare. How might your own beliefs be similar or different from someone from another culture?

RECOMMENDED READINGS

Andrews M, Boyle J 2003 *Transcultural concepts in nursing care*, 4th edn. Lippincott Williams & Wilkins, Philadelphia.

Leininger M, McFarland M 2002 *Transcultural nursing concepts, theories, research and practices*, 3rd edn. McGraw Hill, New York.

Leininger M, McFarland M 2004 *Culture care diversity and universality: a worldwide theory of nursing*, 2nd edn. Jones & Bartletts, Boston.

Omeri A 2003 Meeting diversity challenges: pathway of 'advanced' transcultural nursing practice in Australia. *Contemporary Nurse* 15(3):175–87.

Omeri A, Malcolm P, Ahern M, Wellington B 2002 Meeting the challenges of cultural diversity in the academic setting. *Nurse Education in Practice* 3:5–22.

The author acknowledges Helen Hamilton, consulting editor, who helped prepare this chapter (helenham@bigpond.com).

CHAPTER TWENTY-ONE

Becoming a critical thinker

Steve Parker & Judith Clare

LEARNING OBJECTIVES

At the completion of this chapter, the student will be able to:

- ▲ describe the essential nature of critical thinking;

- ▲ describe the main characteristics of a critical thinker;

- ▲ explain the basic structure of an argument;

- ▲ apply the basic structure of an argument to various areas of nursing practice; and

- ▲ identify resources for further reading and the study of critical thinking.

KEY WORDS
Thinking, reflection, action, evaluation, argument, induction, premise, nursing process, decision making

WHAT IS CRITICAL THINKING?

There are a variety of definitions of critical thinking and, as Richard Paul (1993) suggests, we need to be careful about relying on any one definition. In essence, however, critical thinking refers to the activity of *questioning what is usually taken for granted*.

Whether we are aware of it or not, all behaviour is based on certain values, assumptions and beliefs. These form the basis for our decisions to act in certain ways. In a professional context such as nursing practice, everything that we think, say or do is the result of a complex web of beliefs, values and assumptions that have formed as a result of our life experiences. As we grow up in our family, attend school, participate in religious communities, associate with friends, watch television, read newspapers, and work for various employers, we develop a 'pair of spectacles' through which we understand and interpret the world and all that happens in it. Just as a person who wears glasses eventually becomes unaware that they are even wearing them, so too each of us adjusts to our world-view 'spectacles' until, often, we are completely unaware what values, beliefs and assumptions are influencing us in a specific situation.

Critical thinking means stopping and reflecting on the reasons for doing things the way they are done or for experiencing things the way they are—focusing on what is frequently taken for granted and evaluating the values, beliefs and assumptions that are held, and asking whether or not what is done and thought is justifiable or not. These characteristics of critical thinking imply a self-consciousness of what, how and why we are thinking, with the intention of improving thinking. In short, 'critical thinking is thinking about your thinking while you're thinking in order to make your thinking better' (Paul 1993). Improving thinking is essential because it is intimately related to the many decisions that need to be made each day. The quality of our lives is determined by the quality of our decisions, and the quality of our decisions is determined by the quality of our reasoning (Schick & Vaughn 1995). In particular, '[i]f nurses are to deal effectively with complex change, increased demands and greater accountability, they must become skilled in higher level thinking and reasoning abilities' (Simpson & Courtney 2002).

An important aspect of critical thinking is healthy scepticism. This scepticism is necessary because there are many attempts to persuade people to accept various claims. These attempts to persuade also occur in professional contexts. For example, research reports suggest changes to practice; peers argue that their way of acting is the right one; therapists promote various interventions; administrators argue that certain changes need to be made to the workplace; and so on. Often these claims are contradictory, so they cannot all be acceptable.

Practitioners need to sort through all these, often competing, claims. To accept them all without question will, at best, be highly confusing and, at worst, may endanger the lives of others if actions are based on wrong information or conclusions. To adopt an attitude of healthy scepticism means to cautiously listen to or read the claims that others make, carefully evaluating their legitimacy, and not rushing to accept a conclusion without careful thought.

It is possible, of course, to become too pedantic, resulting in inaction because we are not prepared to accept anything unless it is 100% proven. This is why the scepticism needs to be healthy. There is a limit to what can be known for certain. And part of critical thinking is knowing these limits and making the best evaluation under the circumstances.

THE RELATIONSHIP BETWEEN CRITICAL AND CREATIVE THINKING

Critical thinking is not the same as creative thinking. According to Miller and Babcock (1996), creative thinking is, among other things, more divergent, messy, unpredictable, provocative, spontaneous and playful than critical thinking. They describe critical thinking as selective, orderly, predictable, analytical, judgmental and evaluative.

Creative thinking, although different from critical thinking, is an essential, complementary process to critical thinking. As a practitioner, there are many situations that arise that do not fit with the ideal or that are not predictable. No individual person for whom nurses care ever fits the 'average', because each person and situation is unique. In order to solve problems for these unique situations and individuals, the practitioner needs to be able to develop new approaches and solutions so that all parties have their needs met. Miller and Babcock suggest that:

> Creative thinking is very useful when what we know and what we know how to do are not working, including the rules of reason, common sense, gravity, and routine. The creative thinker is willing to think wildly, without having any idea where her or his path of thinking may lead. Deliberative cognition is temporarily held in abeyance (Miller & Babcock 1996:120).

Because creative thinking is so 'chaotic' it means that it needs to be evaluated to ensure that any conclusions that are reached are appropriate. In this regard, Ruggiero understands the mind to have two phases:

> It both produces ideas and judges them. These phases are intertwined; that is, we move back and forth between them many times in the course of dealing with a problem, sometimes several times in the span of a few seconds (Ruggiero 1998:81).

In the past, critical thinking has often been presented apart from creative thinking. However, in practice, creative and critical thinking go hand-in-hand. Without creative thinking, critical thinking would be dry and mechanical. Without critical thinking, creative thinking would be chaotic and inefficient. As Ruggiero (1998:81) asserts, '[t]o study the art of thinking in its most dynamic form [where creative and critical thinking are intertwined] would be difficult at best'. Consequently, in practice, we need to consider them separately. However, although critical thinking and creative thinking are distinct from each other, they should never be separated.

THE CHARACTERISTICS OF CRITICAL THINKING

So what are the characteristics that a critical thinker will demonstrate? Jacobs et al (1997) have developed a set of observable skills that indicate the presence of critical thinking. These are grouped into categories, as described below.

First, a critical thinker needs the ability to integrate information from all relevant sources by being able to distinguish between relevant and irrelevant data, validate data which are obtained, recognise when data are missing, predict multiple outcomes, and recognise the consequences of actions.

Second, to think critically means to be able to examine assumptions by recognising them when they are present, detect bias, identify assumptions that are not stated, recognise the relationships of action or inaction, and transfer thoughts and concepts to diverse contexts, or develop alternative courses of action.

Third, it is important for the critical thinker to be able to identify relationships and patterns. This includes recognising inconsistencies or fallacies of logic, working out generalisations, developing a plan of action consistent with a model, and, where appropriate, seeking out alternative models.

Jacobs et al offer a definition of critical thinking that incorporates all these characteristics:

> Critical thinking is the repeated examination of problems, questions, issues, and situations by comparing, simplifying, synthesizing information in an analytical, deliberative, evaluative, decisive way (Jacobs et al 1997:20).

Many more examples of various ways of describing the characteristics of critical thinking could be offered. One way of summarising these is to focus on critical thinking as reasoning. The heart of reasoning is the argument. In what follows, the nature of argument will be described, followed by a survey of the ways in which arguments 'appear' in nursing. Suggestions will then be offered regarding the way in which the principles of critical thinking might be applied in these areas. By doing so, the way in which this approach synthesises the skills of critical thinking will become obvious.

WHAT IS AN ARGUMENT?

In colloquial language the word 'argument' is often used for a shouting match between two people who are having a disagreement where the participants are very angry, abusive or physically aggressive. There may be shouting, pointing of fingers, threats, crying, name-calling, and so on.

However, in critical thinking, the term 'argument' does not apply to these situations. In fact, these situations are the very opposite of critical thinking. In critical thinking an argument consists of a conclusion and one or more reasons that are intended to support the conclusion. Figure 21.1 shows the relationship between these parts of an argument. Each reason may or may not have evidence that is intended to support the reason or reasons.

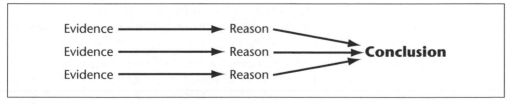

Figure 21.1 Components of an argument

Here is an example of an argument:

Every person has the right to choose how they live their lives. Therefore, a person has the right to choose to practise life-threatening behaviours if they wish.

This is an argument because it has a conclusion ('A person has the right to choose to practise life-threatening behaviours if they wish') and a reason intended to support that conclusion ('Every person has the right to choose how they live their lives'). At this stage, we are not concerned whether this is a good argument or not, only with what makes something an argument. If it were desirable, a person presenting this argument could provide some evidence for the first statement by drawing attention, for example, to various statements of human rights, the constitutions of countries, or discussions about ethics. So an argument needs to have the following:

▲ a conclusion; and

▲ one or more reasons intended to support the conclusion.

WHAT MAKES A SOUND ARGUMENT?

For an argument to be sound, three criteria need to be met. First, the reasons need to be acceptable to the person evaluating the argument. Second, the reasons need to be relevant. And, third, the reasons need to provide adequate grounds for accepting the conclusion. Govier (1992) offers a useful way to remember these three criteria, which she calls the conditions of argument. If the first three letters of the word argument (ARG) are taken on their own, each letter stands for one of the conditions of argument. That is:

A Acceptability
R Relevance
G Grounds

Govier's definitions of each of these conditions is also useful:

▲ *Acceptability*: The premises [reasons] are acceptable when it is reasonable for those to whom the argument is addressed to believe these premises. There is good reason to accept the premises—even if they are not known for certain to be true. And there is no good evidence known to those to whom the argument is addressed that would indicate either that the premises are false or that they are doubtful.

▲ *Relevance*: [Premises are relevant to the conclusion] when they give at least some evidence in favor of the conclusion's being true. They specify factors, evidence, or reasons that do count toward establishing the conclusion. They do not merely describe distracting aspects that lead you away from the real topic with which the argument is supposed to be dealing or that do not tend to support the conclusion.

▲ *Grounds*: The premises provide sufficient or good grounds for the conclusion. In other words, considered together, the premises give sufficient reason to make it rational to accept the conclusion. This statement means more than that the premises are relevant. Not only do they count as evidence for the conclusion, they provide enough evidence, or enough reasons, taken together, to make it reasonable to accept the conclusion (Govier 1992:68–9).

The following example illustrates these criteria:

Nurses must have a practising certificate to be employed as a nurse.
Sue does not have a practising certificate.
Therefore, Sue is not permitted to be employed as a nurse.

Statements 1 and 2 are both reasons, which are intended to support the conclusion in Statement 3. If this is a sound argument, then the reasons must be relevant and acceptable, and they must provide adequate grounds for accepting the conclusion.

Statement 1 is certainly acceptable. Most countries have a requirement that nurses need to be licensed to practice. Statement 2 is hypothetical, so we will assume that it is true for the sake of the discussion. All the reasons, then, are acceptable. The two reasons are also relevant to the issue under consideration.

The next question is whether these reasons provide adequate grounds for accepting the conclusion. We can test this out by asking:

Is it possible to reject the conclusion and still believe the reasons to be true?

In other words, could one believe that Sue could practise and still believe that the two reasons offered are true? In this case, the answer is no. If it is true that a nurse must have a practising certificate to practise, and Sue does not have one, one is 'compelled' to accept the conclusion that Sue cannot practise. This argument, then, is a sound one.

Another example will illustrate a poor argument:

Everyone's hair falls out when undergoing chemotherapy.
Jo is undergoing chemotherapy.
Therefore, Jo's hair will fall out.

First, are the reasons acceptable? Does a person's hair fall out when they are undergoing chemotherapy? Sometimes it does, but not necessarily everyone's. So this reason is not acceptable because, although some people's hair falls out, not everyone's does. For the sake of this discussion, the second reason can be accepted (that Jo is undergoing chemotherapy).

Both of the reasons are relevant, and so the final question is whether the reasons offered provide adequate grounds for accepting that Jo's hair will fall out. The answer is no because the first reason was false. Although it might be true that Jo's hair will fall out, it is not possible to predict it because not everyone's hair does when they are on chemotherapy.

To summarise:

▲ An argument consists of a conclusion, with one or more relevant reasons that are intended to support the conclusion.

▲ Evidence may or may not be offered to support each reason.

▲ A sound argument is one in which the reason(s) are acceptable and provide adequate grounds for accepting the conclusion.

There are a few technical terms that need to be remembered in regard to what has been covered so far.

▲ A *reason* can also be called a *premise*.

▲ The question of whether reasons provide grounds for the conclusion is a question of *validity*. In everyday conversation, the word validity often has a broader meaning. In critical thinking, it is used to refer to the logical relationship between the reasons and the conclusion.

▲ When an argument has reasons that are acceptable and is valid (i.e. the reasons provide adequate grounds for accepting the conclusion) then the argument is said to be *sound*.

It is important to note that an argument can be valid but unsound. For example, the following argument is valid but unsound:

> All nurses are female.
> Jo is a nurse.
> Therefore, Jo is female.

Statement 1 is not true, of course. Some nurses are male. Statement 2 can be assumed to be true. Because Statement 1 is false, we already know that this argument is unsound. But is it valid? Yes it is. If Statement 1 were true, the acceptance of Statement 3 would be unavoidable. This means that the argument is logically valid, but it is not sound—that is, it is not a sound argument.

CRITICAL THINKING IN NURSING

Critical thinking, in essence, means being able to identify the presence of an argument in any form and evaluate it. Once what makes a sound argument, and the questions needed to be asked to evaluate it are known, it is possible to assess any argument that is encountered. Critical thinking means applying to this task thinking which has the characteristics discussed above.

This basic approach can be applied to many areas within nursing. In the following sections some examples of these areas will be surveyed, how the basic framework introduced above applies to that area will be discussed, and some guidelines for thinking critically about issues in the respective area will be offered. The overlaying of the structure of argument onto the various areas in nursing builds on the work of Mayer and Goodchild (1995) in their discussion of critical thinking in psychology.

Clinical practice

In clinical practice, decisions are constantly being made to act in certain ways for the benefit of clients. These actions can be beneficial or have serious consequences for the health and wellbeing of the people a nurse is working for or with. It is essential that these interventions be considered critically. Figure 21.2 illustrates the application of the basic argument framework to clinical practice.

As can be seen, very little alteration is necessary. The equivalent of the conclusion is the particular action that has been, or will be, performed. Each of a nurse's actions should be able to be justified by appealing to an appropriate set of reasons. These reasons, in turn, must be based on high-quality evidence.

In the past, many of the actions and interventions of nurses have been based on tradition, folklore, or no evidence at all. In recent years, however, the developing

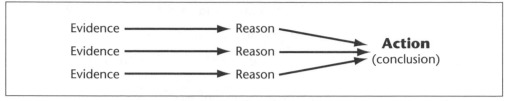

Figure 21.2 The basic argument framework

professional status of nursing has resulted in more concern about the basis for nursing action. There is a growing and strengthening movement called evidence-based practice, which promotes an attitude of thinking critically about what is done by nurses and asking on what basis can what is done be justified.

The increasing interest of consumers in their own healthcare has also had an effect. People are no longer willing to allow health professionals to make all the decisions for them and are demanding higher quality care. The increasing incidence of litigation has also motivated a concern for basing nursing action on high-quality evidence.

On an individual level, a nurse should be able to justify any action performed on behalf of a client. The reasons need to be based on solid evidence. The source of this evidence may take many forms, including personal experience, traditions handed down between 'generations' of nurses, and what is taught during nurse education. However, on their own, these sources of knowledge are not adequate. A formal process for exploring nursing knowledge is needed which allows the testing of ideas and the validation of actions and interventions.

The activity of formal research provides this opportunity. Nursing research will be examined below from a critical thinking perspective. First, however, there are a number of questions that can be asked about practice, which will help nurses think critically about it. When reflecting on an action or intervention, ask the following questions:

▲ What are the reasons for acting or intervening in the way that is planned?

▲ What evidence is available which supports the reasons for acting in this way?

▲ Are the reasons relevant to the issue that is being considered?

▲ Are there other reasons that need to be considered?

▲ Is there any evidence that raises questions about the manner of acting or intervening?

▲ Do the reasons provide adequate grounds for acting in the planned way?

▲ Are there alternative actions or interventions that could be chosen and the reasons still be acceptable in these situations?

The nursing process

The nursing process is a common framework for making practice decisions in nursing; therefore, it will be briefly explored in relation to critical thinking. The steps of the nursing process are:

▲ collection of subjective and objective data;

▲ arrival at a diagnosis of the client's problem(s);

- planning of appropriate nursing interventions in response to the problem(s);

- implementation of the planned intervention(s); and

- ongoing evaluation of the effectiveness of the intervention(s) in relation to the client's problem(s).

The nursing process can be summarised in three 'phases':

1   Diagnosis.

2   Intervention.

3   Evaluation.

Each of these three phases can be understood as an argument (remember the technical meaning of the term argument). Figure 21.3 illustrates this.

The diagnosis is the equivalent of the conclusion in an argument. The data that are collected come from observations of the patient as well as information provided by the client, relatives, friends, past history, and so on. These raw data need to be interpreted and take on meaning in the context of developing a diagnosis. Finally, on the basis of the meaning of the data, a conclusion is arrived at in the form of a diagnosis.

Of course, the description here is somewhat simplistic. The actual process is much richer and more complex than this. However, understanding the process of diagnosis as an argument leads us to ask questions such as the following:

- Are the data collected accurate? If not, how reliable are they?

- Have the data been understood and interpreted correctly?

- Are the data and their interpretation relevant to the diagnosis that has been chosen?

- Does the interpretation of the data provide adequate grounds for arriving at the diagnosis?

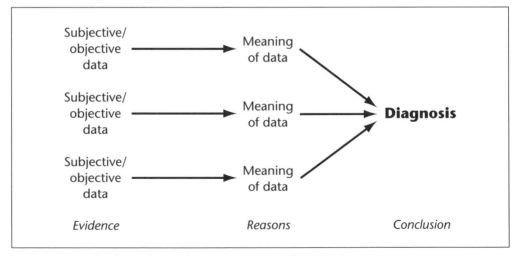

Figure 21.3 The three phases of nursing represented as an argument

▲ Are there any other diagnoses that could possibly fit the data that have been collected? Are any of these more consistent with the data?

A similar process applies to the intervention and evaluation phases. Interventions and evaluation criteria must be justified to support claims of improvement, deterioration or preservation of the status quo. Figures 21.4 and 21.5 illustrate the structure of argument related to these two phases.

Thinking critically about research

The need for nursing research and the current focus on evidence-based practice has been described above. Nursing research provides the evidence nurses need to evaluate the appropriateness of nursing practice, helps to raise new questions for nurses to explore, and provokes new ways of looking at what nurses do.

Nurses may relate to research in three ways. A nurse may be a 'consumer' of research, a researcher, or both. In this discussion, we will be focusing particularly on the role of research consumer.

It has already been argued that nurses must base their practice on high-quality evidence. The results of nursing research form the most significant source of this evidence for nurse practitioners. Nurses must avail themselves of the latest research in their area of practice, and this means that some understanding of the process is important.

Every research project suffers from limitations and flaws of some sort or another. So nurses cannot take a research report and automatically assume that it provides them with the best guidance for practice. The nurse needs to think critically about research reports. Understanding a research report to be an argument assists in thinking critically about the conclusions it draws (Mayer & Goodchild 1995). Mayer and

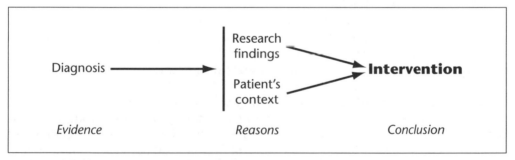

Figure 21.4 The structure of argument: intervention

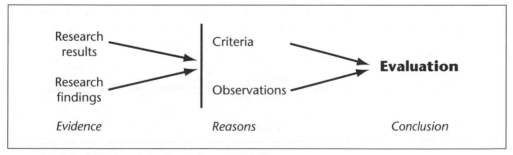

Figure 21.5 The structure of argument: evaluation

Goodchild (1995) discuss the way in which any research can be understood as an argument. Figure 21.6 illustrates this approach.

Given this understanding, it is possible to formulate a number of questions to help think critically about research:

▲ What is the assertion that is being made in the research report? What type of assertion is it? What type of evidence would be needed to be convinced of the truth of the assertion?

▲ What sort of evidence is offered to support the assertion being made? Is the evidence relevant to the assertion being made? Is adequate information provided to convince the reader that the evidence has been collected rigorously?

▲ Does the evidence offered provide adequate grounds for accepting the assertion that is being made? Is it possible to think of any other conclusions that could be drawn from the evidence offered? Are these alternative solutions more reasonable than the assertion made in the report?

▲ Does the theoretical explanation make sense? Are there alternative explanations that make more sense? Does the application of Occam's Razor (the principle that the simplest explanation is most likely to be the right one) make any difference to the likelihood of the explanation being correct?

Asking these questions in relation to any research report heightens one's awareness that the conclusions of research are not always correct, nor is the process in arriving at that conclusion automatically sound. This promotes a careful assessment of new nursing practice proposals and consequent higher levels of safety in practice.

Thinking about ethics

Another essential area of which nurses need to be aware is ethics. Thinking ethically means to be able to justify what is done in terms of ethical principles. All behaviour needs to be ethical. Although there are high-profile issues such as euthanasia, abortion and organ transplantation that demand a great deal of attention, they are, perhaps, not the most important issues for nurses.

Issues such as the style of communicating with a patient, the facilitation of the signing of a consent form, communication with other professional colleagues and patients, the management of work rosters, the provision of childcare for employees, the influencing of clients in choosing treatment options—all need to be considered in ethical terms if the individual nurse is to practise with integrity and fulfil his or her obligations to clients.

Most professional bodies have documented codes of ethics and the nursing profession is no different. For example, the *Code of ethics for nurses in Australia*

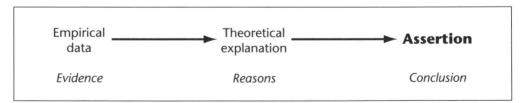

Figure 21.6 Understanding research as an argument

(Australian Nursing Council Inc 1993, revised 2002) contains six value statements for nurses to 'use as a guide in reflecting on the degree to which their practice demonstrates the stated value'. As the Code points out, however, a:

> . . . Code of Ethics is not intended to provide a formula for the resolution of ethical problems, nor can it adequately address the definitions and exploration of terms and concepts which are part of the study of ethics. Nurses are autonomous moral agents and sometimes may adopt a personal moral stance that would make participation in certain procedures morally unacceptable to them.

Because of this, nurses need to develop skills to be able to think through these issues and evaluate various options for practice. Understanding ethical thinking as an argument can help in this task. Figure 21.7 illustrates the components of an ethical argument. Each of these components will now be examined in relation to critical thinking.

The situation

Ethical thinking is often taught using highly controversial case studies that involve an often unresolvable dilemma between competing principles. However, a number of false impressions may be gained from this. One possible false impression is that 'the continued use of controversial examples serves to exaggerate the extent to which morality, as distinct from moral theory, is controversial' (Coope 1996).

In reality, ethical thinking should pervade all activities, and ethical questions about practice should be continually asked. Ethical thinking should be an everyday activity, which may not always be about problems.

Usually, we find ourselves in situations where a decision needs to be made about how to act towards another person. These situations continually occur for nurses. For example, a patient might require a sponge in bed. This may not appear to be a situation where ethical thinking needs to take place. But, as this example is explored below, it will be seen that ethical thinking is fundamental to ensuring that the best care is provided.

The first thing to do when thinking ethically is to be aware of as much about the situation as is possible. Too often assumptions are made on the basis of past experience, but every person is different and has unique needs.

The principles

Everyone has a system of principles (values) which guide their lives and how they act. Some of these will be conscious; others may be unconscious. In healthcare, four principles have been identified as an essential starting point for ethical thinking. They are:

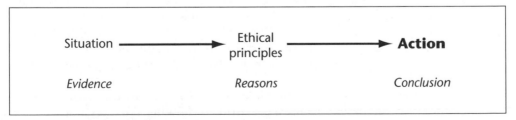

Figure 21.7 The components of an ethical argument

1 *Autonomy*: the right a person has to direct their own life and make their own decisions.

2 *Beneficence*: the responsibility of actively doing good.

3 *Non-maleficence*: the responsibility to actively avoid doing harm.

4 *Justice*: the responsibility to be fair in the way we treat others.

After gaining a knowledge of the situation, the next step is to ask which of the principles (values) are relevant to consider in the particular situation in which the nurse finds themselves. In the example of the person who needs to be washed in bed, the issue of autonomy is clearly relevant. How is autonomy to be ensured in this particular situation? How will the patient be empowered to make their own decisions about their hygiene and the way they wish to maintain it?

The principle of beneficence is also relevant. The whole reason for instituting the patient washing in bed is because it is believed it is good to promote hygiene. It is possible, however, that beneficence may spill over into a denial of the person's autonomy. When this happens, nurses are acting paternalistically—doing what they think is best for the patient—even if the patient does not agree with the nurse. Paternalism needs to be rigorously justified because it overrides a person's fundamental right to autonomy.

Many examples can be found of situations where paternalism occurs: imposing medication on a psychotic individual; or legally enforcing a blood transfusion for a child of a Jehovah's Witness parent. Unfortunately, on many occasions paternalistic attitudes prevail without adequate ethical justification.

Action

Once the situation is understood and the implications of the relevant ethical principles have been thought through, it is necessary to make a decision about how to act. Often this will not be easy. Sometimes ethical principles conflict with each other (such as when beneficence and autonomy conflict). Nurses do not live and practice in an ideal world, and so it is necessary to be satisfied with the best decision that can be made under the circumstances. The point is not that perfect decisions have to be made; that is never possible. It is rather that whatever decisions are made and whatever actions are performed, they have been carefully thought through and can be justified by appeal to accepted ethical principles.

The ethics of critical thinking

Often, when people learn the tools of critical thinking, they become highly critical of others. It is important that critical thinking be viewed primarily as a set of tools applied to one's own thinking. When evaluating the ideas of others, critical thinking skills are used to decide whether an idea is acceptable or should be rejected. Who the other person is, is usually irrelevant. And when critical thinking skills undermine or attack other people, then the purpose of critical thinking is lost. One of the most important distinctions to remember is that between an idea and the person who presents the idea.

The critical thinker always needs to think critically within the framework of well-developed interpersonal relationship skills. Critical thinking skills are not weapons to be wielded to cut another person down to size. They are tools of personal growth, which allow one to travel through an often confusing landscape and keep one's bearings, while providing the best possible quality care for those to whom one is responsible and accountable.

USING SOFTWARE TO PRACTISE REASONING

It takes considerable practice to become accomplished at reasoning and evaluating arguments. There are quite a few software packages available that can help visualise arguments and aid in the process of analysis. One of the best of these is *Reason!Able*, which allows you to create diagrams of arguments and your evaluation. Figure 21.8 shows a diagram, produced by *Reason!Able*, of the argument about hair loss following chemotherapy described above.

You can download a trial version of this software from http://www.goreason. com/.

DEVELOPING CRITICAL THINKING SKILLS

There is no magical solution to actually developing critical thinking skills. An awareness of what critical thinking is and where it can be applied is an appropriate start. Like anything, it requires continual practice. Ultimately, it is about developing a conscious attitude of reflection during daily and professional life. Halpern (1998) suggests a number of attitudes and dispositions that support the development of

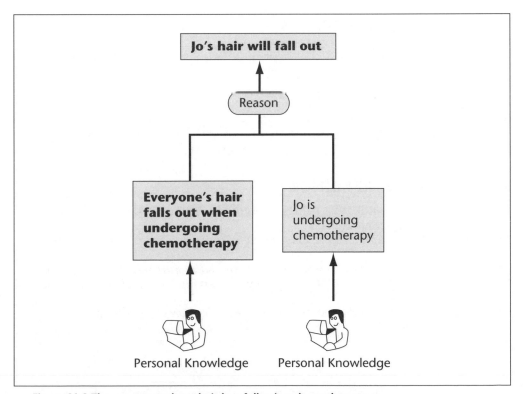

Figure 21.8 The argument about hair loss following chemotherapy

critical thinking. They are: willingness to plan; flexibility; persistence; willingness to self-correct; being mindful ('the habit of self-conscious concern for and evaluation of the thinking process'); and consensus-seeking. As Halpern says:

> No one can become a better thinker just by reading a book. An essential component of critical thinking is developing the attitude and disposition of a critical thinker. Good thinkers are motivated and willing to exert the conscious effort needed to work in a planful manner, to check for accuracy, to gather information, and to persist when the solution is not obvious or requires several steps (Halpern 1998:10–11).

Although it is hard work to develop new skills in critical thinking, the time and energy are well worth the rewards that come with the ability to think clearly.

CONCLUDING REMARKS

Critical thinking is a vital skill to have as a nurse. Nurses are engaged in providing care to people who have a right to high-quality professional conduct and health services. Nurses have a responsibility to make sure that their actions are based on rigorous evidence and can be justified with acceptable reasons. Although developing the skills to think critically may at times be difficult and demanding, thinking critically provides a greater level of confidence and satisfaction as nurses interact with colleagues and it promotes high-quality, safe practice.

REFLECTIVE QUESTIONS

1 How has your understanding of thinking changed as a result of reading this chapter?

2 What areas of your professional life would benefit from applying the principles of critical thinking to them?

3 What will you do now to further develop your skill in critical thinking?

RECOMMENDED READINGS

Bandman E L, Bandman B 1998 *Critical thinking in nursing*, 2nd edn. Appleton & Lange, Norwalk, Connecticut.
Browne M N, Keeley S M 1998 *Asking the right questions*, 5th edn. Prentice Hall, New Jersey.
Miller A, Babcock D E 1996 *Critical thinking applied to nursing*. Mosby, St Louis.
Paul R G, Elder L 2001 *Critical thinking: tools for taking charge of your learning and your life*. Prentice Hall, New Jersey.
Rubenfeld M G 1995 *Critical thinking in nursing: an interactive approach*. J B Lippincott, Philadelphia.

CHAPTER TWENTY-TWO

Using informatics to expand awareness

Moya Conrick

At the completion of this chapter, the reader should:

- ▲ be able to articulate and discuss the major concepts underpinning informatics;

- ▲ be able to critically reflect on informatics as a tool of nursing practice;

- ▲ be able to assess and critically reflect on the automation of nursing and health data;

- ▲ be able to critically evaluate the infostructure requirements for nursing information systems; and

- ▲ be aware of nurses as knowledge workers and be able to analyse knowledge management in nursing to a beginning level.

KEY WORDS
Health informatics, e-health, nursing informatics, knowledge management, current awareness, electronic health records, infostructure

NURSING AND INFORMATION TECHNOLOGY

The development of solutions for health is more difficult than for many other industries because the health sector is complex and fragmented, and involves multiple levels of government, numerous individuals and a large number of private sector organisations. The degree of spending on information infrastructure in healthcare is evidence of a strong belief by policy makers, and others, that information technology will improve patient care and deliver quality health outcomes (Conrick et al 2004). Automation has much to offer healthcare workers and, indeed, the last few years have seen the beginnings of a transformation in healthcare, triggered by a rapid rise in the use of information technology across all areas of healthcare and the rapid increase in the sophistication of information systems. While health administration was an early adopter of information technology, and new technology for diagnostic and treatment purposes is always rapidly embraced, investment in systems to support clinicians lags well behind. Clinicians continue to drown in paperwork and often make decisions based on fragmented, poor-quality data.

Information technology is predicted to improve patient outcomes and reduce errors, because it can deliver timely clinical information quickly and at the point-of-care in a form that can be read and understood. It also empowers clinicians by providing them with the tools of evidence-based decision making with the deployment of knowledge databases and repositories. It is increasingly providing access to more complete, accurate health records that organise patient-specific information from diverse databases (and practitioners). Information technology has and will continue to change the manner in which healthcare workers deliver patient care and how administrators manage their institutions.

Repetitive communications and collecting and manipulating masses of data, the boring tasks that humans dislike, are the forté of computers. As long as appropriate protocols and standards are in place, computers manipulate complex data quickly and are able to communicate seamlessly across the health system. This supports the efficient collection and sharing of comprehensive, quality health information that can be used to improve the delivery of health services across populations. One only has to look at the changes in communications since the development of the internet to realise that information technology has permanently transformed the way in which we communicate. The alpha designations on the telephone, for example, often the source of query as to their function, are now the explosive telecommunications of this emerging century with around 8 billion text messages sent in Australia during 2004. Imagining uses for this type of technology in healthcare is not so difficult and, in the United Kingdom, the National Health Service text messages patients reminders to make them aware of visits, follow-up or changes to appointments.

Information technology has the capacity to reign in the unacceptable levels of errors and adverse events resulting from bad handwriting, as well as mistakes in prescribing and administration of medications. It also has the ability to address the communication failures that account for approximately 70% of causes of sentinel events reported to the Joint Commission for Hospital Accreditation (Leonard et al 2004).

This chapter will expand health professionals' awareness of informatics as a tool of practice and discuss the major issues for nursing in its uptake. It will expand readers' awareness of the use of technology in the collection, use and sharing of digitised health information. There are many branches of health informatics, but it is predominantly nursing informatics that will be perused in this chapter. In such a complex discipline, it is not surprising for confusion in nomenclature to arise and it is pertinent here to discuss the common terms of e-health and health informatics.

HEALTH INFORMATICS OR E-HEALTH

The confusion between the use of the terms e-health and health informatics is recent and has so blurred the lines that the terms are now used interchangeably in some circles. E-health was first introduced to distinguish web-based telehealth activities from videoconferencing. It later described the combined use of electronic communication and information technology in healthcare and encompassed telemedicine and telehealth. In 2003, the special interest group of the Healthcare Information and Management Systems Society defined e-health as:

> . . . [t]he application of the Internet and other related technologies in the healthcare industry to improve the access, efficiency, effectiveness, and quality of clinical and business processes utilised by healthcare organizations, practitioners, patients, and consumers to improve the health status of patients (Healthcare Information and Management Systems Society 2003).

Health informatics on the other hand is seen as an evolving sociotechnical and scientific discipline that deals with the collection, storage, retrieval, communication and optimal use of health-related data, information and knowledge. The discipline utilises the methods and technologies of the information sciences for the purposes of problem solving and decision making—thus, assuring quality healthcare in all basic and applied areas of biomedical sciences for the community it serves (Health Informatics Society of Australia 1998).

The debate is not entered into here and informatics as defined above underpins this chapter. Hopefully, in time, the term 'health' will reemerge with technology (or the 'e') subsumed, but recognised as simply another tool of practice, albeit a very important and dynamic one. In healthcare the use of information technology has caused debate, some of which is quite passionate. In time, parallels will probably be drawn with the following quote, and healthcare workers will wonder what the fuss was about:

> That it will ever come into general use, notwithstanding its value, is extremely doubtful because its beneficial application requires much more time and gives a good bit of trouble, both to the patient and to the practitioner because its hue and character are foreign and opposed to all our habits and associations (*The London Times*, 1834, commenting on the stethoscope).

DRIVERS IN INFORMATICS

The National Health Information Management Group in the paper *Health information development priorities* (2002) highlighted the need for healthcare consumers, providers and funders to have appropriate data available to enable planning, management and monitoring, both at the individual patient or client level, and an aggregated level.

These development priorities have been incorporated into the Commonwealth's Health*Online* strategy, which is at the forefront of national developments that *will have ramifications for all nurses*.

The Health*Online* initiative and other e-health programs have set the Commonwealth, and so all involved in healthcare, on a course that will see the increased delivery of health services using electronic means. Health*Online* sets out a framework for a work program aimed at delivering improved health services through new and innovative ways of managing health information (National Health Information Management Advisory Council 2001). This agenda has brought together the states and territories, most of whom are sponsoring information technology projects.

One of the restraints in the e-health agenda in Australia has been the inadequacy of the mainly copper wire communications network. Sending large amounts of data through the existing network is painfully slow and largely ineffective. In 2004, the Commonwealth committed an investment of $35 million over three years to provide broadband internet access to general practitioners across Australia to ensure that all general practices and Aboriginal-community-controlled health services nationwide have access to high-quality, secure broadband services. Secure e-mail communication between doctors and other health providers, and rapid online delivery of referrals, requests, hospital discharge summaries and test results such as pathology, X-ray and ultrasound images, will be facilitated (Australian Health Information Council 2004). It will also support the National Electronic Health Record—Health*Connect*.

This level of access to broadband technology will enable a level of communications and an interoperability of systems not possible before. However, as with many national initiatives in healthcare, nursing has not been mentioned in this development (other than subsumed in 'Aboriginal communities'), but as the program has developed, so has an understanding that nursing involvement is crucial for the programs to succeed.

INFORMATICS AS A TOOL FOR NURSING

Nurses focus on patients' responses to illness, injury, treatment and care within the context of the patients' family, social structure and location (Conrick et al 2004). In addition, their services are guided by patient risk assessments, which form the basis of preventative nursing interventions. These assessments and interventions include the broader health context of psychosocial, environmental and family/carer considerations, and are crucial to the ongoing health of our community. Nurses are the only professionals who work across health transitions and therefore the continuum-of-care. To effectively and efficiently engage with patients and clients across such diverse practice areas, nurses must use the most efficient and effective tools available to them, and technology is able to provide many of these.

Nurses are found in a diversity of practice areas and geographical settings supporting an increasingly transient community. More and more this is a struggle, particularly in rural and remote Australia, where they are often isolated from other practitioners and must, by necessity, practise alone. The fragmented records of care and inadequate methods of communication are no longer acceptable and, indeed, the general population expects better. Information technology has the potential to support clinicians by providing timely, quality data, and to largely negate the tyranny of distance, through high-speed broadband and satellite access. This is the domain of nursing informatics.

Nursing informatics is:

... a specialty area that integrates nursing science, computer science, and information science to manage and communicate data, information and knowledge in nursing practice settings. It facilitates the integration of data, information and knowledge to support patients, nurses and other providers in their decision-making in all roles and settings, by using information structures, information processes, and information technology (Staggers & Thompson 2002).

As information technology permeates nursing, all nurses must have a working knowledge of informatics and understand what it offers the profession. Nursing input is essential in the development of information systems, and anecdotal evidence suggests that it is a significant factor in the success or failure of these systems.

GATHERING EVIDENCE TO AID DECISION MAKING

It is crucial that clean, quality electronic data are collected for use in practice and for the sharing of quality information across healthcare, because these data are the basis for decision making and provide the evidence for practice at all levels of healthcare. In informatics terms, the gathering of evidence for decision making actually begins with the most basic of language building blocks—that is, data.

The International Standards Organisation defines data as the representation of real world facts, concepts or instructions in a formalised manner suitable for communication, interpretation or processing by human beings or by automatic means (International Standards Organization 1999). Information builds on data and is the output of the data interpretation, organisation and structure (Standards Australia 2003). When information has been synthesised, interrelationships are identified and formalised knowledge is created (Standards Australia 2003). The evidence for use as clinical information and nursing knowledge result from the progressive cognitive or automated processing and manipulation of data, language and knowledge, and in turn governs it. Nurses are recognised as the key collectors, generators and users of patient/client data and information, and the delivery of good nursing care is dependent upon the quality and timeliness of the information available (Hovenga & Hindmarsh 1996a, Currell et al 2002).

THE COLLECTION OF DIGITISED HEALTH INFORMATION

There are three levels at which the collection of digitised health information can be used and shared, according to Mercer (2003). The first level is the service delivery level and most data are generated here (see Fig 22.1). At this level, computer systems capture initial patient care data, but may also exchange data between different systems (e.g. a referral could be generated from the hospital to a community service or from one program to another). Data from this level also form the basis of population surveys. National standards operate here to ensure quality and clean data collection. Mercer describes the second level as the intermediate level, saying that:

... data from the lowest level of the pyramid are often required to be reported, perhaps within a service delivery outlet (total activity counts for a day), or to a regional or area agency or authority (total activity counts for a week, or agency expenditure totals for a financial year) (Mercer 2003:16).

The volume of data reported to the intermediate level will normally be less than the data generated at the service delivery level because not all data that are generated need to be reported. Data may also be aggregated for reporting, or may be reported in the form of individual records for each patient or client.

In the final level, or the national level, data from intermediate levels, or at times directly from the service delivery level, may be reported to national data collection agencies. Alternatively, data from census or surveys may be collected at this level, using data captured from the service providers, patients/clients or the general population (Mercer 2003). Data from intermediate levels, or at times directly from the service delivery level, may be reported to national data-collection agencies, the third level of use and sharing. Alternatively, data from census or surveys may be collected at this level, using data captured from the service providers, patients/clients or the general population. From this it is easy to realise that a breakdown of data collection in any stage has far-reaching ramifications for health.

Data input processes must be rapid and intuitive, without placing any additional burden on the user, or mistakes will follow. While it is unlikely that any method of data collection, other than voice, will be faster than handwritten notes, the benefits of an electronic clinical information system far outweigh any minimal change in work process that might be required.

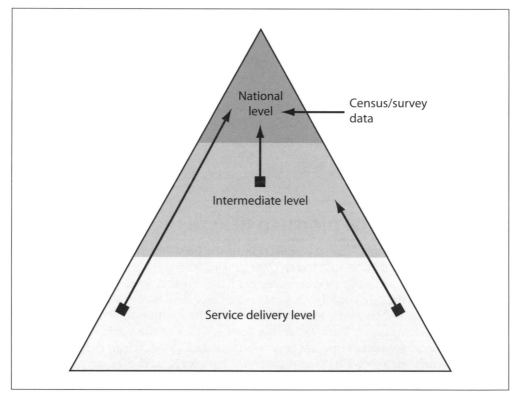

Figure 22.1 Pyramid of reporting activity
Source: Based on N Mercer 2003 *Redevelopment of the AIHW Knowledgebase—Stage 1: scope and issues paper.* AIHW, Canberra.

The most readily realised benefits are those of legibility, error reduction, reduced documentation of redundant data, completeness and cleanness of the data collected, and the ability to use the data for secondary purposes. By eliminating the duplication of services, improving communication and streamlining data collection, clinical information systems can improve care and the outcomes of care, reduce costs and help to offset the effects of a growing worker shortage that is especially hard-felt in nursing.

Indeed the Health*Connect* project echoes this, finding a reduction in the incidence of adverse drug reactions, improved medication management, improved management of diabetes and reduced demand on emergency departments (DMR Consulting 2004a). It is also thought that a total indicative benefits range of $554 million to $604 million per annum might be achieved. This does not consider the value of lives saved or improved quality of life, or the broader economic and social benefits from the Australia-wide implementation of Health*Connect* (DMR Consulting 2004b).

Nursing data, information, knowledge and evidence

It is acknowledged that whereas a medical practitioner may be seen as the major primary care provider, in longitudinal care, nurses embrace the concept of continuity-of-care as both an aim and a philosophy that affects the delivery of care (Conrick et al 2004). Continuity always involves transitions on the part of individuals, such as wellness to illness, home to hospital, and the gaps they may encounter along the way. In nursing, these transitions usually involve practice that deals with populations who have complex health issues. During times of transition, the nurse is very often the health professional most involved in evaluation, planning and delivering the changes in care that may be required (Conrick et al 2004). If patient care is not consistently and accurately recorded, the possible adverse effects on patient care, nursing practice and the development of nursing knowledge may be quite significant (Currell et al 2002).

If progress is to be made on the electronic exchange of data and information, as outlined in the Health*Online* strategy, nurses must decide how the 'natural language' text and oral data that are used in nursing can be entered into a computerised documentation system and translated, through the design of the computer software, into a database capable of supporting nationally agreed, consistent terms (Walker et al 2003). Without some type of organisation or classification, differences in language can be quite marked from hospital to hospital, and this is, of course, increased between states and territories, resulting in inappropriate interpretation of the record and the key process of nursing care being measured in different ways (Conrick 2005).

The development of a health information infrastructure in electronic format must (ultimately) be capable of supporting machine-readable terminology, as this will ensure that data can be readily accessed electronically. Nursing must be active in determining how health concepts are defined by computer software to ensure standardisation and accurate communication, meaning that a computer used by a nurse in one area is using the same concept (with the same meaning) when interacting with a computer used by a health practitioner elsewhere.

In national projects such as the Commonwealth's Health*Connect*, the development of classifications and terminologies is a priority, because they enable the standardised collection of machine-readable health information to:

▲ provide for the measurement of clinical care outcomes and support an evidence-based approach to client assessment—evaluating care outcomes for individuals requires the capacity to organise patient-based information from a variety of service delivery settings in both public and private sectors;

▲ flow into case management and decision support software;

▲ facilitate coordinated care across sectors (acute care, emergency, other ambulatory and community health settings, non-acute settings);

▲ improve the monitoring of safety and quality in healthcare;

▲ enable statistical analysis and reporting of health information for decision making, policy development, service administration and financial management, and health research; and

▲ enable standardised indicator development (Walker et al 2003).

Defining the language of practice is also necessary so that all care settings are using the same unique terms. These factors are critical if service providers are to continuously improve safety, enhance the quality of health and healthcare, and to base their practice on evidenced-based research (Walker et al 2003). If language collection and definition can be achieved, it will enable activities such as outcomes research and benchmarking based on valid, consistent and reliable data. It will also underpin the development of nursing archetypes (discussed later in this chapter).

Current health projects, such as Health*Connect* and within it Medi*Connect*, focus on automating the capture, exchange, transmission and collection of health data from the Australian population. This is not possible now because, in Australia, no clinical data are coded other than hospital data collected under the ICD10 AM (International Classification of Diseases, Australian Modifications). These data are currently coded and aggregated post hoc, limiting its use for clinical decision making at the point of care and constraining communications (Walker et al 2003).

The patient's health record, whether electronic or paper, should contain a complete record of nursing work. In fact, this is the only place that it can be captured, but frequently the care given and outcomes of nursing care are poorly reported. The lack of structure of nursing data also means that they are infrequently used to support nursing practice because retrieval from patients' records is very difficult (Conrick 2005). These problems have existed for a long time, but it is still sobering to read recent studies that indicate that fragmented, disorganised, and inaccessible clinical information continues to adversely affect the quality of healthcare and compromises patient safety (Gahart et al 2004). To provide better care for patients, it is essential that all clinicians and others involved in a patient's care can accurately communicate treatment plans, assessments, patient diagnoses and symptoms.

Information technology enables the sharing and storage of data not possible with paper-based records and other current means of communication. However, it must be done in an appropriate, specific and accurate manner, and the only way to achieve this is the use of standard, accepted, relevant terminology or terminologies that both the senders and receivers of information can understand. In an electronic environment, standard reference terminologies are required, and nursing has developed an International Reference Terminology for this purpose. Such terminologies communicate information well, but at a higher level, and they are not suited for counting information units for statistical purposes. In order to both communicate health information, and to count it accurately (for burden of disease studies, epidemiology, public health initiatives, resource planning and so forth), both classifications and terminologies are needed (Walker et al 2003).

While humans communicate with each other using 'natural language', computers cannot; they need to be told what things are and how they are related to each other, and this is achieved through use of terminologies. Despite the considerable terminologies work that is underway in Australia and internationally, little has been done to identify those that will be acceptable to Australian nurses. Nurses, as they should, have rejected language classification systems that were inadequate or inappropriate, but with the implementation of electronic health records, consensus on language classification must be achieved. One of the most difficult problems has been finding an appropriate terminology(ies) that represents the spectrum of nursing practice, while making sense to both the user and the computer. There are several datasets that appear to have some merit and that are in use elsewhere, and they must be trialled in Australia.

Workforce challenges

Other than the state of its data, there are a number of factors that have the potential to undermine the use of technology to support nursing. Nursing workflow issues are some of the most important of these and they must be understood if nurses' information requirements are to be realised. Consideration of these issues is also necessary for nurses to work seamlessly across the continuity-of-care with individual patients or groups of patients or in interdisciplinary care teams. Although substantial investment may be expended on technology, this will not assure success, as nurses will not willingly use tools incompatible with their work or communication processes; and nor should they. Imposing information systems is also futile, as this usually results in the collection of sporadic, poor-quality data on which nurses base decision making or which they abstract as evidence for nursing outcomes.

Investment in information technology infrastructure also requires an investment in the health workforce to ensure that nurses have the skills required to effectively use the information and technology, and to enter the technology debate. Few universities offer sufficient informatics education to their undergraduate or postgraduate students, and nurses not recently qualified are likely to have minimal 'training' at work or may have undertaken self-education because of a particular interest in the field. A comprehensive national health informatics education framework is required to address this crucial issue, and this is something that the Commonwealth is now contemplating.

Computer skills are just as essential to nurses in the twenty-first century as pencil and paper were in the eighteenth and nineteenth centuries. However, as technology changes, computer skills must be updated and this requires a systematic program of ongoing education, training and skills development. Currently, there is little information available on the information management and computing skill base of the nursing workforce, making it difficult to assess nurses' education needs. However, low computer literacy levels in nursing have been alluded to in the literature and discussed in other forums (e.g. in the 'think tank' of 2003) (Commonwealth of Australia 2003b).

If nurses cannot evaluate systems and define technology needs, then others will continue doing this for them. Indeed, there are many vendors currently implementing or developing nursing systems that are targeted specifically for local use and, in fact, this is a selling point for their product. Nursing is at risk of continuing service delivery in a fragmented manner that is unable to traverse locations or geographical settings. It will perpetuate and exacerbate funding and retention issues, and thwart nursing's ability to achieve quality, cost-effective patient outcomes on a state-wide or national basis. In terms of the Australian Health Information Council's (AHIC) vision for Australia's health and its perceived 'opportunity to create one of the world's best healthcare systems' (Coats 2004), these are major issues.

THE STORAGE AND USE OF DIGITISED HEALTH INFORMATION

Healthcare organisations will continue to invest heavily in clinical information systems because they envisage an improvement in patient safety, reduced variability of care, and increased staff efficiency. This is because of the quality of data available for decision making. Nursing work is information intensive, with nurses processing information for multiple purposes: to create a greater awareness of patient needs; to guide practice; report observations; and document patient care. Although it is estimated that nurses spend at least 20% of their time processing written information and up to a further 30% engaging in verbal communication (Hovenga & Hindmarsh 1996b), currently across practice the highest recording rate of outcomes documentation is just 13%, with some practice areas failing to capture outcomes at all (Kennedy 2004). This leaves a huge gap in the continuity-of-care, but it also has ramifications for nursing knowledge and evidence for nursing practice.

Electronic health records

Many anecdotal reports about the problems of paper health records abound, and the literature also documents many of these. The following list typifies some of these:

▲ fragmentation of information and data;

▲ illegible;

▲ no linkages to underlying data;

▲ no information or data management;

▲ no decision support capabilities;

▲ competition for access;

▲ inaccessibility of information; and

▲ missing data.

Electronic health records (EHRs) help to negate most of these difficulties and create an awareness of the holistic needs of the patient because information is readily available from multiple sources. Appropriate and timely information at the point-of-care improves decisions about what type of care is provided and how it is delivered, reducing risk and improving the quality and outcomes of care (Conrick 2005). An EHR is defined as the longitudinal collection of personal health information concerning a single individual, entered or accepted by healthcare providers, and stored electronically. The information is organised primarily to support continuing, efficient and quality healthcare, and is stored and transmitted securely. The EHR contains information that is:

▲ *retrospective*: an historical view of health status and interventions;

▲ *concurrent*: a 'now' view of health status and active interventions; and

▲ *prospective*: a future view of planned health activities and interventions (Standards Australia 2003).

Health records serve not only as archival records, but may be viewed as diaries of diagnostic discoveries, observations made and care provided (Conrick et al 2004). A by-product of the rigorous collection and recording of health status data, and nursing activity data into a point-of-care EHR, would be the capacity to perform post-hoc analyses on these data to determine the effectiveness and efficiency of nursing activity in real-world settings. It would also feed data into a quality improvement cycle and form the basis of evidence-based decision making in clinical practice. It is for many of these reasons that the states have embarked on the deployment of EHRs and the Commonwealth is introducing Health*Connect,* which it feels has the ability to improve the quality and safety of healthcare through a longitudinal, national health information network, based on a computerised summary EHR.

Under Health*Connect*, a person's health-related information will be collected in a standard, electronic format at the point of care (such as a care centre or a hospital) and exchanged via a secure network, between the healthcare providers authorised by the consumer to access this information (Commonwealth of Australia 1999b). The access issue is a difficult one and currently opinion is divided between an opt-in or an opt-out system. Many clinicians and some governments believe that the record will be fragmented and almost useless if a patient can decide to withhold information about a visit, whereas consumers see it as their right. New South Wales is trialling an opt-out model as part of their Health*Connect* trial, based on the Canadian and United Kingdom experience, which saw expenses blow out with the opt-in option. On balance, the opt-in strategy seems no different from the current system in which the patient has the right to attend multiple practitioners and institutions and the paper record is not accessible outside the individual organisation.

People who participate in Health*Connect* will have full control over their personal health information; they will have viewing rights, but will be unable to write on their personal record. At some stage a free text area may be available to enable participants to record their personal health information. For example, a log of blood-sugar-level results for the day may be recorded, which may be of great value across the continuum-of-care. Another positive outcome is the production of event summaries, which would be automatically generated at the time of discharge, and this has already demonstrated its worth in a trial in the Katherine region of the Northern Territory, in which a number of health consumers trialled Health*Connect*. The Commonwealth will provide $128.3 million over the next four years for the implementation of Health-*Connect* as a major platform for reforming healthcare delivery in Australia (Commonwealth of Australia 2004). The implementation of Health*Connect* will include the integration of Medi*Connect* as the medicines component of Health*Connect*, and this will be discussed later in this chapter.

In EHRs, clinicians will be able to use documentation more effectively and efficiently because of its higher quality and accessibility. All information will be available, removing errors related to missing and inaccessible data, although Health*Connect* may pose a problem because of access protocols. Network speed and hardware specifications that facilitate rapid login and ready access are necessary, as are searching capabilities for the end user. Data collection for management decision making, quality and statistical reporting must be an output of data collected during the routine clinical workflow, rather than an additional task (Conrick et al 2004).

To realise the positive outcomes from EHR, systems must be designed around best-practice workflow of the end user. They must be comprehensive in their scope, with all major components of the clinical process including all clinical orders (medications, diagnostic orders and specialty consults), nursing care and outcomes documentation available in an electronic records format (Conrick et al 2004). Self-population of multiple components and fields in the record will then eliminate duplicate data entry. They must enable once only and point-of-care entry that eliminates transcription errors and clinical systems that provide decision support to aid in the decision making of all clinicians. This information made available through clinical decision support systems assists clinicians to gather evidence for decision making and to prevent adverse events.

Clinical decision support

Clinical decision support systems (CDSSs) are usually built around alerting systems, based on rules of logic. The alerting system can notify clinicians immediately or may generate alerts over time, after relating data from multiple sources (Lyons & Richardson 2003). Broad categories of decision support systems include formatting tools, decision modelling, advisory and knowledgebase systems. They provide strategies to analyse, evaluate, develop and select effective solutions to complex problems in complex environments. Nurses are able to quickly access sources of evidence to assist with the provision of quality care, as the evidence can be locally sorted in policy and procedure manuals, for example, or it can be retrievable from wide-ranging sources such as journal databases or professional collaborative networks (Conrick et al 2004).

To date, much of the development work on electronic decision support systems has been fragmented and uncoordinated, leading to problems of accessibility, scalability, duplication and lack of integration with existing systems. The Commonwealth has begun a nationally coordinated approach for developments in the area and are perusing a national governance structure to provide direction and coordination (Commonwealth of Australia 2003a). In the United Kingdom, 'The Map of Medicine™', a fast and intuitive decision support system, has been trialled and demonstrates the capabilities of CDSSs.

The Map™ is a clinical knowledge system that visually combines specialist knowledge with best practice, making the resources of medical information available to all clinical staff. It is designed to support interaction across disciplines, help improve the use of clinical resources and underpin professional development (Medic to Medic 2004). Clinical knowledge is organised into more than 300 patient 'journeys' in all major diagnostic areas and 'maps' clinical process throughout the healthcare system, starting from initial patient presentation in the general practitioner's surgery or the accident and emergency unit. The Map™ is customisable to local clinical needs in the healthcare organisation and is designed to integrate into every aspect of modern healthcare, from diagnosis through to education and training. The developers describe a virtual 'desktop consultant' for healthcare professionals to use when the patient's journey leads them into unfamiliar territory (Medic to Medic 2004). Nurses in this project have remarked on the ways that the system has changed their process of decision making, from isolation to shared decision making. They report a sense of empowerment and a vision for the future.

No matter the advances in decision support systems, the nurse must still exercise and use clinical judgment in the context of the problem, as well as the recommendations of the decision support tool, and nursing must be responsible for nursing needs. The Map™ represents just one example of electronic clinical decision support, but just as important to the clinician is awareness of potential errors, which can also be built into these systems. Another type of clinical decision support can be built into medications management systems, in which data from clinical systems provide an alerting service. These systems demonstrate the worth of clinical decision support in very tangible ways.

Medications management

Medications management is an ongoing concern in most countries and medication errors are responsible for considerable morbidity. In Australia, misuse, underuse, overuse, and reactions to therapeutic drugs, result in 140,000 hospital admissions every year, with the inappropriate use of medicines costing approximately $380 million per year in the public hospital system alone (Australian Institute of Health and Welfare 2002a). Meadows (2002) has found that clinical information systems can assist in reducing medication errors through sophisticated medication management solutions. Apart from legibility, prescribing safety is enhanced with online access to decision support databases carrying patient drug history, scientific drug information guideline reference, and patient-specific information. Such specific information includes discharge summaries, surgical procedure summaries, laboratory data and investigation reports. In addition, decision support and prompts can be built in to catch errant orders (Ong 2002).

Technology enables doctors, pharmacists and nurses to make prescribing, dispensing and administration decisions based on knowledge of previous prescriptions, the current medications regime and previous medication reactions. These types of medications systems also provide consumers with the opportunity to become active participants in their medication management, which has demonstrated to improve outcomes. The area for greatest gains, however, may be at the hospital interface, where quick access to a patient's medication record could be life saving. Barcode-enabled point-of-care medication management systems that can also combine with computerised provider-order-entry systems, replacing handwritten prescribing, are designed to improve efficiency and reduce medication and other errors in the clinical setting. Bar codes on inpatients' identification bands assist with administration tasks, with alerts warning of allergies or interactions. According to the Australian Council for Safety and Quality in Health Care (2002), 'the evidence suggests that careful implementation of computerised prescribing with clinical decision support systems should be a priority'.

The Commonwealth government has also found substantial benefits of their Medi*Connect* trial, which has now been subsumed under Health*Connect*. This trial linked the medications record of patients to doctors, pharmacists and hospitals (DMR Consulting 2004a, 2004b), creating an electronic consumer medication record. It was constructed by drawing together personal medicine information held in differ-ent medical practices, pharmacies and hospitals. Prescription, over-the-counter and complementary (alternative) medicines information was added to patient records, as were allergies. The trials demonstrated a potential for significant improvements in health outcomes and savings.

Another use of information technology has also demonstrated the capability to reduce costs by improving health communications and outcomes, and this is e-health.

Gathering and sharing information using e-health

E-health is healthcare provided to the consumer over distance, and managed by moving the information two ways with the use of communications technologies. E-health clinical uses include but are not limited to: diagnosis from radiological images; reviewing laboratory findings; interviewing, assessing and monitoring patients in rural and remote locations; consulting with specialist health professionals; and education and continuing education.

There are two main forms of e-health, including the store-and-forward (e.g. e-mail and images from radiology, pathology or dermatology can be sent electronically for a consultant to view when convenient). The transmission may be rapid, but does not need to be synchronous. The other form of e-health is synchronous communication, such as a telephone consultation. The telephone has always been a tool of nursing, and telephone triage is well established in some countries.

Real-time interactive systems include videoconferencing, videophones and specialised e-health units that combine videoconferencing capability with medical peripheral devices, such as electronic stethoscopes, sphygmomanometers or endoscopes, and are particularly successful using broadband technology (Greenberg et al 2003). While high bandwidths are useful but not essential for education, training and some consultations, such as telepsychiatry, they are necessary for telesurgery, radiology, ultrasonography, still images, cardiac telemonitoring and consultations requiring a very clear image. E-health saves patients displacement from their communities, and has enabled timely, cost-effective general and specialist care across the vast distances of our country.

Gathering evidence with patient dependency systems

Patient dependency systems (PDSs) are commonly used and were adopted solely as administrative decision-making tools to provide appropriate staff expertise and staff-to-patient allocation. More recently, nurse managers have used PDSs to match patient needs with the available nursing resources. Although nursing acuity systems have been discussed for many years and there are several in use, few studies evaluate their use in practice, and those that do focus on validity and reliability, and cross-checking the relationships between nursing dependency, diagnosis-related groups (DRGs), and length of hospital stay (LOS) (Victorian Government Health Services 2004).

Donaldson and Conrick (2004) demonstrated the ability of value adding to a PDS system (in this case PAIS) and for it to acquire a clinical function. The PAIS system produces timely data that are important in understanding acuity profiles and specific activities associated with patients from homogenous DRGs. These data lend themselves to active variance analysis and the flagging of the indicators that might suggest variance, which in turn, improves decision making, leading to more comprehensive care planning and may achieve a more optimal LOS. This method is applicable in developing or reviewing existing clinical pathways, and is effective for all

DRGs where there is a sufficient patient population to validate the data (Donaldson & Conrick 2004). Although this is not an automated pathway production program for the clinician, it is invaluable for providing evidentiary support and an awareness of all issues when making decisions regarding the inclusion of particular tasks in the clinical pathway (Donaldson & Conrick 2004).

When this method is incorporated into information systems, it could also form the basis for clinical decision support. Using 'live' data analysis, instead of retrospective clinical audit, enables active variance analysis, and the flagging of specific indicators in patients' conditions might preempt variance during an episode of care. The availability of this information may prompt appropriate intervention earlier, rather than later, resulting in better care planning and possibly optimal LOS.

Using data in clinical practice improvement

The real value of the adoption and use of clinical systems, EHRs, intelligent decision support and care planning is the ability to share clinical nursing information between systems (Conrick et al 2004). This information needs to be processable by the receiving computer system so that it is understood at the level of formally defined nursing domain concepts. This requires four prerequisites: a standardised EHR reference model; a service interface model; terminologies; and domain-specific concept models (for open EHR). The latter requires the development and adoption of nursing-domain-specific archetypes (constraint models discussed later), templates and agreed terminologies.

This infostructure will enable nurses to engage in effectiveness research using techniques such as the clinical practice improvement cycle (CPIC), which is designed to develop data-driven, analytically based protocols to achieve desirable outcomes, at the lowest essential cost over the continuum of care (Horn 2001). Information technology provides nurses with the tools to gather evidence for evaluation, comparison and the improvement of nursing service delivery relative to patient outcomes. Nurses collect data on outcomes, treatments and care activities, as well as patient signs and symptoms based on nursing assessments. Ideally, this can be achieved as a secondary function of routine documentation of care via a clinical information system (Conrick et al 2004). The use of standardised data enables studies that compare different practices in any number of organisations for specific patient cohorts and leads to the development of evidence-based clinical guidelines. These in turn can be incorporated in decision support systems and positively influence future care and clinical decision making. The cycle is completed when the results of improved practices are again evaluated.

However, clinical and nursing systems that enable the use of data-mining software and the adoption of methods such as CPIC must include or have access to sufficient demographic data to enable data aggregation across systems for specific patient cohorts. This will enable the undertaking of 'virtual' randomised clinical trials to evaluate and assess homogeneous patients and their outcomes relative to treatment and care options provided (Conrick et al 2004).

A national strategic approach for involvement in relevant international research and development would be possible with the development of a nursing information framework that would provide appropriate data for nursing research and evaluation. As standardised data are collected and used, automation would enable consensus on admission health status and nursing-sensitive outcome measures that would facilitate the automation of practice evaluation. It would also provide a foundation for the development of clinical decision support systems that would enable patients to be provided with the best possible evidence-based nursing care.

SEARCHING FOR AND SHARING KNOWLEDGE

Information and knowledge are the currency of the information technology revolution, but in today's environment of evidence-based healthcare, it is not possible for any healthcare provider to absorb all the knowledge required to maintain best practice. Nurses are true knowledge workers, using information and knowledge to support and inform all areas of their practice. Although the knowledge is an individual conative process, and as such cannot be managed by external processes, information technology makes it possible for knowledge to be captured in forms that can be stored and shared.

The health record should be the vehicle for comparing information and sharing knowledge, but the lack of standardisation of the existing paper records makes nursing data almost impossible to abstract. The use of electronic data capture and storage will change this, provided nurses are responsible for the development of such systems. The exchange of digitised information across settings using electronic knowledgebases, and being able to research that knowledge, is extremely important to nursing and to the outcomes of patient care.

Managing evidence and knowledge

It is accepted that a distributed national EHR system such as Health*Connect* needs to be underpinned by an appropriate, standardised architecture that defines how patient information is structured, stored and managed, so it can be securely stored and safely used by healthcare providers (Conrick et al 2004). The South Brisbane Health*Connect* trial is assessing the *open*EHR architecture for this task. Fundamental to *open*EHR is the use of 'archetypes' or electronically generated documents that provide a relatively simple means for clinicians to specify the structure, content and context of clinical information, without becoming involved in how programmers might represent the information within an EHR system. When implemented with appropriate software, these archetypes are used to manage clinical information and knowledge in an EHR system. In other words, this technology will, for the first time, enable nursing to articulate what it is that nurses do and will store this knowledge in an accessible knowledgebase. Nursing archetypes must be based on evidence, and the content and upkeep of the database is something for which all nurses must take responsibility.

Another type of knowledgebase is one that stores evidence-based nursing information and resources that are used by nurses on a daily basis to inform their practice (Conrick et al 2004). Much of this is already available in the form of journals, books and other types of peer-to-peer communications. A cursory surf of the worldwide web reveals a broad range of electronic health information that is extremely difficult and time consuming to sift through, and is dynamic—forever changing, expanding and shifting (Conrick 2002). A well-developed knowledgebase could organise this knowledge into a searchable form, and perhaps facilitate interactive peer-to-peer exchange, collective intelligence networking, debate, smart sharing, learning and discussion to support individuals and their organisations. The knowledgebase should have tools such as smart browsers that only search particular types of sites or those with particular content. Networks of nurses interested in specific clinical or management problems can form 'virtual communities' to exchange knowledge, enabling skills development and shared learning, promoting best practice ideals and more informed decisions. This would improve productivity, effectiveness and efficiency of practice, increase satisfaction in the clinical area, and the sharing of evidence-based decision making resources and tools, information and experiences.

The Australian Institute of Health and Welfare (2004a) has developed another type of knowledgebase, which is also internet-based. This is a 'registries store' and provides the contents of the national health, community services and housing assistance data dictionaries. Various groups and their associated national information management groups develop the contents of the knowledgebase. It also stores details of national minimum data sets (or agreed national data collections) and national information models, and also provides links between these metadata components.

The current knowledgebase is undergoing redevelopment because of the pressures and issues facing national data development. The redevelopment provides for an opportunistic expansion of the database beyond the scope of the national data dictionaries. It will, in future, include other national metadata content and reflect changes in user expectations and needs, the international standard used to underpin the knowledgebase structure, and changes in technology and web-browser software and so forth (Australian Institute of Health and Welfare 2004a). The redevelopment provides an opportunity to consider these issues and to determine how a national metadata registry can best support the national data development work programs, many of which are crucial to supporting nursing work and communications between nurses and others in an electronic world.

Current awareness tools

'Current awareness' is a timely topic with worker shortages, reduced time and information overload being facts of life. Dynamic resource tools for 'knowledge and awareness discovery' enable the user to use the internet to access, read and retrieve material from library catalogues, online databases and resources from millions of sites. The internet has an expansive range of quantity and quality of materials available to support nursing. It also has a great deal of rubbish, and accessing the material stored there can be difficult and frustrating because of the variable nature of the resources available, and the challenge in locating them (Conrick 2002).

Although the internet is referred to as 'the web', it really consists of two webs. The first is the surface web that can be accessed by regular search engines. The second is the deep web, which consists of a sizeable proportion of government resources, databases and similarly structured materials not written in hypertext mark-up language (html)—the language of the surface web. It is estimated that the deep web is 500 times larger than the surface web, it is highly specialised, 95% fee free and is the largest growth category on the web (Conrick 2002).

Awareness tools come in many forms, offer many current awareness resources including e-mail alerts, table of content alerts and e-mail, all of which arrive in a timely fashion and can be read either online or offline. There are custom alerting services that will monitor the internet for the latest information to be posted to the web, based on the user's customised search algorithm. These alerting systems enable immediate awareness of these new resources, as they send e-mail alerts to the subscriber's computer, mobile telephone or personal digital assistant (PDA). Specific subject-based mailing lists, bulletin boards, message boards and forums have been available for many years and provide one of the easiest ways of remaining current. List finders such as CataList and Delphi Forum assist in finding the most appropriate of these. Weblogs (Blogs) and News aggregators are perhaps the fastest growing tools on the internet and offer huge amounts of current information and knowledge. The internet provides easy access to health information on almost any topic imaginable that is evidence-based and maintains currency. Nurses have access to the latest developments in patient care, particularly for patients with complex or multiple problems; they also have timely access to a solid base of the most recent evidence on which to base decision making.

Decision making is only possible with high-quality communication and, characteristically, nurses working across the continuity of care or with complex patients do not have all the information on which to base decisions or an awareness of their patients to deliver seamless care. Nursing event summaries and nursing referrals are of critical importance to nursing communications, and the continuity of care.

Nursing event summaries

Nurses have never been good at communicating outside of the institution, and nursing discharge summaries, if provided, are often not timely and the content leaves much to be desired. Nursing event summaries should contain all the information required by the receiving clinician to enable seamless and continuous care and sufficient information for ongoing decision making. However, other pressures on the discharging clinician often mean that discharge summaries are given a low priority. Automated systems event summaries can be developed by a computer with no other involvement from the discharging clinician other than to press the 'go' button as part of the discharge. Anecdotal evidence suggests that this is one of the most positive aspects of the Katherine Health*Connect* trial. However, on a larger scale, discharge summary systems are reliant on many different sources systems, feeding data to the clinical repository, and where these will come from remains unclear.

CONCLUDING REMARKS

The nursing profession is an amalgamation of diverse practitioners working in many settings. Information technology will significantly redefine the way in which nurses work and the boundaries of practice, as it provides access to quality, timely data, information and knowledge. Nurses are key participants and the largest stakeholder group in healthcare; therefore, nursing will be most impacted by the introduction of any technology.

As new technology is developed and implemented, personnel and organisations have to adjust, and sometimes the adjustment is major. Technology has much to offer the clinician, but the acceptance of informatics requires more than mere buy-in or passive agreement because change is inevitable. It demands ownership by leaders willing to accept responsibility for making change happen in all of the areas they influence or control and an atmosphere of ownership by all nurses. Substantial changes to health education are required in both course design and content, and incentives for informatics education must be tangible for this to occur. Without these structures, nursing's approach to informatics will continue to be fragmented, duplication of effort will continue, and the workforce capacity in informatics will remain very low.

Systems will fail because of either apathy or ignorance, and the projected improvement in clinical care and health outcomes will not eventuate.

Underpinning the real value of the adoption and use of clinical systems, EHRs, intelligent decision support and automated care planning, is the ability to share clinical nursing information between clinicians and systems. The ability to access knowledge from formerly inaccessible places (in departments or the minds of staff and in information repositories) will greatly change healthcare delivery, the boundaries of healthcare and how decisions in healthcare are made. Nursing concepts must be valid, be embedded in evidence, exist in searchable knowledgebases and be available for nurses to make decisions on a strong base of knowledge. Knowledge management has the capacity to have a major impact on the knowledge levels of nurses, with nursing acquiring the capacity to engage in quality improvement cycles based on clean, quality data. This will result in high-level decision making, based on the best available information at the point of care resulting in improved outcomes.

Information technology has the capacity to take nurses into the future as informed, aware knowledge workers ready to meet the challenges. It has the capacity to change nursing as never before, and perhaps the profession will not be recognisable to us in 15 years' time. Whether or not nursing rises to the challenge depends on nursing's and nurses' commitment to the ownership of the process.

REFLECTIVE QUESTIONS

Choose one or more of the following areas of healthcare and then answer the four questions that follow:

- clinical;

- management;

- research; and/or

- education.

1 What is the problem(s) for which technology is the solution?

2 Whose problem is it?

3 How is technology the solution?

4 What problems could using the technology create?

RECOMMENDED READINGS

Commonwealth of Australia research reports. Department of Health and Ageing. Canberra. Accessed 15 December 2004. Available from: http://www.healthconnect.gov.au/atoz.htm.

Conrick M 2002 Looking for a needle in a haystack: searching the internet for quality resources. *Contemporary Nurse* 12(1):49–58.

Conrick M, Hovenga E, Cook R, Laracuente T, Morgan T 2004 *A framework for nursing informatics in Australia: a strategic paper* (commissioned national research report). HISA-NIA, Department of Health and Ageing, Melbourne. (Also available online through Nursing Informatics Australia and www.hisa.org.au.)

Graves J, Corcoran S 1989 The study of nursing informatics. *Image: Journal of Nursing Scholarship* 21(4):227–31.

Walker S, Frean I, Scott P, Conrick M 2003 *Classifications and terminologies in residential aged care: an information paper*. Department of Health and Ageing, Canberra.

CHAPTER TWENTY-THREE

Connecting clinical and theoretical knowledge for practice

Jane Conway & Margaret McMillan

LEARNING OBJECTIVES

Those who have read this chapter should be able to:

- ▲ appreciate the interaction between clinical practice and classroom-based learning activities;

- ▲ identify strategies that maximise learning opportunities in a range of contexts;

- ▲ explore strategies for acquiring knowledge-ABILITY;

- ▲ view themselves as autonomous, action-oriented learners; and

- ▲ appreciate the interaction between lifelong learning and professional development.

KEY WORDS
Transition, graduate, accountability, lifelong learning, curriculum, clinical learning, clinical decision making

THE CLINICAL AREA: THE SITE OF NURSING PRACTICE

Nursing programs globally recognise that the clinical area is an important, if not the most important, area for practice professions such as nursing (Melia 1987, Bartle 2000, Campbell 2003).The value of clinical experience to nursing practice, and hence to nursing students, cannot be overemphasised. Definitions of clinical teaching and learning invariably include some notion that clinical practice is the place where students apply theory in practice, or where contradictions between theory and practice, and nursing and educational values, are highlighted (Melia 1987, Bartle 2000, Campbell 2003). The clinical environment is, in fact, where students begin to develop professional identities as nurses.

The role of the professional nurse has changed from being a person who practised modified medicine to a person who appreciates the dynamic and evolving nature of nursing, and is able to use the skills of inquiry, critical thinking, problem solving and reflective practice. Clinical practice provides the stimulus for students and practitioners alike to use these skills in order to recognise best practice and, if necessary, enhance and modify existing practice. This chapter is designed to encourage students to view clinical and on-campus learning as one entity—a continuum of development and lifelong learning that has the unifying goal of achieving and maintaining competence within the complexities of contemporary practice.

The transition from student to graduate requires the development of the ability to critically examine our own and others' practice and be accountable for our own actions. These abilities are often linked to the idea of being a lifelong learner (Buchan 1998, Royal College of Nursing Australia 1998, Australian Government 2002), and are seen as increasingly important to professional nursing practice in the twenty-first century. Our capacity to respond appropriately and effectively in nursing practice is dependent upon the extent to which we connect clinical and theoretical knowledge.

Figure 23.1 depicts the interrelationship between clinical practice knowledge and the theoretical knowledge embedded in nursing-specific frameworks within nursing curricula. This diagram indicates that clinical activity and on-campus learning are interdependent.

In writing about the development of registered nurses, Benner (1984) has identified that the ability to integrate theory and practice to the point of being able to generalise is essential to development from novice (newly qualified nurse) to more advanced levels of nurse. However, Benner also acknowledges that there are particular challenges in being able to transfer concepts across clinical contexts. Effective clinicians are aware that *context* is the crucial moderator in nursing practice, and have developed mechanisms for managing situations contextually rather than seeking to manage all situations in the same way. Such ability to transfer core concepts across situations and modify actions according to context is an indication of 'expert' nursing practice (Benner 1984). Expanding upon this, we believe there is a need for learners to be able to transfer concepts between the learning cultures typical of on-campus and clinical environments.

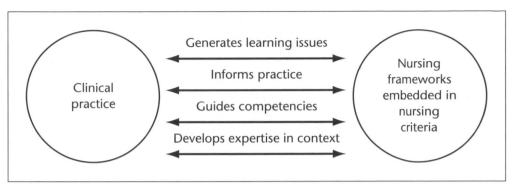

Figure 23.1 The interrelationship between practice and curriculum in nursing programs

In 1994, Dale argued that experiential knowledge (the knowledge that arises from the integration and subsequent analysis of theory in practice) is not adequately developed in nursing students. Thus, without clinical learning experiences which provide the opportunity to integrate classroom theory in 'real life' practice situations, nursing students have little opportunity to develop the lifelong learning skills of critical thinking and reflective practice considered important to professional practice (Benner et al 1996). Now, a decade on from Dale's work, the changing nature of health service delivery presents additional challenges to both clinicians and students. In literature related to contemporary health service delivery, it is widely acknowledged that reduced average lengths of stay, an ageing clientele, increased throughput and acuity, developments in healthcare and educational technology, and increasing numbers of learners requiring clinical experience, impact on the clinical learning milieu (Baker 2004, McMillan et al 2004). It is imperative that learners capitalise on events in both clinical and on-campus settings that foster their ability to critically analyse situations, identify underpinning knowledge and ideas, and critique their own professional development.

CONNECTING CLINICAL AND THEORETICAL LEARNING TO BECOME A KNOWLEDGE-ABLE NURSE

We recognise that, for many student nurses, clinical practice is the goal of nursing education.

Clinical educators, lecturers and clinicians often declare that they have a shared goal of ensuring quality education for nursing students. However, each of these sectors of the nursing community has what, at times, may seem to students to be very different definitions of nursing. This results in what students may perceive as a lack of alignment between experiences in education and health service sectors.

Much of this perceived lack of alignment has been attributed to what students and clinicians may hear described as the theory–practice gap. According to Howatson-Jones (2003), undergraduate nursing education programs have the dual purposes of preparing students for both vocational and educational areas. It is our view that nursing education has a single unifying focus—to assist people to be nurses. Being a nurse requires the ability to actively respond with nursing interventions, to think about the clinical judgments made and the consequences of action taken, and to develop a capacity to articulate that thinking to others.

The principles that underpin learning in the clinical area are used in on-campus learning activities. These are transferable across clinical and theoretical learning contexts.

Nursing has emerged as a distinct entity with curricula that emphasise nursing as a discipline distinguished from others (Duffy et al 1995, Greenwood 1996). Contemporary nursing curricula include discipline-specific knowledge, and integrate knowledge from other disciplines to inform the practice of nursing. This differs from previous practices of modifying knowledge from other disciplines to suit nursing situations. Thus, nursing education serves both an epistemological and political purpose, and students should be able to articulate and conceptualise the nature of their discipline and apply their thinking to actual practice.

The overarching structure of all nursing courses is the nursing curriculum, which determines both the outcomes which should be achieved and the processes by which these will be achieved. Nursing education programs include both on-campus and clinical learning experiences, which provide students with opportunities to practise the skills of nursing, to develop and demonstrate their knowledgebase about nursing, and to acquire academic skills that support communication of their thinking about nursing. Increasingly, nursing curricula use problem-based teaching strategies to encourage development of the knowledge, skills and behaviours of effective clinicians. This type of learning fosters exploration of 'real life' situations to enhance critical thinking and clinical decision making (Conway & Little 2003).

Figure 23.2 demonstrates the continual process of conceptualisation and reconceptualisation of nursing, which occurs through situation deconstruction, analysis and reconstruction. These enquiring and processing skills are essential to professional practice and the development of knowledge.

The curriculum should cause students to think about what they do as nurses, why they do what they do, and how they might do it differently. It is these enquiry skills that will cause the student to generate knowledge about nursing. For this reason it is important that the nursing curriculum raises questions such as: 'What is nursing?' 'What does it mean to nurse?' 'Whom do nurses nurse?' 'Where do nurses nurse?' 'Is nursing the same as caring?' and so on, as well as helping students to learn the task-oriented content of how to nurse.

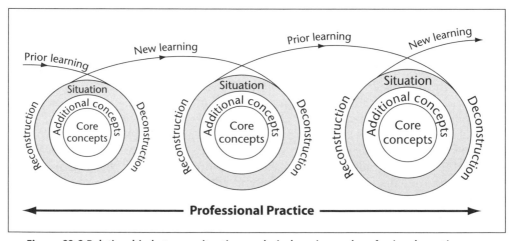

Figure 23.2 Relationship between situation analysis, learning and professional practice

Conceptualising or thinking about nursing needs to both direct and emerge from practice. It is a process of enquiry in which students work with concepts and form networks of concepts that frame and impact on their practice. It is not our intention to give the impression that qualified nurses should only think about nursing. The goal of nursing programs is to develop a graduate who can apply concepts to practice, manage complex nursing situations, and accept accountability for practice. Of course, this also demands skills in doing nursing activities.

However, we believe that students should be aware that nursing is about the ability to analyse situations and respond appropriately. How we interpret and analyse situations depends upon how we think about them. As our thinking about nursing develops, the meaning we give to situations changes and learning occurs. We then take this learning with us to the next situation and create new meanings and new, experiential knowledge.

Experiential knowledge is not merely being exposed to an experience. It is that which emerges when the experience is structured to achieve learning as an outcome of the experience. Therefore, students should use the theoretical base developed from on-campus, university-based activities to frame the clinical experience so that learning, rather than merely experiencing, occurs. Students should ask themselves: 'What is it that I want to achieve from this learning experience and how does this relate to my ability to practise nursing?'

Clinical learning experiences provide nursing students with the opportunity to begin to develop the skills of identifying general principles of practice, transferring these across contexts, and modifying actions based on principles of management. While clinical experience clearly is a powerful motivator for students to learn *how to* nurse, the literature suggests that clinical experiences are an important part of the transfer of learning from the classroom to the practice setting. Thus, *how* we think about nursing practice shapes *what* we learn from practice. *Being a nurse* requires the ability to integrate the knowledge, skills and attitudes of nursing into who we are and how we practise (Thorne & Hayes 1997).

Now, more than ever before, contemporary health service delivery demands that nurses demonstrate the full suite of skills representative of the knowledge-ABLE worker. The knowledge-ABLE worker aspires to enhance patient and staff safety, minimise adverse circumstances, promote partnership initiatives, focus on 'fitness-to-function' and acknowledge that health service delivery is dependent upon multiprofessional team effort. Thus, the student nurse as a knowledge-ABLE learner sees connections between clinical and theoretical knowledge of nursing within a broader framework of learning that integrates his or her experience and the outcomes of education for a knowledge-ABLE worker.

Table 23.1 presents the elements of contemporary health service challenge and desired knowledge-ABLE worker responses. The table indicates that although the factors that impact on health service delivery and healthcare work can be viewed in isolation, nurses, as knowledge-ABLE workers, require a multifaceted education to respond meaningfully to the challenges in contemporary health service provision.

HOW TO BEST DEVELOP KNOWLEDGE-ABILITY

Classroom-based learning activity provides us with the opportunity to explore, in a relatively safe environment, what we know, what we do and who we are as nurses,

Table 23.1: Worker response to a changing health service

Health service challenges	Knowledge-ABLE worker responses
Fragmented patient experience/changing health patterns/chronicity and consumerism	Contributors to systems review
Technology: increased emphasis on clinical and information systems interface	Effective managers of consumer expectations, competing value systems, and tensions in resource allocation
Changing workforce: unaligned skill mix and case mix	Procedurally competent, information fluent personnel
Inappropriate structures and process	Coordinators of throughput and care processes
Changing professional roles and functions	Participants in networked organisation and healthcare teams
Overcoming rigidity in professional frameworks and knowledge bases	Personnel who focus on consumer needs and outcomes rather than profession-specific outcomes

so that we are more prepared for professional practice situations. Clinical learning activity provides us with the opportunity both to test out what we have learnt in practice and to confront new situations from which we can further our learning. However, we can only learn if we are prepared to do so. It is important that we value learning as much as we value what we have learnt. It is our ability to question ourselves and our practice that enhances our professional development.

In order to learn we need to develop the process skills for lifelong learning (Maslin-Prothero 2001, Griffitts 2002, Armstrong et al 2003). These process skills are the basis of learning and are transferable across disciplines. In the case of nursing, nursing knowledge provides specific content which, when processed, results in nursing action. That is to say, when we become nurses we have developed general learning skills and we demonstrate our use of these through being able to 'think and act like a nurse'. In order to be lifelong learners in relation to nursing practice, we need to become what has been termed 'reflective practitioners'(Brookfield 1993, Johns 2000). We need to reflect about what we do as nurses, how we respond as nurses and individuals, and what we would do again in a similar situation. We then need to act when a similar situation occurs. The skills of reflective practice unite theoretical and clinical concepts.

In Figure 23.3 Gibbs (1988) provides a useful framework for situation analysis that is both thought-oriented and action-oriented, allows for consideration of the affective aspects of nursing experience and provides opportunity to explore how the learner as a reflective practitioner felt about the experience. Such an approach is particulary useful in nursing as it acknowledges human and emotional, as well as intellectual, domains of decision making.

Little (1996) has developed a framework of questions that are applicable in both classroom and clinical learning situations. These questions provide a useful guide to developing lifelong learning skills, yet are equally important questions for clinical decision making. The framework recognises that learning is inherently a personal experience and places emphasis on the subjective nature of learning (Griffitts 2002). In

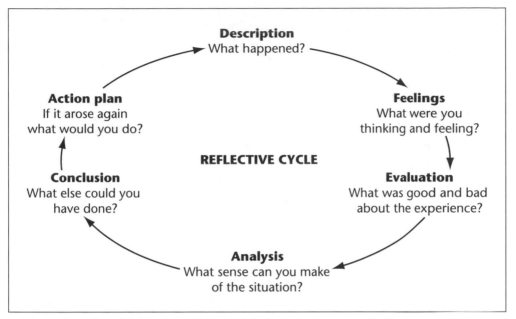

Figure 23.3 The reflective cycle
Source: G Gibbs 1988 *Learning by doing: a guide to teaching and learning methods.* Further
Education Unit, Oxford Polytechnic, Oxford.

order to be accountable for their practice, nurses need to become subjectively engaged
in that practice.

Little's approach consists of the sets of questions, related to a range of areas, in
the box below.

Little's (1996) framework of questions

Situation/analysis or decision making

- What information do I have?
- What further information do I need?
- What options/alternatives do I have?
- What should I prioritise?
- What action/s should I take?
- Why?
- Can I justify this action (lawfully, ethically, effectively, theoretically)?

The learning process

- What do I already know?
- How do I know it?
- What do I need to know?

- Where will I find it?
- What resources can I use?
- How will I know I know?
- Why should I learn it?

Perceptions

- What are my feelings?
- What are my beliefs about the situation?
- What are my assumptions?
- How have I derived these beliefs/assumptions?
- How do my feelings/beliefs:
  —affect my interpretation?
  —affect my response?
  —relate to espoused professional values?

Learning processes

- What is the validity of my source?
  —legislation
  —data based on research
  —opinion
  —practice
  —expertise
  —experience
- What is the currency of the knowledge, skills, behaviour?
- What is the support for this view?
  —political/ideological
  —cultural
- What other ideas/concepts/skills does it relate to?
- How does it relate to my view of the world (current understanding)?
- Why do I hold this belief/assumption?
- What are alternative beliefs/assumptions?

The situation revisited

- How does my learning relate to/apply in this situation?
- How does my learning relate to/affect my original ideas?
- What gaps/misconceptions did my learning identify?
- What ideas/skills did my learning confirm?
- What response would I give now in the situation?

Reflection on:

- Situation analysis:
  - —How well did I use the data?
  - —How well did I define the situation in need of a response?
  - —How comprehensive were my alternatives?
  - —How well can I justify my response?

The learning process:

- How valid/relevant were my sources?
- How comprehensive were my sources?
- How effective was my learning?

The group process:

- How well did I contribute?
- What was my role in the groups?
- How effective was each member's contribution?
- Did the group remain on task?
- Did the group attend to process (i.e. how people were feeling/responding/behaving)?

This framework of questions is useful because it encourages us to look at situations in context and to appreciate that, as learners and professionals who make sound clinical judgments, we are required to interact effectively with others, provide reasoning and support for our actions and decisions, and be aware that we are accountable for our own learning and practice actions.

KNOWLEDGE-ABILITY AS ACTIVE LEARNING

While both Gibbs' and Little's frameworks are relevant to a number of practice disciplines, including nursing, there is potential for nurses to utilise the 'learning' components of models such as these selectively and to overlook the critical elements related to action. In responding to the needs of individuals and communities, nursing is both reactive and proactive. As both the guardians of and visionaries for nursing's future, it is important that students be given the opportunity to develop the skills to critically evaluate the nursing practice they observe and to create and consider alternatives to this practice. The imagination of possibilities can only occur when nurses think about nursing. In other words, each of us has a professional responsibility to conceptualise in context. We need to think about what needs to be done for the client and how this impacts on the care situation. There needs to be a relationship established between theory, judgment and action-taking.

Ultimately, professional accountability is related to actions, not a capacity to generate ideas. Although theory is important, because it provides a framework for the work nurses do, it is of little consequence unless it results in effective nursing actions. Conversely, practice can become meaningless unless we seek to understand it through conceptualising the practice of nursing. Such integration of theory and practice leads to our moving beyond *becoming* nurses to *being* nurses who integrate our knowing, doing and being to produce what is meaningful, client-focused management of situations. Being reflective practitioners means that we are, both personally and professionally, constantly transformed and emancipated from our previous ways of thinking and acting (Brookfield 1993, Cranton 1994, Friere 1972, Mezirow 1985).

We agree that the primary aim of nursing education is to prepare nurses:

> . . . to be more responsive to societal needs, more successful in humanizing the highly technological milieus of health care, more caring and compassionate, more insightful about ethical and moral issues, more creative, more capable of critical thinking and better able to bring scholarly approaches to client problems and issues and to advocate ethical positions on behalf of clients (Bevis & Watson 1989:1).

We are also concerned that the attitude that clinical and classroom learning are separate entities may result in the mistaken perception that there is an insurmountable division between the theoretical and practical aspects of nursing. Students of nursing need to be encouraged to develop skills in reflective practice and situation analysis, not for the purpose of intellectualising or rationalising nursing practice, but for the purpose of identifying and maintaining excellence in clinical practice and meeting the goals of nursing identified by Bevis and Watson. Figure 23.4 represents what we perceive to be the relationships between context and lifelong learning processes and curriculum and improved practice. Achieving improved practice requires the process skills of lifelong learning and reflective practice.

The knowledge-ABLE nurse develops awareness that the range of factors that impact upon nursing extend beyond the immediate client care situation. Organisational theorists have developed PETS—a schema for examining these political, economic, sociocultural and technological factors. When nurses seek to enhance their knowledge-ABILITY, they should reflect upon the extent to which these factors shape what constitutes nursing service delivery. Figure 23.5 provides an example of the application of PETS to delivery of nursing services.

Invariably, when nursing students, qualified nurses and their employers are asked to evaluate nursing education, they feel that the time in clinical placements was

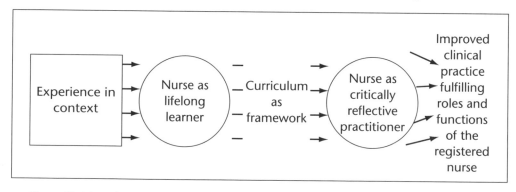

Figure 23.4 An educational equation for improved nursing practice

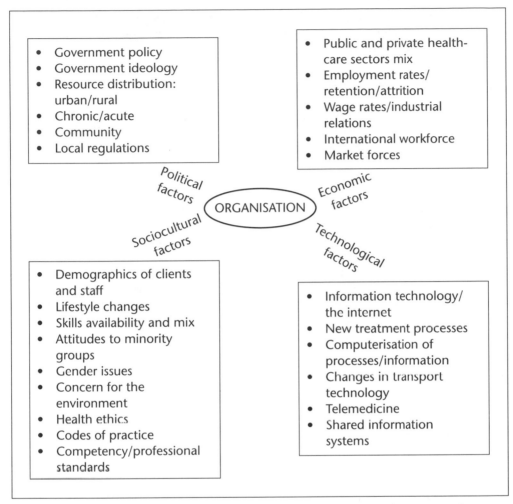

Figure 23.5 Application of the PETS framework to explore professional change in nursing

inadequate and suggest that there needs to be an increase in clinical time (Madjar et al 1997). However, it may well be that an increase in *quality* of the clinical experience is preferable to an increase in *quantity* of clinical placements (Conway & McMillan 2000). We believe that while clinical educators, lecturers and unit staff share in structuring the clinical experience, students are also accountable for ensuring that they gain a quality clinical experience. This accountability for self-learning links closely with the principles of adult learning and ongoing professional development (Maslin-Prothero 2001, Herrick et al 1998).

Chun-Heung and French (1997) report that, despite the emphasis on skills such as critical thinking, problem solving and reflective practice in on-campus learning experiences, in clinical settings students are encouraged to operate routinely and are not challenged to reflect upon their practice in a way that creates intellectual challenge.

Each student has a responsibility to integrate theory and practice experiences. With their colleagues in practice and education, students should seek intellectual challenge.

A useful framework for this can be reflective practice models, which facilitate full particpation in learning experiences. Underpinning reflective practice is a capacity to intellectualise and evaluate performance in context.

GAINING THE MOST FROM EXPERIENCE

In order to optimise learning it is important that each experience be approached as a way of linking theory and practice, and as an opportunity for further learning and generation of new perspectives. Increasingly, nurses are required to engage in roles beyond that of direct patient caregiver and engage in 'systems level intervention', such as contributor in multidisciplinary teams, researcher and manager, through which they facilitate quality patient care. At the very least, students need to think about how the roles and functions that registered nurses perform have shaped, and been shaped by, the practice situation.

Nursing students should explore roles other than direct caregiver. In most nursing programs the primary emphasis is placed on providing clinical experience in a range of settings (e.g. mental health, acute care and the community). However, it is unclear whether students are encouraged to explore a range of nursing roles and functions while in those settings (Conway & McMillan 2000). In order to prepare for the diversity of practice, students themselves should analyse each situation and try to determine what nursing roles and competencies are applicable. For example, students should ask themselves:

▲ What is the role of the registered nurse here? Is the registered nurse in this context a 'direct caregiver' or a 'care facilitator'?

▲ Does the role require skills as a clinician, supervisor, researcher, educator, manager or communicator, or a combination of these?

▲ If I were to be asked to manage this person's situation, what would I do and why?

▲ What nursing activities are most important and why?

▲ What knowledge base is required for sound clinical decision making?

▲ Where does this knowledge come from?

▲ How do I know what I know?

▲ What more could I know?

▲ How could I find out about this?

▲ How has my response to this situation been shaped by my beliefs about what practice is?

Asking questions such as these encourages us to explore the diverse roles and functions of nurses and to differentiate between the roles of registered nurses and other levels of nurses.

In order to maintain effectiveness as clinicians, nurses need to learn continually from a range of situations. In order to achieve this, it is essential that someone facilitate their learning towards *nursing* outcomes. Learners often seek, indeed need, external support, guidance and assessment (Brennan & Hutt 2001, Maslin-Prothero 2001). Thus the clinical educator, the university lecturing staff and other personnel can provide feedback and support to students or peers.

Clinical educators and preceptors in practice settings have been reported to fulfil many roles which seemingly mirror the roles of nurses, including practitioner, administrator, teacher, counsellor, problem solver, manager, assessor, advocate, guide and facilitator (Hart 1987, cited in Conway & McMillan 2000, Maslin-Prothero & Owen 2001).

The current trend in education to view educators as 'facilitators' rather than 'givers' of learning has been well recognised in nursing education literature. It implies that nurses as educators are increasingly adopting a more student-centred, collaborative model of education, which views nursing as a client-centred mutual interaction (Bevis & Krulik 1991). Moreover, the nurse as educator needs to model the way students or peers are expected to approach learning, as well as modelling exemplary nursing practice.

Clinical experiences provide the opportunity for students to observe and participate in nursing practice. Inherent in the notion of effective practice is the ability to make sound clinical judgments based on assessments and reassessments, to collaborate with others, to provide meaningful feedback to colleagues about performances, and to establish and maintain professional relationships. Clinical experiences acclimatise students to the real world of practice and its culture, providing preparation for the reality of practice which is dynamic and replete with novel situations.

Specifically, we have observed that students and clinicians in the clinical setting are often confused about when students should be observing another's practice and when they should be actively participating in the provision of client care. Understandably, students and clinicians alike want to be opportunistic and seize what they perceive to be limited practice learning opportunities and may, with the very best of intentions, place themselves and the client at risk because they are dealing with situations that are new to them. Our advice would be for the student to always consider the need for optimal client outcomes to be sure of the core objectives and concepts of the clinical placement, and determine the relationship between these goals and the activity to be performed. If the learning experience is highly desirable, students need to seek advice from the clinical educator about the scope of the student's practice and the need for close supervision.

When students are invited to perform care with which they do not feel comfortable, they might tell the qualified nurse that they are too busy or have other things to do. Sometimes the nurse, who has made an effort to give the student a meaningful learning experience, may interpret this response as disinterest in nursing. In situations such as these, we would suggest that students recognise the nurse's offer as a way to enhance their learning. The student should explain their situation to the senior nurse on duty, confirm that the qualified nurse is ultimately responsible for the client's care and engage in the activity as far as possible.

THE IMPORTANCE OF OTHER RESOURCES IN LEARNING

We have already made substantial reference to the reciprocity between theoretical and practical frameworks for learning, and identified the importance of focused experiences related to nursing in either classroom or clinical settings.

Classroom learning provides opportunities to explore options and alternatives, to justify thinking and to learn from examples drawn from practice. It also gives students opportunities to develop the 'scholarly approaches' referred to by Bevis and Watson (1989:1). An amplified enquiry approach is needed. Skills in clinical judgment are encouraged through the student developing nursing intervention strategies built upon explicit relationships between thought, judgment and action. Knowing about the person for whom students are caring requires a focus on our ability to acquire, recall and process information from a range of sources including, but not confined to, the immediate care situation.

While this is important learning, in our experience, it is also essential that student nurses are able to access, retrieve and use information from reputable sources, to draw conclusions about implications of ideas for nursing practice, and to communicate these in writing. Increasingly nursing programs are integrating these skills into the core nursing program and instructing students in information literacy and writing skills. Information literacy and fluency is required in both learning and practice settings.

Additional support in informative literacy and academic writing skills is available to students. Generic assistance to students ranges from short courses to individual consultations to assist in essay writing, including analysing and interpreting questions, planning, structuring and writing essays, referencing and assistance with mathematics for drug calculations. Students also benefit from spending time with the librarian, learning how to use the library effectively, to conduct literature searches, and use databases to access resources (McNeil et al 2003, National Advisory Council on Nurse Education and Practice 1997).

While we encourage the use of these support services, we would caution students that they do not provide discipline-specific information. That is to say, staff of these units can assist you in structuring your writing, ensure your grammar and punctuation are correct and inform you about referencing, but they cannot provide the ideas for your work because they do not 'think and act like nurses'. It is important that students seek assistance from lecturing and library staff who are aware of current issues and debates in nursing, to clarify questions and check their understanding of aspects of nursing.

Perhaps the most effective strategy we have seen students use in on-campus learning is the peer learning group, which provides students with a forum for discussion and clarification of their ideas, mutual assistance and support. We would encourage all students to participate in such a learning group. Your nursing department may already provide a web-based support service (such as 'Blackboard' or 'Web CT'), which perhaps you can ask about. This need not necessarily be on campus. The internet has made it possible to access a number of resources, including other students via the worldwide web. Of course, users should be cautious about disclosing personal information and should check the validity of any information obtained via 'the net'.

CONCLUDING THOUGHTS

Nursing has not fully appreciated the integration of thinking and doing to create informed action, and has historically tended to 'compartmentalise thinking from doing' (Pearson 1992:219). Discussion of the separation of thinking and doing does little to promote integration of on-campus and clinical learning activity. Students should view their learning to be nurses as occurring in two distinct yet interdependent contexts, the classroom and the clinical setting.

While there is increasing emphasis on the development of cognitive abilities in nursing students as well as the nature of contemporary practice, this should not lead to what has been labelled as a dichotomy between clinical skills and theoretical knowledge. Despite claims made by some authors that emphasis on theoretical knowledge in nursing results in a devaluing of clinical skills and, consequently, a devaluation of clinical practice (Bjork 1995, Elzubeir 1995), practical and theoretical nursing knowledge are inevitably and infinitely intertwined.

The past few decades have provided evidence that there is a paradigm shift in education, which now views learning as the construction of meaning in context rather than what to learn and how to do things (Ford & Profetto-McGrath 1994, Leder 1993, Townsend 1994). Nurse education is about the ability—indeed flexibility—to examine situations, deconstruct them from a number of perspectives, and reconstruct them around core concepts essential to nursing practice.

Contemporary nursing practice demands that nurses question and justify decisions in context, and emphasises the ability to think about nursing as well as the ability to perform nursing actions to best manage nursing situations. The challenge for students is to develop an integrated approach to practice which values thoughtful, highly skilled and efficient action, and to continue with lifelong learning and professional development—that is, to be knowledge-ABLE rather than simply knowledgable.

REFLECTIVE QUESTIONS

1 How can you become more responsible and accountable for your own learning?

2 How can you plan and evaluate your ongoing professional development?

3 Who can assist you with meeting these needs?

4 What are the factors that influence the extent to which espoused theory of nursing service delivery can be applied in the contemporary clinical practice?

RECOMMENDED READINGS

Benner P, Tanner C A, Chesla C A 1996 *Expertise in nursing practice: caring clinical judgement and ethics.* Springer, New York.

Lipe S, Beasley S 2003 *Critical thinking in nursing: a cognitive skills workbook.* Lippincott, Philadelphia.

Palmer A M, Burns S, Bulman C 1994 *Reflective practice in nursing: the growth of the professional practitioner.* Blackwell, Oxford.

REFERENCES

Abbey J C 1978 Bio-instrumentation: twentieth century slave. *Nursing Clinics of North America* 13(4):631–40.

Aber C S, Hawkins J 1992 Portrayal of nurses in advertisements in medical and nursing journals. *Image: Journal of Nursing Scholarship* 24:289–93.

Aboriginal and Torres Strait Islander Commission 2000 *Health framework summary*. Accessed 20 January 2004. Available from: http://www.atns.net.au.

Ackroyd S, Bolton S 1999 It is not Taylorism: mechanisms of work intensification in the provision of gynaecological services in a NHS hospital. *Work Employment and Society* 13(2):369–87.

Adamson B, Kenny D T, Wilson-Barnett J 1995 The impact of perceived medical dominance on the workplace satisfaction of Australian and British nurses. *Journal of Advanced Nursing* 21(1):172–83.

Ahmad M, Alasad J 2004 Predictors of patients' experiences of nursing care in medical-surgical wards. *International Journal of Nursing Practice* 10(5):235–41.

Allan J D, Hall B A 1988 Challenging the focus on technology: a critique of the medical model in a changing health care system. *Advances in Nursing Science* 10:22–34.

Allen D G, Allman K K M, Powers P 1991 Feminist nursing research without gender. *Advances in Nursing Science* 13(3):49–58.

Alligood M, Marriner-Tomey A eds 2002 *Nursing theory: utilization and application*, 2nd edn. Mosby, St Louis.

Alspach G 1993 Nurses as victims of violence (editorial). *Critical Care Nurse* 13(5):13–14, 17.

American Association of Colleges of Nursing 2002 *Annual state of the schools* Accessed 14 February 2003. Available from: http://www.aacn.nche.edu/media/annual report02.pdf.

Anderson L M, Scrimshaw S C, Fullilove M I, Fielding J E, Normand J 2003 Culturally competent healthcare systems: a systematic review. *American Journal of Preventive Medicine* 24(3S):68–79.

Anderson M 2004 Lesson from a postcolonial-feminist perspective: suffering and the path to healing. *Nursing Inquiry* 11(4):238–46.

Andrews B, Simmons P, Long I, Wilson R 2002 Identifying and overcoming the barriers to Aboriginal access to general practitioner services in rural New South Wales. *Australian Journal of Rural Health* 10:196–201.

Angell D (undated) *Vivian Bullwinkle*. Available from: http://www.angellpro.com.au/Bullwinkel.htm.

Antrobus S 2004 Why does nursing need political leaders? *Journal of Nursing Management* 12(4):227–8.

Armstrong M L, Johnston B A, Bridges R A, Gessner B A 2003 The impact of graduate education on reading for lifelong learning. *Journal of Continuing Education in Nursing* Thorofare, 34(1):19–25.

Aronowitz R A 1998 *Making sense of illness*. Cambridge University Press, Cambridge.

Arthur H, Wall D, Halligan A 2003 Team resource management: a programme for troubled teams. *Clinical Governance* 8(1):86–91.

Atkins S 2000 Developing underlying skills in the move towards reflective practice.

REFERENCES

In S Burns & C Bulman (eds) *Reflective practice in nursing: the growth of the professional practitioner,* 2nd edn, pp 28–51. Blackwell Science, Oxford.

Atwell A 2004 Discharge planning and multidisciplinary teamwork: an interprofessional battlefield? *Journal of Interprofessional Care* 18(1):79–80.

Australasian Nurses' Journal 1903 (editorial). March(1):1.

Australian Bureau of Statistics 2001 *Census population and housing Australia.* Accessed 10 January 2005. Available from: http://www.abs.gov.au.

Australian College of Midwives Incorporated (Victorian Branch) 1999 *Reforming midwifery: a discussion paper on the introduction of Bachelor of Midwifery Programs into Victoria.* Australian College of Midwives Inc, Melbourne.

Australian Council for Safety and Quality in Health Care 2002 *Second national report on patient safety improving medication safety.* Third report to the 'Australian health ministers' conference', Canberra.

Australian Government 2002 *National review of nursing education 2002: nursing regulation and practice.* Commonwealth of Australia, Canberra.

——2004a. Accessed 1 December 2004. Available from: http://health.gov.au/internet/wcms/publishing.nsf/Content/ruralhealth-policy-heal.

——2004b. Accessed 1 December 2004. Available from: http://www.health.gov.au/internet/wcms/publishing.nsf/Content/ruralhealth-studying-in.

——2004c. Accessed 1 December 2004. Available from: http://www.health.gov.au/internet/wcms/publishing.nsf/Content/ruralhealth-scholarship.

——2004d. Accessed 1 December 2004. Available from: http://www.hecs.gov.au/pels.htm.

Australian Health Information Council 2004 *Health workforce health informatics capacity building: national statement 2004.* Department of Health and Ageing, Canberra (in press).

Australian Institute of Family Studies 2002 *Introducing the longitudinal study of Australian children.* Australian Institute of Family Studies, Melbourne.

Australian Institute of Health and Welfare 1998 *Health in rural and remote Australia.* AIHW, Canberra.

——2000 *Australia's Health 2000: the seventh biennial report of the Australian Institute of Health and Welfare.* AIHW, Canberra.

——2002a *Australian hospital statistics 1999–00.* AIHW, Canberra.

——2002b *Australia's Health,* pp 215, 270–4. AIHW, Canberra.

——2002c *Australia's Health 2000.* Accessed 20 January 2005. Available from: http://www.AIHW.gov.au.

——2003 *Nursing labour force 2002.* AIHW, Canberra.

——2004a *Knowledgebase redevelopment.* AIHW, Canberra.

——2004b *Rural, regional and remote health: a guide to remoteness classifications.* AIHW, Canberra.

——2004c *Rural, regional and remote health: a study on mortality.* AIHW, Canberra.

Australian Legal Information Institute 2000 Council for Aboriginal Reconciliation Archive, *Members of Council 1991–2000.* Available from: http://www.austlii.edu.au/au/other/IndigLRes/car/2000/16/appendices04.htm.

Australian Nursing and Midwifery Council 2000 *National competency standards for the registered nurse,* 3rd edn. Available from: http://www.anmc.org.au/website/.

——2005 *Competency standards.* Available from: http://www.anmc.org.au/?event=-1,query=website/National%20Standards.

Australian Nursing Council Inc 1993 *Code of ethics for nurses in Australia,* revised 2002. ANCI, Canberra.

——1998 *ANCI national competency standards for the registered nurse*, 2nd edn. ANCI, Canberra.

Australian War Memorial (undated) *Nurse survivors of the* Vyner Brooke. Available from: http://www.awm.gov.au/encyclopedia/nurse_survivors/bullwinkel.htm.

Baker J 1996 Shared record keeping in the multidisciplinary team. *Nursing Standard* 10(26):39–41.

Baker K 2004 Issues from the health perspective. Keynote address to NSW Clinical Placement Forum, Sydney, 22 September.

Baly M E 1987 The Nightingale nurses: the myth and reality. In C Maggs (ed) *Nursing history: the state-of-the-art*. Croom Helm, New Hampshire.

Barger-Lux M J H, Heaney R P 1986 For better or worse: the technological imperative in health care. *Social Science Medicine* 22(12):1313–20.

Barker M 1989 *Nightingales in the mud: the digger nurses of the Great War*. Allen & Unwin, Sydney.

Barnard A 1996 Technology and nursing: an anatomy of definition. *International Journal of Nursing Studies* 33:433–41.

——1997 A critical review of the belief that technology is a neutral object and nurses are its master. *Journal of Advanced Nursing* 26:126–31.

——1998 Understanding technology in contemporary surgical nursing: a phenomenographic examination. Unpublished PhD thesis, University of New England, Armidale.

——2000a Alteration to will as an experience of technology and nursing. *Journal of Advanced Nursing* 31(5):1136–44.

——2000b Technology and the Australian nursing experience. In J Daly, S Speedy & D Jackson (eds) *Contexts of nursing: an introduction*, pp 163–76. MacLennan & Petty, Sydney.

——2002 Philosophy of technology and nursing. *Nursing Philosophy* 3:15–26.

Barnard A, Cushing A 2001 Technology and historical inquiry in nursing. In R Locsin (ed) *Advancing technology, caring and nursing*, pp 12–21. Auburn House, Westport.

Barnard A, Sandelowski M 2001 Technology and humane nursing care: (ir)reconcilable or invented difference? *Journal of Advanced Nursing* 34:367–75.

Barone S H, Roy C 1996 The Roy adaptation model in research: rehabilitation nursing. In P H Walker & B Neuman (eds) *Blueprint for use of nursing models: education, research, practice, and administration*, pp 64–75. National League for Nursing, New York.

Bartle J 2000 Clinical supervision: its place within the quality agenda. *Nursing Management* 7(5):30–3.

Barum B S 1998 Leadership: can it be holistic? In E C Hein *Contemporary leadership behaviour. Selected readings*. Lippincott, New York.

Bashford A 1997 Starch on the collar and sweat on the brow: self-sacrifice and the status of work for nurses. *Journal of Australian Studies* 67:74.

Bassett C 2002 Nurses' perceptions of care and caring. *International Journal of Nursing Practice* 8(1):8–15.

Baum F 2002 *The new public health*, 2nd edn. Oxford University Press, Melbourne.

Baumann A, Deber R, Silverman B, Mallette C 1998 Who cares? Who cures? The ongoing debate in the provision of health care. *Journal of Advanced Nursing* 28(5):1040.

Baumgardner J, Richards A 2003 The number one question about feminism. *Feminist Studies* 29(2):448–54.

BBC World Service, Tuesday 22 August 2000, Who wants to live forever? Available from: 20http://www.bbc.co.uk/worldservice/people/highlights/000822_116.shtml.

REFERENCES

Beare P, Meyers J 1994 *Principles and practice of adult health nursing*. Mosby, St Louis.

Beauchamp T, Childress J 2001 *Principles of biomedical ethics*, 5th edn. Oxford University Press, New York.

Beck C 1999 Quantitative measurement of caring. *Journal of Advanced Nursing* 30(1):24.

Begany T 1994 Your image is brighter than ever. *RN* 57:28.

Benner P 1984 *From novice to expert: excellence and power in clinical nursing*. Addison Wesley, Menlo Park, California.

——1991 The role of experience, narrative, and community in skilled ethical comportment. *Advances in Nursing Science* 14(2):1–21.

——ed 1994 *Interpretive phenomenology: embodiment, caring, and ethics in health and illness*. Sage, Thousand Oaks, California.

Benner P, Hooper-Kyriakidis P, Stannard D 1999 *Clinical wisdom and interventions in critical care: a thinking-in-action approach*. W B Saunders, Philadelphia.

Benner P, Tanner C A, Chesla C A 1996 *Expertise in nursing practice: caring clinical judgment and ethics*. Springer, New York.

Benner P, Wrubel J 1989 *The primacy of caring: stress and coping in health and illness*. Addison Wesley, Menlo Park, California.

Bent K N 1993 Perspectives on critical and feminist theory in developing nursing praxis. *Journal of Professional Nursing* 9(5):296–303.

Berriot-Salvadore E 1993 The discourse of medicine and science. In N Z Davis & A Farge (eds) *A history of women in the west: Vol. 3 Renaissance and enlightenment paradoxes*. Belknap Press, Cambridge, Massachusetts.

Bessant G 1980 Rural schooling and the rural myth in Australia. *Comparative Education* 14:121–32.

Bevis E 1978 *Curriculum building in nursing*. Mosby, St Louis.

Bevis E, Krulik T 1991 Nationwide faculty department: a model for a shift from diploma to baccalaureate education. *Journal of Advanced Nursing* 16(3):362–70.

Bevis E O, Watson J 1989 *Toward a caring curriculum: a new pedagogy for nursing*. National League for Nursing, New York.

Biedermann N 2004 *Tears on my pillow: Australian nurses in Vietnam*. Random House, Sydney.

Bishop A, Scudder J 1990 *The practical, moral, and personal sense of nursing: a phenomenological philosophy of practice*. State University of New York Press, Albany.

Bjork I T 1995 Neglected conflicts in the discipline of nursing: perceptions of the importance and value of practical skill. *Journal of Advanced Nursing* 22:6–12.

Black A 2003 *Guild and state: European political thought from the twelfth century to the present*. Transaction Publishers, New Jersey.

Black F ed 1992 *Primary nursing: an introductory guide*. King's Fund Centre, London.

Blendon R J, Schoen C, DesRoches C M, Osborn R, Scoles K L, Zapert K 2002 Inequalities in health care: a five-country survey. *Health Affairs* 21:182–91.

Blue I, Fitzgerald M 2002 Interprofessional relations: case studies of working relationships between registered nurses and general practitioners in rural Australia. *Journal of Clinical Studies* 11:314–21.

Bolton S C 2000 Who cares? Offering emotion work as a 'gift' in the nursing labour process. *Journal of Advanced Nursing* 32(3):580–6.

Bonawit V 1989 The image of the nurse: the community's perception and its implications for the profession. In G Gray & R Pratt (eds) *Issues in Australian nursing 2*, pp 163–74. Churchill Livingstone, Melbourne.

Borbasi S-A 1996 Living the experience of being nursed: a phenomenological text. *International Journal of Nursing Practice* 2(4):222–8.

REFERENCES

Borbasi S, Jones J, Gaston C 2004 Leading, motivating and supporting colleagues in nursing practice. In J Daly, S Speedy & D Jackson (eds) *Nursing leadership*, pp 167–81. Churchill Livingstone, Sydney.

Boss B J 1989 Presidential address: specialty nursing. *Journal of Neuroscience Nursing* 21(4):213–15.

Boud D, Keogh R, Walker D 1985 *Reflection: turning experience into learning*. Kogan Page, London.

Boughn S 2001 Why women and men choose nursing. *Nursing and Health Care Perspectives* 22(1):14–24.

Bowd D G 1968 *Lucy Osburn: founder of the Nightingale system of nursing at Sydney Hospital*. Hawkesbury Press, Windsor.

Bowers L 1989 The significance of primary nursing. *Journal of Advanced Nursing* 14:13–19.

Boykin A, Schoenhofer S O 2001 *Nursing as caring: a model for transforming practice*. Jones & Bartlett, Publishers, National League for Nursing Press, Sudsbury, Massachusetts.

Boyle M V 2002a Sailing twixt Scylla and Charybdis. *Women in Management Review* 17(3/4):131–41.

——2002b You wait until you get home: emotional regions, emotional process work and the role of off-stage support. Paper presented at the 'Third emotions in organisational life conference', Bond University, Gold Coast.

Brackman Keane C 1969 *Essentials of nursing: a medical-surgical text for practical nurses*. W B Saunders, Philadelphia.

Braithwaite J, Westbrook M 2004 A survey of staff attitudes and comparative managerial and non-managerial views in a clinical directorate. *Health Services Management Research* 17:141–66.

——2005 Rethinking clinical organisational structures: an attitude survey of doctors, nurses and allied health staff in clinical directorates. *Journal of Health Services Research & Policy* 10(1):10–17.

Brennan A M, Hutt R 2001 The challenges and conflicts of facilitating learning in practice: the experiences of two clinical nurse educators. *Nurse Education in Practice* 1(4):181–8.

Brennan S 1998 Nursing and motherhood constructions: implications for practice. *Nursing Inquiry* 5(1):11–17.

Bridges J 1990 Literature review on the images of the nurse and nursing in the media. *Journal of Advanced Nursing* 15:850–4.

Briggs D 1991 Critical care nurses' roles—traditional or expanded/extended. *Intensive Care Nursing* 7:223–9.

Briles J 1994 *The Briles report on women in healthcare: changing conflict to collaboration in a toxic workplace*. Jossey-Bass, San Francisco.

Brink P J, Wood M J 1993 Basic steps in planning nursing research. Jones & Bartlett, Boston.

Brockett M, Bauer M 1998 Continuing professional education: responsibilities and possibilities. *Journal of Continuing Education in the Health Professions* 18:235–43.

Brodie J A 1984 Response to Dr J Fawcett's paper. *Image: Journal of Nursing Scholarship* 16(3):87–98.

Bronfenbrenner U 1979 *The ecology of human development*. Harvard University Press, Cambridge, Massachusetts.

Brookfield S 1993 On impostorship, cultural suicide and other dangers: how nurses learn critical thinking. *Journal of Continuing Education in Nursing* 24(5): 197–205.

Brown C R 1998 Gender segmentation in the paid work force: the case of nursing. Unpublished PhD thesis. Griffith University, Brisbane.

Brown J 1992 Nurses or technicians? The impact of technology on oncology nursing. *Canadian Oncology Nursing Journal* 2:12–17.

Brown M S, Ohlinger J, Rusk C, Delmore P, Ittmann P, Group C 2003 Implementing potentially better practices for multidisciplinary team building: creating a neonatal intensive care unit culture of collaboration. *Pediatrics* 111(4 Pt 2):482–8.

Brunt H J 1985 An exploration of the relationship between nurses' empathy and technology. *Nurse Administration Quarterly* 9:69–78.

Brykczynska G ed 1997 *Caring: the compassion and wisdom of nursing*. Arnold. London.

Bubeck P E 1995 *Care, gender and justice*. Clarendon Press, Oxford.

Buchan J 1998 Nurses off the peg. *Nursing Standard* 13(1):23–4.

Buchanan T 1997 Nursing our narratives: towards a dynamic understanding of nurses in literary texts. *Nursing Inquiry* 4(2):80–7.

——1999 Nightingalism: haunting nursing history. *Collegian* 6(1):28–33.

Bullough B, Bullough V 1972 A brief history of medical practice. In E Friedson & J Lorber (eds) *Medieval men and their work*, pp 86–102. Aldine-Atherton, Chicago.

Bulter A, Garvey A 2003 Professional issues: the more things change . . . *The Lamp* 60(6):24–5.

Burbridge G N 1935 *Lecture for nurses*. Infectious Diseases Hospital, Melbourne.

Buresh B, Gordon S 2003 *From silence to voice: what nurses know and must communicate to the public*. Cornell University Press, New York (first published in 2000 by the Canadian Nurses' Association).

Burley M, Harvey D 1993 Nurses and their small rural communities. In conference proceedings of the 'Nursing the country conference of the Association for Australian Rural Nurses Inc', pp 149–58. Warrnambool, Victoria.

Burns N, Grove S K 2005 *The practice of nursing research: conduct, critique and utilization*, 5th edn. Elsevier/Saunders, St Louis.

Burton A J 2000 Reflection: nursing's practice and education panacea? *Journal of Advanced Nursing* 31(5):1009–17.

Burton B 2004 News: Australia's contribution to global health fund provokes dismay. *British Medical Journal* 328:486.

Bush A, van Holst Pellekaan S 1995 Footprints: a trail to survival. In G Gray & R Pratt (eds) *Issues in Australian nursing*, pp 219–33. Churchill Livingston, Melbourne.

Bushy A 2002 International perspectives on rural nursing: Australia, Canada, USA. *Australian Journal of Rural Health* 10(2):104–11.

Caffrey R, Caffrey P 1994 Nursing: caring or codependent? *Nursing Forum* 29(1):12–17.

Calne S 1994 Dehumanisation in intensive care. *Nursing Times* 90:31–3.

Cameron C, McKenzie F, Warnock L, Farquhar D 2000 Impact of a nurse led multidisciplinary team on an acute medical admissions unit. *Health Bulletin* 60(6):512–14.

Campbell S L 2003 Cultivating empowerment in nursing today for a strong profession tomorrow. *Journal of Nursing Education* 42(9):423.

Campinha-Bacote J 1999 A model and instrument for addressing cultural competence in health care. *Journal of Nursing Education* 38:203–7.

Canadian Institute of Health Information 2003. Accessed 20 January 2005. Available from: http://www.cihi.ca.

Caplan G, Brown A 1997 Post-acute care: can hospitals do better with less? *Australian Health Review* 20(2):43–52.

Capra F 1982 *The turning point: science, society and the rising culture*. Simon & Schuster, New York.

REFERENCES

Carnevali D L 1985 Nursing perspectives in health care technology. *Nursing Administration Quarterly* 9:10–18.

Carpenter M 1977 The new managerialism and professionalism in nursing. In M Stacey, M Reid, C Heath & R Dingwall (eds) *Health and the division of labour*, pp 165–91. Croom Helm, London.

Carper B 1978 Fundamental patterns of knowing in nursing. *Advances in Nursing Science* 1:13–23.

Carter S, Garside P, Black A 2003 Multidisciplinary team working, clinical networks, and chambers: opportunities to work differently in the NHS. *Quality & Safety in Health Care* 12(1):25–8.

Castles S 1999 Globalisation, multicultural citizenship and transnational democracy. In G H Hage & R Couch (eds) *The future of Australian multiculturalism: reflections on the 20th anniversary of Jean Martin's The Migrant Presence*. NSW Research Institute for Humanities, University of Sydney, Sydney.

Castles S, Foster W, Iredale R, Withers G eds 1998 *Immigration and Australia: myths and realities*. Allen & Unwin, Sydney.

Ceci C 2004a Gender, power, nursing: a case analysis. *Nursing Inquiry* 11(2):72–81.

——2004b Nursing, knowledge and power: a case analysis. *Social Science & Medicine* 59:1879–89.

Cesario S, Morin K, Santa-Donato A 2002 Evaluating the level of evidence of qualitative research. *Journal of Obstetrics, Gynecology and Neonatal Nursing* 31:531–7.

Chan P, Fischer S, Steward T, Hallett D, Hynes-Gay P, Lapinsky S, MacDonald R, Mehta S 2001 Practising evidence-based medicine: the design and implementation of a multidisciplinary team-driven extubation protocol. *Critical Care* 5:349–54.

Cheek J 1995 Nurses, nursing and representation: an exploration of the effect of viewing positions on the textual portrayal of nursing. *Nursing Inquiry* 2: 235–40.

Cheek J, Rudge T 1995 Only connect . . . feminism and nursing. In G Gray & R Pratt (eds) *Scholarship in the discipline of nursing*. Churchill Livingstone, Melbourne.

Chiarella M 2000 Silence in court: the devaluation of the stories of nurses in the narratives of health law. *Nursing Inquiry* 7(3):191–9.

Chinn P 1989 Awake, awake. *Advances in Nursing Science* 11(2):1.

Chinn P, Jacobs M K 1983 *Theory and nursing: a systematic approach*. Mosby, St Louis.

——1987 A model for theory development in nursing. *Advances in Nursing Science* 1(1):1–11.

Chinn P L, Maeve M K, Bostick C 1997 Aesthetic inquiry and the art of nursing. *Scholarly Inquiry for Nursing Practice* 11(2):83–100.

Chinn P L, Watson J eds 1994 *Art and aesthetics in nursing*. National League for Nursing, New York.

Chun-Heung L, French P 1997 Education in the practicum: a study of the ward learning climate in Hong Kong. *Journal of Advanced Nursing* 26(3):455–62.

Clark G 1989 To be or not to be—it's time to market nursing's image. In G Gray & R Pratt (eds) *Issues in Australian nursing 2*, pp 175–92. Churchill Livingstone, Melbourne.

Cloyes K 2002 Agonizing care: care ethics, agonistic feminism and a political theory of care. *Nursing Inquiry* 9(3):203–14.

Coats A 2004 *Report from the chair. AHIC e-bulletin*. Australian Health Information Council, Canberra.

Cochrane A L 1972 *Effectiveness and efficiency: random reflections on health services*. Nuffield Provincial Hospitals Trust, London.

Cockrill P 1999 *Healing the heart: 60 years of Alice Springs Hospital 1939–1999*.

Alice Springs Hospital's 60th Anniversary Reunion organising committee, Alice Springs.

Cohen I B 1984 Florence Nightingale. *Scientific American* March:128–36.

Cohen J S 1991 Two portraits of caring: a comparison of the artists, Leininger and Watson. *Journal of Advanced Nursing* 16:899–909.

Collins Y 1999 The provision of hospital care in country Victoria 1840s to 1940s. Unpublished PhD thesis. Department of History of Philosophy and Science, University of Melbourne, Melbourne.

Collins Y, Kippen S 2003 The 'Sairey Gamps' of Victorian nursing? Tales of drunk and disorderly wardsmen in Victorian hospitals between the 1850s and the 1880s. *Health and History* 5:42–64.

Committee of Inquiry into Allegations Concerning the Treatment of Cervical Cancer at National Women's Hospital and into Other Related Matters 1988 *The report of the committee of inquiry into allegations concerning the treatment of cervical cancer at National Women's Hospital and into other related matters.* Auckland.

Commonwealth Department of Veterans Affairs 2000 *The Sinking of the* Centaur. Available from: ttp://www.dva.gov.au/media/publicat/2003/centaur/index.htm.

Commonwealth of Australia 1999a *A new agenda for multicultural Australia.* Accessed 20 January 2005. Available from: http://www.immigration.gov.au/multicultural/inc/publication.

——1999b Health*Connect*. Department of Health and Ageing. Canberra. Accessed 15 December 2004. Available from: http://www.healthconnect.gov.au/.

——2002 *National review of nursing education 2002: our duty of care.* Commonwealth of Australia, Canberra.

——2003a *National electronic decision support taskforce report (final).* Department of Health and Ageing, Canberra.

——2003b *Report on the health information workforce capacity think tank.* Department of Health and Ageing, Canberra.

——2004 *Budget papers*. Canberra. Accessed 20 October 2004. Available from: http://www.health.gov.au/internet/wcms/publishing.nsf/Content/health-budget2003-index1.htm.

Compact Oxford English dictionary 2004. Available from: http://www.askoxford.com/concise_oed/research.

Coney S 1988 *The unfortunate experiment*. Penguin Books, Auckland.

Conrick M 2002 Looking for a needle in a haystack: searching the internet for quality resources. *Contemporary Nurse* 12(1):49–58.

——2005 The international classification for nursing practice: a tool to support nursing practice? *Collegian* (in press).

Conrick M, Hovenga E, Cook R, Laracuente T, Morgan T 2004 *A framework for nursing informatics in Australia: a strategic paper.* HISA–NIA, Department of Health and Ageing, Melbourne.

Conway J, Little P 2003 Adopting PBL as an institutional approach: considerations and challenges. *Journal of Excellence in College Teaching* 11(2):11–26.

Conway J, McMillan M 2000 Maximising learning opportunities. In J Daly, S Speedy & D Jackson (eds) *Contexts of nursing: an introduction*, pp 238–52. MacLennan & Petty, Sydney.

Coope C 1996 Does teaching by cases mislead us about morality? *Journal of Medical Ethics* 22(1):46–52.

Cooper M C 1993 The intersection of technology and care in the ICU. *Advances in Nursing Science* 15(3):23–32.

Cornia G 1999 Liberalization, globalization and income distribution. UNU/WIDER Working paper No. 157. Cited in Poverty and health in Australia: an edited version of the Doctors Reform Society submission to the Senate Inquiry into Poverty and Financial Hardship, 2003. *New Doctor* Autumn:80.

Cotton A 2001 Private thoughts in public spheres: issues in reflection and reflective practices in nursing. *Journal of Advanced Nursing* 36(4):512–19.

Council of Australian Governments (undated) *Trans-Tasman Mutual Recognition Arrangement*. Available from: http://www.coag.gov.au/recognition.htm#ttmra.

Courtney M, Edwards H, Smith S, Finlayson K 2002a The impact of rural clinical placement on student nurses' employment intentions. *Collegian* 9:12–18.

Courtney M, Yacopetti J, James C, Walsh A, Finlayson K 2002b Comparison of roles and professional development needs of nurse executives working in metropolitan, provincial, rural or remote settings in Queensland. *Australian Journal of Rural Health* 10:202–8.

Cox H, Hickson P, Taylor B 1991 Exploring reflection: knowing and constructing practice. In G Gray & R Pratt (eds) *Towards a discipline of nursing*, pp 373–89. Churchill Livingstone, Melbourne.

Cramer J 1992 Remote area community health services. In F Braum, D Fry & I Lennie (eds) *Community health: policy and practice in Australia*, pp 235–48. Pluto Press, Sydney.

——1994 Finding solutions to support remote area nurses. *Australian Nursing Journal* 2:21–5.

Crane S 1991 Implications of the critical paradigm. In G Gray & R Pratt (eds) *Towards a discipline of nursing*, pp 391–411. Churchill Livingstone, Melbourne.

Cranton P 1994 *Understanding and promoting transformative learning: a guide for educators of adults*. Jossey-Bass, San Francisco.

Craven R F, Hirnle C J eds 2003 *Fundamentals of nursing: human health and function*, 4th edn. Lippincott, Philadelphia.

Crookes P A 1992 The politics of health care. In J Boddy & V Rice *Health: perspectives and practices*, pp 216–32. Dunmore Press, Palmerston North.

Crookes P A, Davies S eds 1998 *Research into practice: essential skills for reading and applying research in nursing and health care*. Bailliere Tindall, Edinburgh.

——eds 2004 *Essential skills for reading and applying research in nursing and health care: research into practice*, 2nd edn. Bailliere Tindall, Sydney.

Crowell D M 2000 Building spirited multidisciplinary teams. *Journal of Perianesthesia Nursing* 15(2):108–14.

Cuff H E, Gordon Pugh W T 1924 *Practical nursing including hygiene and dietetics*. William Blackwood, Edinburgh.

Currell R, Wainwright P, Urquhart C 2002 *Nursing record systems: effects on nursing practice and health care outcomes*. Cochrane Library Update Software, Oxford.

D'Antonio P 1997 Toward a history of research in nursing. *Nursing Research* 4(2):105–10.

Dale A 1994 The theory–theory gap: the challenge for nurse teachers. *Journal of Advanced Nursing* 20:521–4.

Darbyshire P 1985 Bedpans or broomsticks? *Nursing Times* 81:44–5.

——1994a Understanding caring through arts and humanities: a medical/nursing humanities approach to promoting alternate experiences of thinking and learning. *Journal of Advanced Nursing* 19(5):856–63.

——1994b Understanding the life of illness: learning through the art of Frida Kahlo. *Advances in Nursing Science* 17(1):51–9.

——1995 Reclaiming 'Big Nurse': a feminist critique of Ken Kesey's portrayal of Nurse Ratched in *One flew over the cuckoo's nest*. *Nursing Inquiry* 2(4): 198–202.

Daski I 2000 The road to professionalism in nursing: case management or practice based in nursing theory. *Nursing Science Quarterly* 13(1):74–9.

REFERENCES

David B A 2000 Nursing's gender politics: reformulating the footnotes. *Advances in Nursing Science* 23(1):83–94.

Davies B 1991 The concept of agency: a feminist poststructuralist analysis. *Social Analysis* 30:42–53.

Davies C 1995 *Gender and the professional predicament in nursing.* Open University Press, Buckingham.

——2004 Political leadership and the politics of nursing. *Journal of Nursing Management* 12:235–41.

Davies C, Sharp P 2000 The assessment and evaluation of reflection. In S Burns & C Bulman (eds) *Reflective practice in nursing: the growth of the professional practitioner,* 2nd edn, pp 52–78. Blackwell Science, Oxford.

Davis R, Thurecht R 2001 Care planning and case conferencing. Building effective multidisciplinary teams. *Australian Family Physician* 30(1):78–81.

Davison G 2000 *The use and abuse of Australian history.* Allen & Unwin, Sydney.

Dawson S 2000 *Whistleblowing: a broad definition and some issues for Australia.* Working Paper 3/2000. Victoria University of Technology. Available from: http://www.uow.edu.au/arts/sts/bmartin/dissent/documents/Dawson.html.

Deeble J S 1999 Medicare: Where have we been? Where are we going? *Australian New Zealand Journal of Public Health* 23:563–70.

Delacour S 1991 The construction of nursing: ideology, discourse and representation. In G Gray & R Pratt (eds) *Towards a discipline of nursing,* pp 413–33. Churchill Livingstone, Melbourne.

Demerouti E, Bakker A B, Nachreiner F, Schaufeli W B 2000 A model of burnout and life satisfaction amongst nurses. *Journal of Advanced Nursing* 32(2): 454–64.

Dendaas N 2004 The scholarship related to nursing work environments: where do we go from here? *Advances in Nursing Science* 27(1):12–21.

Denzin N K, Lincoln Y S 2000 eds *Handbook of qualitative research,* 2nd edn. Sage, Thousand Oaks, California.

Department of Employment, Education, Training and Youth Affairs 1998 *Review of higher education financing and policy (final report): learning for life* (DEETYA Publication No. 6055HERE 98A). AGPS, Canberra.

Department of Human Services 2000 *Victorian secondary school nursing program: consultation paper.* DHS, Melbourne.

——2001 *Best start: evidence base summary.* Community Care Division, DHS, Melbourne. Available from: www.beststart.vic.gov.au.

——2004a *Continuity of care: a communication protocol for Victorian maternity services and the Maternal and Child Health Service.* Community Care Division, DHS, Melbourne. Available from: www.health.dhs.vic.gov.au/commcare/.

——2004b *Cultural diversity guide.* Policy and Strategic Projects Division, DHS, Melbourne. Available from: www.dhs.vic.gov.au/mulitcultural/.

Department of Human Services and Health 1994 *Nursing education in Australian universities: report of the national review of nurse education in the higher education sector, 1994 and beyond.* AGPS, Canberra.

Department of Immigration and Multicultural and Indigenous Affairs 2002 *Refugee and humanitarian issues: Australia's response.* Accessed 20 January 2005. Available from: http://www.immi.gov.au/refugee/publications/refhumiss.htm.

——2003 *Review of settlement services for migrants and humanitarian entrants.* Accessed 20 January 2005. Available from: http://www.dima.gov/settle/settle-review/execum1.htm.

Devine E C, Cook T D 1986 Clinical and cost saving effects of psychosocial educational interventions with surgical patients: a meta-analysis. *Research in Nursing and Health* 9:89–105.

342

REFERENCES

DeVries R G B, Barroso R 2000 *Midwives among the machines: recreating midwifery in the late 20th century*. Accessed 14 September 2000. Available from: http://www. stolaf.edu/people/devries/docs/midwifery.html.

DeVries S, Dunlop M, Goopy S, Moyle W, Sutherland-Lockhart D 1995 Discipline and passion: meaning, masochism and mythology in popular medical romances. *Nursing Inquiry* 2(4):203–10.

Dickens C 1843 *The life and adventures of Martin Chuzzlewit*. Chapman & Hall, London.

——1910 *Martin Chuzzlewit*. Macmillan, New York.

Dickoff J, James P 1984 Toward a cultivated but decisive theoretical pluralism. In M McGee (ed) *Theoretical pluralism in nursing science*. University of Ottawa Press, Ottawa.

DiMauro N M 2000 Continuous professional development. *Journal of Continuing Education in Nursing* 31(2):59–62.

Dion X 2004 A multidisciplinary team approach to public health working. *British Journal of Community Nursing* 9(4):149–54.

DMR Consulting 2004a *Benefits realisation framework*. Department of Health and Ageing, Canberra. Accessed 20 February 2004. Available from: http://www. healthconnect.gov.au/research/benefits.htm.

——2004b *Indicative benefits report*. Department of Health and Ageing, Canberra. Accessed 20 February 2004. Available from: http://www.healthconnect.gov.au/ research/benefits.htm.

Dobson R 1999 Global health gap widens says World Bank. *British Medical Journal* 319(7208):470.

Dock L L, Stewart I M 1920 *A short history of nursing*. Putnam, New York.

Doering L 1992 Power and knowledge in nursing: a feminist poststructuralist view. *Advances in Nursing Science* 14(4):24–33.

Doherty M K, Russell R L eds 1996 *The life and times of Royal Prince Alfred Hospital, Sydney, Australia*. New South Wales College of Nursing, Sydney.

Donahue P 1996 *Nursing: the finest art*. Mosby, St Louis.

Donaldson P, Conrick M 2004 *The effectiveness of using a patient dependency system to develop and audit clinical pathways*. HIC2004. HISA, Brisbane.

Donaldson S K, Crowley D M 1978 The discipline of nursing. *Nursing Outlook* February:113–20.

Donnelly C 2003 Leadership: professional, inspirational or dysfunctional? *Journal of Nursing Management* 11(2):65–7.

Dowd T, Johnson S 1995 Remote area nurses—on the cutting edge. *Collegian* 2:36–40.

Droogan J, Cullum N 1998 Systematic reviews in nursing. *International Journal of Nursing Studies* 35:13–22.

Duckett S J 2004 *The Australian health care system*, 2nd edn. Oxford University Press, Melbourne.

Duffield C, Lumby J 1994 Caring nurses: the dilemma of balancing costs and quality. *Australian Health Review* 17(2):72–83.

Duffy N, Foster C, Kuiper R, Long J, Robison L 1995 Planning nurses' education for the 21st century. *Journal of Advanced Nursing* 21:772–7.

Duke S 2000 The experience of becoming reflective. In S Burns & C Bulman (eds) *Reflective practice in nursing: the growth of the professional practitioner*, 2nd edn, pp 137–55. Blackwell Science, Oxford.

Duncan P A A 1992 Media portrayals of nursing versus the actual work of nurses. Unpublished PhD thesis. Syracuse University, New York State (UMI order number PUZ 9303654).

Dunlop M 1986 Is a science of caring possible? *Journal of Advanced Nursing* 11(3):661–70.

REFERENCES

Dunn A 1985–86 Images of nursing in the nursing and popular press. *Bulletin of the Royal College of Nursing (UK) History of Nursing Group* 6:2–8.

Durdin J 1991 *They became nurses: a history of nursing in South Australia 1836–1980.* Allen & Unwin, Sydney.

Dye T R, Harrison B C 2005 *Power and society: an introduction to the social sciences,* 10th edn. Thomson Wadsworth, Belmont, California.

Dyson J 1996 Nurses' conceptualizations of caring attitudes and behaviours. *Journal of Advanced Nursing* 23:1263–9.

Eckermann A, Dowd T, Martin M, Nixon L, Gray R, Chong E 1996 *Binaj Goonj: bridging cultures in Aboriginal health.* University of New England Press, Armidale.

Edgecombe G 2004 Child and family nursing and early intervention. *Contemporary Nurse* 18(1):143–4.

Edgecombe G, Hope M, Ward M 2004 *Because you're a nurse—I thought I would come and see you: a participatory action research project of Victoria's secondary school nursing program.* RMIT University, Melbourne.

Edgecombe G, Rogers P, Kimberley S, Jackson C, Myers D, Mancini V, Needham P, White S, Marsh G, Stewart M 2001 *Maternal and child health New Initiatives Projects Evaluation (NIPE).* Department of Human Services, Melbourne.

Edwards S D 1999 The idea of nursing science. *Journal of Advanced Nursing* 29(3):563–9.

Ehrenreich B, English D 1973 *Witches, midwives, and nurses.* Writers and Readers Co-operative, London.

——1979 *For her own good: 150 years of experts' advice to women.* Pluto, London.

Ekstrom D N 1999 Gender and perceived nurse caring in nurse–patient dyads. *Journal of Advanced Nursing* 29(6):1393–1401.

Elliott D 2003a Assessing instrument psychometrics. In Z Schneider, D Elliott, G LoBiondo-Wood & J Haber (eds) *Nursing research: methods, critical appraisal and utilisation,* 2nd edn, pp 331–48. Mosby, Sydney.

——2003b Research and professional practice. In Z Schneider, D Elliott, G LoBiondo-Wood & J Haber (eds) *Nursing research: methods, critical appraisal and utilisation,* 2nd edn. Mosby, Sydney.

——2003c Searching literature sources. In Z Schneider, D Elliott, G LoBiondo-Wood & J Haber J (eds) *Nursing research: methods, critical appraisal and utilisation,* 2nd edn, pp 38–51. Mosby, Sydney.

Elzubier M 1995 Education and debate: nursing skills and practice. *British Journal of Nursing* 4(18):1087–92.

Emden C 1991 Becoming a reflective practitioner. In G Gray & R Pratt (eds) *Towards a discipline of nursing,* pp 335–54. Churchill Livingstone, Melbourne.

Emden C, Young W 1987 Theory development in nursing: Australian nurses advance global debate. *Australian Journal of Advanced Nursing* 4(3):22–40.

Emerald Hill Rate Books 1864–81 Microfilm 1864–81. Port Phillip City Collection, South Melbourne Council.

Epps R, Sorensen T 1993 Introduction. In T Sorensen & R Epps (eds) *Prospects and policies for rural Australia,* pp 1–6. Longman, Melbourne.

Ersser S 1997 *Nursing as a therapeutic activity: an ethnography.* Avebury, Aldershot.

Ersser S, Tutton S eds 1991 *Primary nursing in perspective.* Scutari Press, London.

Erturk Y 2004 Considering the role of men in gender agenda setting: conceptual and policy issues. *Feminist Review* 78(1):3–21.

Eunson B 2005 *Conflict management: communicating in the 21st century.* John Wiley & Sons, Brisbane.

Evans A, Ali S, Singleton C, Nolan P, Bahrami J 2002 The effectiveness of personal education plans in continuing professional development: an evaluation. *Medical Teacher* 24(1):79–84.

Evans J 2004 Men nurses: a historical and feminist perspective. *Journal of Advanced Nursing* 47(3):321–8.

Evans M 1997 *Introducing contemporary feminist thought*. Blackwell Publishers, Oxford.

Fagin C, Diers D 1983 Nursing as a metaphor. *New England Journal of Medicine* 309:116–17.

Fair G, Hartery T 2001 Medical dominance in multidisciplinary teamwork: a case study of discharge decision-making in a geriatric assessment unit. *Journal of Nursing Management* 9(1):3–11.

Fairman J 1992 Watchful vigilance: nursing care, technology and the development of intensive care units. *Nursing Research* 41:56–60.

——1996 Response to tools of the trade: analysing technology as object in nursing. *Scholarly Inquiry for Nursing Practice: An International Journal* 10:17–21.

——1998 The nurse–technology relationship in the context of the history of technology. *Nursing History Review* 6:129–46.

Fairman J, D'Antonio P 1999 Virtual power: gendering the nurse–technology relationship. *Nursing Inquiry* 6:178–86.

Fairman J, Lynaugh J 1998 *Critical care nursing: a history*. University of Pennsylvania Press, Philadelphia.

Falk Rafael A 1996 Power and caring: a dialectic in nursing. *Advances in Nursing Science* 19(1):3–17.

——1998 Nurses who run with the wolves: the power and caring dialectic revisited. *Advances in Nursing Science* 21(1):29–42.

Fargason C A, Haddock C C 1992 Cross-factional, integrative team decision making: essential for qi in health care. *Quality Review Bulletin* 157–63.

Fassett D, Gallagher M R 1998 *Just a head: stories in a body*. Allen & Unwin, Sydney.

Fawcett J 1984 The meta-paradigm of nursing: present status and future refinements. *Image: Journal of Nursing Scholarship* 16(3):84–6

Fealy G M 2004 'The good nurse': visions and value in images of the nurse. *Journal of Advanced Nursing* 46(6):649–56.

Feenberg A 1999 *Questioning technology*. Routledge, New York.

Ferre F 1995 *Philosophy of technology*. University of Georgia Press, London.

Fiedler L 1988 Images of the nurse in fiction and popular culture. In A Jones (ed) *Images of nurses: perspectives from history, art, and literature*, pp 100–12. University of Pennsylvania Press, Pennsylvania.

Field J, FitzGerald M 1989 Therapeutic nursing: emerging imperatives for nursing curricula. In R McMahon & A Pearson (eds) *Nursing as therapy*, pp 93–111. Stanley Thornes, Cheltenham.

Fineman S 1993 ed *Emotion in organizations*. Sage, London.

Firth-Cozens J 2001 Multidisciplinary teamwork: the good, bad, and everything in between (comment). *Quality in Health Care* 10(2):65–6.

Fitter M 1987 The impact of new technology on nurses and patients. In R Payne & J Firth-Cozens (eds) *Stress in health professions*, pp 211–29. John Wiley & Sons, London.

FitzGerald M 1991 Change in the ward: making things happen. *Nursing Times* 87(30):25–7.

——1994 Lecturer practitioners: creating the environment. In J Lathlean & B Vaughan (eds) *Unifying nursing theory and practice*, pp 55–70. Butterworth Heinemann, Oxford.

——1995 The experience of chronic illness in rural Australia. Unpublished PhD thesis. University of New England, Armidale.

Flaskerud J H, Halloran E J 1980 Areas of agreement in nursing theory development. *Advances in Nursing Science* 3(1):1–7.

Ford J S, Profetto-McGrath J 1994 A model for critical thinking within the context of curriculum as praxis. *Journal of Nurse Education* 33(8):341–4.

Forth G, Critchett J, Yule P eds 1998 *The biographical dictionary of the western district of Victoria.* Hyland House, Melbourne.

Foss C 2002 Gender bias in nursing care? Gender-related differences in patient satisfaction with the quality of nursing care. *Scandinavian Journal of Caring Sciences* 16(1):19–26.

Foucault M 1970 *The order of things: an archaeology of the human sciences.* Tavistock, London.

——1972 *The archaeology of knowledge* (translated by Sheridan Smith AM). Tavistock, London.

——1978 *The history of sexuality, volume one.* Pantheon, New York.

——1980 Two lectures. In C Gordon (ed) *Power/knowledge,* pp 78–108. Pantheon Books, New York.

——1983 Afterword: the subject and power. In H Dreyfus & P Rabinow *Michel Foucault: beyond structuralism and hermeneutics,* 2nd edn, pp 208–26. University of Chicago Press, Chicago.

Fragar L, Gray E J, Franklin R J, Petrauskas V 1997 *A picture of health? A preliminary report of the health of country Australians.* Australian Agricultural Health Unit, Moree.

Francis D 1995 The reflective journal: a window to pre-service teachers' practical knowledge. *Teaching and Teacher Education* 11(3):229–41.

Freshwater D 2002 *Therapeutic nursing: improving patient care through self-awareness and reflection.* Sage, Thousand Oaks, California.

Freudenberg N 2000 Health promotion in the city: a review of current practice. *Annual Review of Public Health Nursing* 21:473–503.

Friedman A, Phillips M 2002 The role of mentoring in the CPD programmes of professional associations. *International Journal of Lifelong Education* 21(3): 269–84.

Friere P 1972 *The pedagogy of oppression.* Penguin, Harmondsworth.

Fuller J, Harris E, Nutbeam N, Harris M 2004 UK health inequalities: the class system is alive and well. *Medical Journal of Australia* 181(10):583–4.

Gaff-Smith M 2003 *Midwives of the black soil plains.* Triple D Books, Wagga Wagga.

——2004 *Riverina midwives—from the mountains to the plains.* Triple D Books, Wagga Wagga.

Gahart M, Barsoum G, Dievler D, Khan S, Price R, Sanchez Y et al 2004 *HHS's efforts to promote health information technology and legal barriers to its adoption.* Institute of Medicine, Washington DC.

Gair G, Hartery T 2001 Medical dominance in multidisciplinary teamwork: a case study of discharge decision-making in a geriatric assessment unit. *Journal of Nursing Management* 9(1):3–11.

Galbally F 1978 *Migrant services and programs: report of the review of post-arrival programs and services to migrants (Galbally report),* vols 1 and 2. AGPS, Canberra.

Gallagher R ed 1995 Team building. In P S Yoder Wise (ed) *Leading and managing in nursing,* pp 275–99. Mosby, St Louis.

Gamarnikow E 1978 Sexual division of labour: the case of nursing. In A Kuhn & A M Wolpe (eds) *Feminism and materialism.* Routledge & Kegan Paul, London.

REFERENCES

Garbett R, McCormack B 2002 A concept analysis of practice development. *NT Research* 7(2):87–100.

Garrett P, Lin V 1990 Ethnic health policy and service development. In J Reid & P Trompf (eds) *The health of immigrant Australia: a social perspective*. Harcourt Brace Jovanovich, Sydney.

Gattuso S, Bevan C 2000 Mother, daughter, patient, nurse: women's emotion work in aged care. *Journal of Advanced Nursing* 31(4):892–9.

Gaze H 1987 Man appeal. *Nursing Times* 83(20):24–7.

Georges J M, McGuire S 2004 Deconstructing clinical pathways: mapping the landscape of health care. *Advances in Nursing Science* 27(1):2–12.

Gherardi S 1994 The gender we think, the gender we do in our everyday organizational lives. *Human Relations* 47(6):591–601.

Gibbs G 1988 *Learning by doing: a guide to teaching and learning methods*. Further Education Unit, Oxford Polytechnic, Oxford.

Gibson J M 1998 Using the Delphi technique to identify the content and context of nurses' continuing professional development needs. *Journal of Clinical Nursing* 7:451–9.

Gillan G 1988 Foucault's philosophy. In J Bernauer & D Rasmussen (eds) *The final Foucault*. MIT Press, London.

Godden J 1997 'For the benefit of mankind': Nightingale's legacy and hours of work in Australian nursing, 1868–1939. In A M Rafferty, J Robinson & R Elkan (eds) *Nursing history and the politics of welfare*. Routledge, London.

Goffman I 1959 *Presentation of the self in everyday life*. Overlook Press, New York.

Goold S 2001 Transcultural nursing: can we meet the challenge of caring for the Australian indigenous person? *Journal of Transcultural Nursing* 12:94–9.

Gortner S R 1983 The history and philosophy of nursing science and research. *Advances in Nursing Science* January:1–8.

Govier T 1992 *A practical study of argument*, 3rd edn. Wadsworth, Belmont, California.

Gray G, Pratt R eds 1991 *Towards a discipline of nursing*. Churchill Livingstone, Melbourne.

Gray J, Forsstrom S 1991 Generating theory from practice: the reflective technique. In G Gray & R Pratt (eds) *Towards a discipline of nursing*. Churchill Livingstone, Melbourne.

Greenberg M, Espense M, Becker C, Cartwright J 2003 Telehealth nursing practice: SIG adopts teleterms. *Viewpoint* February:8–10.

Greene A D, Latting J K 2004 Whistle-blowing as a form of advocacy: guidelines for the practitioner and organization. *Social Work* 00378046, 49(2):1–13.

Greenhalgh J, Vanhanen L, Kyngas H 1998 Nurse caring behaviours. *Journal of Advanced Nursing* 27(5):927–32.

Greenhalgh T 1997 *How to read a paper: the basics of evidence based medicine*. BMJ Publishing, London.

Greenwood J ed 1996 *Nursing theory in Australia: development and application*. Harper Educational, Sydney.

——1998 The role of reflection in single and double loop learning. *Journal of Advanced Nursing* 27:1048–53.

Grehan M 2004 From the sphere of Sarah Gampism: the professionalisation of nursing and midwifery in the colony of Victoria. *Nursing Inquiry* 11(3):192–201.

Griffin M L 2003 Using critical incidents to promote and assess reflective thinking in preservice teachers *Reflective Practice* 4(2):207–20.

Griffitts L 2002 Geared to achieve with lifelong learning. *Nursing Management* 33(11):22–4.

REFERENCES

Grimshaw P 1994 Gendered settlements. In P Grimshaw, M Lake, A McGrath & M Quartly (eds) *Creating a nation*. McPhee Gribble, Melbourne.

Grosz E 1990 Conclusion: a note on essentialism and difference. In S Gunew (ed) *Feminist knowledge: critique and construct*. Routledge, London.

——1993 Bodies and knowledges: feminism and the crisis of reason. In L Alcroff & E Potter (eds) *Feminist epistemologies*, pp 187–216. Routledge, New York.

——1994 *Volatile bodies: toward a corporeal feminism*. Allen & Unwin, Sydney.

Habermas J 1971 *Knowledge and human interest* (translated by J J Shapiro). Beacon Press, Boston.

Hadfield L 1991 Violence in the accident and emergency department: differences across the Atlantic (guest editorial). *Journal of Emergency Nursing* 15(5):269–70.

Hage G H, Couch R eds 1999 *The future of Australian multiculturalism: reflections on the 20th anniversary of Jean Martin's The Migrant Presence*. NSW Research Institute for Humanities, University of Sydney, Sydney.

Hagell E I 1989 Nursing knowledge: women's knowledge. A sociological perspective. *Journal of Advanced Nursing* 14:226–33.

Halimi K 2002 Afghan refugees: the ugly truth. *Annals of Emergency Medicine* 39:200–2.

Hallam J 1998 From angels to handmaidens: changing constructions of nursing's public image in post-war Britain. *Nursing Inquiry* 5:32–42.

Halpern D 1998 *Critical thinking across the curriculum: a brief edition of thought and knowledge*. Lawrence Erlbaum Associates, Mahweh, New Jersey.

Hancock P 1999 Reflective practice: using a learning journal. *Nursing Standard* 13(17):37–40.

Hanna L 2001 Continued neglect of rural and remote nursing in Australia: the link with poor health outcomes. *Australian Journal of Advanced Nursing* 9:36–45.

Hansen H F 1958 *Study guide: a review of practice nursing*. W B Saunders, Philadelphia.

Harding A, Lloyd R, Greenwell H 2001 *Financial disadvantage in Australia 1990–2000: the persistence of poverty in a decade of growth*. The Smith Family National Centre for Social and Economic Modelling (NATSEM), Sydney.

Harding A, Szukalska A 2000 *Financial disadvantage in Australia: 1999*. The Smith Family National Centre for Social and Economic Modelling (NATSEM), Sydney.

Harding S 1980 Value laden technologies and the politics of nursing. In S F Spicker & S Gadow (eds) *Nursing: images and ideals*, pp 49–75. Springer, New York.

Hardy S, Garbett R, Titchen A, Manley K 2002 Exploring nursing expertise: nurses talk nursing. *Nursing Inquiry* 9(3):196–202.

Harris M, Telfer B 2001 The health needs of asylum seekers living in the community. *Medical Journal of Australia* 175:589–92.

Harvey D 1989 *The condition of postmodernity*. Basil Blackwell, Oxford.

Harvey J 1997 The technological regulation of death: with reference to the technological regulation of birth. *Sociology* 31(4):719–36.

Hayman R 1997 *Nietzsche: Nietzsche's voices*. Phoenix, London.

Hays R B, Veitch P C, Cheers B, Crossland L 1997 Why doctors leave rural practice. *Australian Journal of Rural Health* 5:198–203.

Health Informatics Society of Australia 1998 *Definition of health informatics*. Accessed 6 October 2004. Available from: www.hisa.org.au.

Health Workforce Advisory Committee 2003 *The New Zealand health workforce future directions: recommendations to the Minister of Health*. HWAC, Wellington.

Healthcare Information and Management Systems Society 2003 *Definition of eHealth*. Accessed 20 November 2004. Available from: www.HIMSS.org. 2005.

Hearn J 1993 Emotive subjects: organizational men, organizational masculinities and the (de)construction of 'emotions'. In S Fineman (ed) *Emotion in organizations.* Sage, London.

Heath H 1998 Keeping a reflective practice diary: a practical guide. *Nurse Education Today* 18:592–8.

Heath P 2002 Introduction. In *National review of nursing education: our duty of care 2002.* Commonwealth of Australia, Canberra.

Hegney D 1996 The windmill of rural health: a Foucauldian analysis of the discourses of rural nursing in Australia, 1991–1994. Unpublished PhD thesis. Southern Cross University, Lismore.

——1997a Defining rural and rural nursing. In L Siegloff (ed) *Rural nursing in the Australian context*, pp 25–44. Royal College of Nursing Australia, Canberra.

——1997b Extended, expanded, multi-skilled or advanced practice? *Collegian* 4:22–7.

——1997c Rural nursing practice. In L Siegloff (ed) *Rural nursing in the Australian context*, pp 34–44. Royal College of Nursing, Canberra.

——1997d Rural nursing practice. In L Siegloff (ed) *Rural nursing in the Australian content*, pp 25–44. Royal College of Nursing Australia, Canberra.

——1998 The advanced practice role of the rural nurse: challenging the culture of nursing, pharmacy and medicine. In conference proceedings of 'The cultures in caring, 4th biennial Australian rural and remote health scientific conference', pp 1.200–1.228. Toowoomba Hospital Foundation, Toowoomba.

——2000 Rural nursing in Australia. In A Bushy *Orientation to nursing in the rural community*, pp 203–17. Sage, Thousand Oaks, California.

Hegney D, McCarthy A, Rogers-Clark C, Gorman D 2003a Why nurses are resigning from rural and remote Queensland health facilities. *Collegian* 9:33–9.

Hegney D, Pearce S, Rogers-Clark C, Martin-McDonald K 2005a Close, but still too far. The experiences of people with cancer commuting from a provincial town to a major city for radiotherapy treatment. *European Journal of Cancer Care* 14:75–82.

Hegney D, Pearson A, McCarthy A 1997 *The role and function of the rural nurse in Australia.* Royal College of Nursing, Canberra.

Hegney D, Plank A, Parker V 2003b Nursing workloads: the results of a study of Queensland nurses. *Journal of Nursing Management* 11:307–14.

——2003c Workplace violence in nursing in Queensland. *International Journal of Nursing* 9:261–8.

Hegney D, Plank A, Watson J, Raith L, McKeon C 2005b Patient education and consumer medicine information. *Journal of Clinical Nursing* 14:855–62.

Hektor L 1994 Florence Nightingale and the women's movement: friend or foe? *Nursing Inquiry* 1:38–45.

Helman C 1994 *Culture, health and illness*, 3rd edn. Butterworth Heinemann, London.

Henderson A 1994 Power and knowledge in nursing practice: the contribution to Foucault. *Journal of Advanced Nursing* 20(5):935–9.

——2001 Emotional labour and nursing: An under-appreciated aspect of caring work. *Nursing Inquiry* 8(2):130–8.

Henderson R F 1975 *Poverty in Australia: first main report of the Commission of Inquiry into Poverty.* AGPS, Canberra.

Henderson S 2003 Power imbalance between nurses and patients: a potential inhibitor of partnership in care. *Journal of Clinical Nursing* 12(4):501–8.

Henderson V 1964 The nature of nursing. *American Journal of Nursing* 64(8):62.

——1985 The essence of nursing in high technology. *Nursing Administration Quarterly* 9(4):1–9.

Hennessy D, Spurgeon P 2000 *Health policy and nursing.* Macmillan Press, London.

REFERENCES

Hepworth S, Fitter M 1981 *Nurses' attitudes to computers in hospitals* (No. Memo No. 419, MCR/ESCR). University of Sheffield, Sheffield.

Herrick C A, Jenkins T, Carlson J 1998 Using self-directed learning modules: a literature review. *Journal of Nursing Staff Development* 14(2):73–80.

Hertzman C 2001 Health and human society. *American Scientist* 89(6):538–44.

Hicks C 1997 The research–practice gap: individual responsibility or corporate culture? *Nursing Times* 93(39):38–9.

——1999 Incompatible skills and ideologies: the impediment of gender attributions on nursing research. *Journal of Advanced Nursing* 30(1):129–39.

Higgins Y, Jones C 2004 *Baby take a walk in the park*. City of Darebin, Melbourne. Available from: www.darebin.vic.gov.au.

Hill D W, Summers R 1994 *Medical technology: a nursing perspective*. Chapman & Hall, Melbourne.

Hiraki A 1992 Tradition, rationality, and power in introductory nursing textbooks: a critical hermeneutics study. *Advanced Nursing Science* 14(3):1–12.

Hobart Town Courier newspaper 1837.

Hodge B 1993 Uncovering the ethic of care. *Nursing Praxis in New Zealand* 8(2):13–22.

Hofstadter R 1963 *Anti-intellectualism in American life*, pp 233–71. Alfred A Knopf, New York.

Holden R J 1991 In defence of Cartesian dualism and the hermeneutic horizon. *Journal of Advanced Nursing* 16(11):1375–81.

Hollinger R 1994 *Postmodernism and the social sciences: a thematic approach*. Sage, London.

Holly M L 1984 *Keeping a personal professional journal*. Deakin University Press, Geelong.

Holman C D J 1991 *Building the future of community and child health services*. Health Department of Western Australia, Perth.

Holmes C 1997 Why we should wash our hands of medical soaps. *Nursing Inquiry* 4:135–7.

Holmes C A 1995 Postmodernism and nursing. In G Gray & R Pratt (eds) *Scholarship in the discipline of nursing*, pp 351–70. Churchill Livingstone, Melbourne.

Holmes C A, Warelow P J 2000 Nursing as normative praxis. *Nursing Inquiry* 7(3):175–81. Reprinted with comments in P Reed (ed) 2003 *Nicoll's perspectives on nursing theory*, 4th edn. Lippincott, Williams & Wilkins, Philadelphia.

Holmes D, Gastaldo D 2002 Nursing as means of governmentality. *Journal of Advanced Nursing* 38(6):557–65.

Holter J M 1988 Critical theory: a foundation for the development of nursing theories. *Scholarly Inquiry for Nursing Practice: An International Journal* 2(3):223–32.

Hoover J 2002 The personal and professional impact of undertaking an educational module on human caring. *Journal of Advanced Nursing* 37(1):79–86.

Horn S 2001 Quality, clinical practice improvement, and the episode of care. *Managed Care Quarterly* 9(3):10.

Houghton K, Strong P 2004 *Women in business in rural and remote Australia—growing regional economies*. Rural Industries Research and Development Corporation, Australian Government, Canberra.

Hovenga E, Hindmarsh C 1996a *Queensland Health—PAIS validation study report*. Queensland Health, Brisbane.

——1996b *Queensland Health—PAIS validation study: results and issues for nursing cost capture*. 'Eighth Casemix conference', Sydney.

Howatson-Jones I L 2003 Difficulties in clinical supervision and lifelong learning. *Nursing Standard* 17(37):37.

REFERENCES

Humphreys J 1999 Rural health status: what do statistics show that we don't already know? *Australian Journal of Rural Health* 7:60–3.

Humphreys J S, Lyle D, Wakerman J, Chalmers E, Wilkinson D, Walker J, Simmons D, Larson A 2000 Roles and activities of the Commonwealth Government university departments of rural health. *Australian Journal of Rural Health* 8:120–33.

Humphreys J, Rolley F 1991 *Health and health care in rural Australia.* University of New England, Armidale.

Humphreys J S, Rolley F 1993 Neglected factors in planning rural health services. In K Malko (ed) *A fair go for rural health—forward together*, pp 47–54. University of New England, Armidale.

Hunter K 1988 Nurses: the satiric image and the translocated ideal. In A Jones (ed) *Images of nurses: perspectives from history, art, and literature*, pp 113–27. University of Pennsylvania Press, Pennsylvania.

Huntington A 1996 Nursing research reframed by the inescapable reality of practice: a personal encounter. *Nursing Inquiry* 3(3):167–71.

Huntington A D, Gilmour J A 2001 Re-thinking representations, re-writing nursing texts: possibilities through feminist and Foucauldian thought. *Journal of Advanced Nursing* 35(6):902–8.

International Council of Nurses 1973 *Ethical concepts applied to nursing.* ICN, Geneva.

——2004a *ICN on health and human rights. Nursing matters.* Accessed 20 January 2004. Available from: http://www.icn.ch/matters_humanrights.htm.

——2004b *Nurses: working with poor; against poverty. Information and action tool kit.* ICN, Geneva.

International Standards Organization 1999 ISO 2382–4. *Information technology—vocabulary—Part 4: organization of data.* ISO, Geneva.

Irigaray L 1993 *Je, tu, nous: toward a culture of difference.* Routledge, New York.

Ivancevich J M, Matteson M T 1993 *Organisational behaviour and management.* Irwin, Boston.

Jackson D 1995 Constructing nursing practice: country of origin, culture and competency. *International Journal of Nursing Practice* 1(1):32–6.

——1997 Feminism: a path to clinical knowledge development. *Contemporary Nurse* 6(2):85–91.

——2003 Culture, health and social justice. *Contemporary Nurse* 15(3):347–8.

Jackson D, Borbasi S 2000 The caring conundrum: potential and perils for nursing. In J Daly, S Speedy & D Jackson (eds) *Contexts of nursing: an introduction.* MacLennan & Petty, Sydney.

Jackson D, Clare J, Mannix J 2002 Who would want to be a nurse? Violence in the workplace—a factor in recruitment and retention. *Journal of Nursing Management* 10(1):13–20.

Jackson D, Mannix J, Daly J 2001 Retaining a viable workforce: a critical challenge for nursing. *Contemporary Nurse* 11(2–3):163–72.

Jackson D, Raftos M 1997 In uncharted waters: confronting the culture of silence in a residential care institution. *International Journal of Nursing Practice* 3(1): 34–9.

Jacobs P M, Ott B, Sullivan B, Ulrich Y, Short L 1997 An approach to defining and operationalizing critical thinking. *Journal of Nursing Education* 36(1):19–22.

Jameson F 1984 Postmodernism: or the cultural logic of late capitalism. *New Left Review* 146:53–92.

Jamieson M, Griffiths R, Jayasuriya R 1998 Developing outcomes for community nursing: the Nominal Group Technique. *Australian Journal of Advanced Nursing* 16(1):14–19.

Jamrozik K, Weller D P, Heller R F 2005 Rural health turned upside-down. *Medical Journal of Australia* 182(4):152–3.

Janiszewski Goodin H 2003 The nursing shortage in the United States of America: an integrative review of the literature. *Journal of Advanced Nursing* 43(4): 335–50.

Jefferies H, Chan K K 2004 Multidisciplinary team working: is it both holistic and effective? *International Journal of Gynecological Cancer* 14(2):210–11.

Jenkins E 1989 Nurses' control over nursing. In G Gray & R Pratt (eds) *Issues in Australian nursing 2*. Churchill Livingstone, Melbourne.

Jenkins V, Fallowfield L, Poole K 2001 Are members of multidisciplinary teams in breast cancer aware of each other's informational roles? *Quality in Health Care* 10(2):70–5.

Jennings B M 1986 Nursing science: more promise than threat. *Journal of Advanced Nursing* 11(5):505–11.

Johansson P, Oleni M, Fridlund B 2002 Patient satisfaction with nursing care in the context of health care: a literature review. *Scandinavian Journal of Caring Sciences* 16(4):337–44.

Johns C 1998 Opening the doors of perception. In C Johns & D Freshwater (eds) *Transforming nursing through reflective practice*, pp 1–20. Blackwell Science, London.

——2000 *Becoming a reflective practitioner: a reflective and holistic approach to clinical nursing, practice development and clinical supervision*. Blackwell Science, London.

——2001 Reflective practice: revealing the [he]art of caring. *International Journal of Nursing Practice* 7(4):237–45.

Johnson D E 1961 The behavioural system model for nursing. In J P Riehl & C Roy (eds) *Conceptual models for nursing practice*, 2nd edn. Appleton Century Crofts, New York.

Johnson J L 1993 Toward a clearer understanding of the art of nursing. Unpublished doctoral dissertation. University of Alberta, Edmonton.

——1994 A dialectical examination of nursing art. *Advances in Nursing Science* 1(1):1–14.

——1996 The perceptual aspect of nursing art: sources of accord and discord. *Scholarly Inquiry for Nursing Practice: An International Journal* 10(4):307–27.

Johnson P 1994 *Feminism as radical humanism*. Allen & Unwin, Sydney.

Johnston C, Cooper P 1997 Patient-focused care: what is it? *Holistic Nursing Practice* 11(3):1–7.

Johnstone M 1998 *Determining and responding effectively to ethical professional misconduct: a report to the Nurses Board of Victoria*. RMIT, Melbourne.

——1999 *Bioethics: a nursing perspective*, 3rd edn. Harcourt/Saunders, Sydney.

——2002 Poor working conditions and the capacity of nurses to provide moral care. *Contemporary Nurse* 12(1):7–15.

——2004a *Bioethics: a nursing perspective*, 4th edn. Churchill Livingstone/Elsevier Australia, Sydney.

——2004b Leadership ethics in nursing and health care domains. In J Daly, S Speedy & D Jackson (eds) *Nursing leadership*, pp 89–102. Churchill Livingstone, Sydney.

—— 2004c Patient safety, ethics and whistleblowing: a nursing response to the events at the Campbelltown and Camden Hospitals. *Australian Health Review* 28(1): 13–19.

Johnstone M, Da Costa C, Turale S 2004 Registered and enrolled nurses' experiences of ethical issues in nursing practice. *Australian Journal of Advanced Nursing* 22(1):31–7.

Johnstone M-J 1994 *Nursing and the injustices of the law*. W B Saunders/Bailliere Tindall, Sydney.

Jones A 1988a *Images of nurses: perspectives from history, art, and literature*. University of Pennsylvania Press, Pennsylvania.

——1988b *The white angel* (1936): Hollywood's image of Florence Nightingale. In A Jones (ed) *Images of nurses: perspectives from history, art, and literature*, pp 221–42. University of Pennsylvania Press, Pennsylvania.

——2001 Time to think: temporal considerations in nursing practice and research. *Journal of Advanced Nursing* 33(2):150–8.

Jones M 2004 Case report. Nurse prescribing: a case study in policy influence. *Journal of Nursing Management* 12:266–72.

Jong K E, Vale P J, Armstrong B K 2005 Rural inequalities in cancer care and outcome. *Medical Journal of Australia* 182(1):13–14.

Joy E A, Wilson C, Varechok S 2003 The multidisciplinary team approach to the outpatient treatment of disordered eating. *Current Sports Medicine Reports* 2(6):331–6.

Kalisch B, Kalisch P 1983a An analysis of the impact of authorship on the image of the nurse presented in novels. *Research in Nursing and Health* 6:17–24.

——1983b Heroine out of focus: media images of Florence Nightingale. Part 1: popular biographies and stage productions. *Nursing & Health Care* 4:181–7.

——1984 An analysis of news coverage of maternal-child nurses. *Maternal-Child Nursing Journal* 13:77–90.

Kalisch B, Kalisch P, McHugh M 1982 The nurse as a sex object in motion pictures. *Research in Nursing & Health* 5:147–54.

Kalisch P, Kalisch B 1987 *The changing image of the nurse*. Addison-Wesley, Menlo Park, California.

Kalisch P, Kalisch B, Scobey M 1983 *Images of nurses on television*. Springer Publishing Company, New York.

Kampen N 1988 Before Florence Nightingale: a prehistory of nursing in painting and sculpture. In A Jones (ed) *Images of nurses: perspectives from history, art, and literature*, pp 6–39. University of Pennsylvania Press, Pennsylvania.

Kane D, Thomas B 2000 Nursing and the 'f' word. *Nursing Forum* 35(2):17–25

Kapborg I, Bertero C 2003 The phenomenon of caring from the student nurse's perspective: a qualitative content analysis. *International Nursing Review* 50(3):183–92.

Katz S 1995 Disciplinary texts: rhetoric and the science of old age in the late nineteenth century and early twentieth century. *Australian Cultural History* 14:109–26.

Kawachi I, Kennedy B 1999 Income inequality and health: pathways and mechanisms. *Health Services Research* 34:215–27.

Keating D P, Hertzman C eds 1999 *Developmental health and the wellbeing of nations—social, biological and educational dynamics*. Guildford Press, New York.

Keleher H 2004 Public and population health: strategic responses. In H Keleher & B Murphy (eds) *Understanding health: a determinants approach*. Oxford University Press, Melbourne.

Keleher H, Murphy B eds 2004 *Understanding health: a determinants approach*. Oxford University Press, Melbourne.

Kelly A 1985 The construction of masculine science. *British Journal of Sociology of Education* 6:33–154.

Kelly B 1977 *A background to the history of nursing in Tasmania*. Privately published.

Kelly N R, Shoemaker M, Steele T 1996 The experience of being a male student nurse. *Journal of Nursing Education* 35(4):170–4.

Kelly-Thomas K J 1998 *Clinical and nursing staff development, current competence, future focus*. Lippincott, New York.

Kemmis S 1985 Action research and the politics of reflection. In D Boud, R Keogh & D Walker (eds) *Reflection: turning experience into learning*. Kogan Page, London.

Kennedy M 2004 *Nursing language: the international classification for nursing practice*. Nursing Informatics, HIC2004, HISA, Brisbane.

Kenny A, Duckett S 2003 Educating for rural nursing practice. *Journal of Advanced Nursing* 44(6):613–22.

Keyes E 2000 Mental health status in refugees: an integrative review of current research. *Issues in Mental Health Nursing* 21:397–410.

Khabir A 1999 World Bank predicts development for next century. *The Lancet* 354(9183):1005.

Khamis V 1998 Psychological distress and well-being among traumatized Palestinian women during Intifada. *Social Science and Medicine* 19:1033–41.

Kieser A 1989 Organisational, institutional and societal evolution: medieval craft guilds and the genesis of formal organisations. *Administrative Science Quarterly* 34(4):540–64.

Kiger A 1993 Accord and discord in students' images of nursing. *Journal of Nursing Education* 32:309–17.

King I 1981 *A theory for nursing: systems, concepts, process*. Wiley, New York.

——1987 King's theory of goal attainment. In R R Parse (ed) *Nursing science: major paradigms, theories and critiques*, pp 107–113. W B Saunders, Philadelphia.

King K, Norsen L 1994 The care/cure, nurse/physician dichotomy doesn't do it anymore. *Image: Journal of Nursing Scholarship* 26(2):89.

Kinkle S 1993 Violence in the ED: how to stop it before it starts. *American Journal of Nursing* 93(7):22–4.

Kitson A L 1987 Raising standards of clinical practice—the fundamental issue of effective nursing practice. *Journal of Advanced Nursing* 12(3):321–9.

Kitson A 2004 Drawing out leadership. *Journal of Advanced Nursing* 48(3):211.

Kitwood T 1997 On being a person. In T Kitwood (ed) *Dementia reconsidered: the person comes first*, pp 7–19. Open University Press, Milton Keynes.

Kleffel D 1991 Rethinking the environment as a domain of nursing knowledge. *Advances in Nursing Science* 15:307–15.

Kleinman A 1980 *Patients and healers in the context of culture: an exploration of the borderland between anthropology, medicine and psychiatry*. University of California Press, Berkeley.

Kralik D, Koch T, Wootton K 1997 Engagement and detachment: understanding patients' experiences with nursing. *Journal of Advanced Nursing* 26(2):399–407.

Kramer M 1974 *Reality shock*. Mosby, New York.

Krause E A 1996 *Death of the guilds: professions, states and the advance of capitalism 1930 to the present*. Yale University Press, New Haven.

Kreger A 1991 Report on the national nursing consultative committee project: enhancing the role of rural and remote area nurses (unpublished).

Kritek P B 1985 Nursing diagnosis in perspective: response to a critique. *Image: Journal of Nursing Scholarship* 17(1):3–8.

Kuhn T S 1970 *The structure of scientific revolutions*. University of Chicago Press, Chicago.

Lafferty P M 1997 Balancing the curriculum: promoting aesthetic knowledge in nursing. *Nurse Education Today* 17:281–6.

Lampshire & Rolfe 1993 *The realities of rural district nursing: a study of practice issues and education needs—Loddon–Mallee Region*. Victorian In-service Nurse Education and Department of Health and Community Services, Victoria.

——1996 *Postgraduate and continuing education for Victorian rural nurses:*

issues and further directions. Committee for Rural Health Education Victoria, Melbourne.

Land and Water Australia 2004 *Australia's farmers: past, present and future.* Australian Government, Canberra.

Larsson G, Peterson V, Lampic C, von Essen L, Sjoden P 1998 Cancer patients and staff ratings of the importance of caring behaviours and their relations to patient anxiety and depression. *Journal of Advanced Nursing* 27(4):855–64.

Lasswell H 1958 *Politics: who gets what, when, how.* World Publishing Company, New York.

Lather P 1991a *Feminist research in education: within/against.* Deakin University Press, Geelong.

——1991b *Getting smart: feminist research and pedagogy with/in the postmodern.* Routledge, London.

Latimer J 1998 Organising context: nurses' assessments of older people in an acute medical unit. *Nursing Inquiry* 5(1):43–57.

Lawler J 1991 *Behind the screens: nursing, somology and the problem of the body.* Churchill Livingstone, Melbourne.

Lawrence G 1987 *Capitalism and the countryside: the rural crisis in Australia.* Pluto Press, Sydney.

Lawrence G, Williams C 1990 The dynamics of decline: implications for social welfare delivery in Australia. In T Cullen, P Dunn & G Lawrence (eds) *Rural health and welfare in Australia.* Centre for Welfare Research, Wagga Wagga.

Leder D 1984 Medicine and pardigms of embodiment. *Journal of Medicine and Philosophy* 9:29–43.

Leder G 1993 Constructivism: theory for practice? The case of mathematics. *Higher Education Research and Development* 12(1):5–20.

Leftwich R 1993 Care and cure as healing processes in nursing. *Nursing Forum* 28(3):13–17.

Leininger M 1984 *Care: the essence of nursing and health.* Slack, New Jersey.

——1986 Care facilitation and resistance factors in the culture of nursing. *Topics in Clinical Nursing* 8(2):1–12.

——1991a Becoming aware of types of health practitioners and cultural imposition *Journal of Transcultural Nursing* 2(2):32–9.

——1991b *Culture care diversity and universality: a theory of nursing.* National League for Nursing Press, New York.

——1995 *Transcultural nursing concepts, theories, research and practices,* 2nd edn. McGraw Hill, New York.

Leininger M, McFarland M 2002 *Transcultural nursing concepts, theories, research and practices,* 3rd edn. McGraw Hill, New York.

Lenkman C, Gibbins R 1994 Multidisciplinary teams in the acute care setting. *Holistic Nursing Practice* April:81–7.

Leonard M, Graham S, Bonacum D 2004 The human factor: the critical importance of effective teamwork and communications in providing safe care. *Quality and Safety in HealthCare* 13(Suppl 1):i85–i90.

Leslie G, Finn J 2003 Evidence-based nursing. In Z Schneider, D Elliott, G LoBiondo-Wood & J Haber J (eds) *Nursing research: methods, critical appraisal and utilisation,* 2nd edn, pp 91–107. Mosby, Sydney.

Leuning C J, Swiggum P D, Balmore Wegert H M, McCullough-Zander K 2002 Proposed standards for transcultural nursing. *Journal of Transcultural Nursing* 13(1):40–6.

Levine M 1971 Holistic nursing. *Nursing Clinics of North America* 6(2):253–63.

Liaschenko J, Peter E 2004 Nursing ethics and conceptualizations of nursing: profession, practice and work. *Journal of Advanced Nursing* 46(5):488–95.

Liberman R P, Hilty D M, Drake R E, Tsang H W H 2001 Requirements for multidisciplinary teamwork in psychiatric rehabilitation. *Psychiatric Services* 52(10):1331–42.

Lifton R 1990 Foreword. In H M Weinstein *Psychiatry and the CIA: victims of mind control*, pp ix–xiv. American Psychiatric Press, Washington DC.

Lipson J G, Omidian PA 1997 Afghan refugee issues in the US social environment. *Western Journal of Nursing* 19(1):110–26.

Little P 1996 Questions for learning. Unpublished workshop material. PROBLARC. University of Newcastle, Newcastle.

Locsin R 1995 Machine technologies and caring in nursing. *Image: Journal of Nursing Scholarship* 27:201–3.

——1998 Technologic competence as caring in critical care. *Holistic Nursing Practice* 12:50–6.

——ed 2001 *Advancing technology, nursing and caring*. Auburn House, Westport.

Loftus L A, McDowell J 2000 The lived experience of the oncology clinical nurse specialist. *International Journal of Nursing Studies* 37:513–21.

Long L, Hobbs W, Mander T 1999 Primary nursing in the haematology ward: Does it make a difference? Research Paper Series No. 1. University of Adelaide Department of Clinical Nursing, Adelaide.

Lotringer S 1989 *Foucault live (interviews, 1966–84)*. Semiotext(e), New York.

Lovekin D 1991 *Technique, discourse and consciousness: an introduction to the philosophy of Jacques Ellul*. Associated University Press, New Jersey.

Lovett J 1993 Foreword. In T Sorensen & R Epps (eds) *Prospects and policies for rural Australia*, pp vii–ix. Longman, Melbourne.

Lumby J 1991 Threads of an emerging discipline: praxis, reflection, rhetoric and research. In G Gray & R Pratt (eds) *Towards a discipline of nursing*, pp 461–83. Churchill Livingstone, Melbourne.

——2000 Theory generation through reflective practice. In J Greenwood (ed) *Nursing theory in Australia: development and application*, 2nd edn, pp 330–48. Pearson Education Australia, Sydney.

——2001 *Who cares? The changing health care system*. Allen & Unwin, Sydney.

Lumley J 1987 Assessing technology in a teaching hospital: three case studies. Paper presented at the 'Technologies in health care: policies and politics conference', Canberra.

Lundgren B, Houseman C 2002 Continuing competence in selected health care professions. *Journal of Allied Health* 31(4):232–40.

Lundy C 1996 Nursing beyond Fordism. *Employee Responsibilities and Rights Journal* 9(2):163–71.

Lupton D 1998 *The emotional self*. Sage, London.

——2003 *Medicine as culture*, 2nd edn. Sage Publications, London.

Lyons A, Richardson S 2003 Clinical decision support in critical care nursing. *AACN Clinical Issues* 14(3):295–301.

Lyotard J-F 1984 *The postmodern condition: a report on knowledge*. Manchester University Press, Manchester.

MacGinley M R 1996 *A dynamic of hope: institutes of women religious in Australia*. Crossing Press for the Institute of Religious Studies, Sydney.

MacGuire J 1991 Quality of care assessed: using the senior monitor index in three wards for the elderly before and after a change to primary nursing. *Journal of Advanced Nursing* 16:511–20.

Mackay B 2003 General practitioners' perceptions of the nurse practitioner role: an exploratory study. *The New Zealand Medical Journal* 116(1170). Available from: http://www.nzma.org.nz/journal/116-1170/356/.

Mackintosh C 1997 A historical study of men in nursing. *Journal of Advanced Nursing* 26:232–6.

Macklin J 1991 *The Australian health jigsaw: integration of health care delivery*. Background Paper No. 1, Department of Health, Housing and Community Services, Canberra.

——1992 *The future of general practice*. Issues Paper No. 3, Department of Health and Housing, Canberra.

Madge S, Khair K 2000 Multidisciplinary teams in the United Kingdom: problems and solutions. *Journal of Pediatric Nursing* 15(2):131–4.

Madjar I, McMillan M, Sharkey R, Elwin C, Cadd A 1997 *Project to review and examine expectations of beginning registered nurses in the workforce, 1997*. New South Wales Nurses' Registration Board, Sydney. Available from: http://nursesreg. health.nsw.gov.au/corporate-services/hprb/nrb_web/exp_brns/exp_brns.pdf.

Manthey M 1980 *The practice of primary nursing*. Blackwell, Boston.

Marmot M 2000 Social determinants of health: from observation. *Medical Journal of Australia* 172:379–82.

Marrow C E, Macauley D M, Crumbie A 1997 Promoting reflective practice through structured clinical supervision. *Journal of Nursing Management* 5:77–82.

Marshall B 2004 Health promotion in action: case studies from Australia. In H Keleher & B Murphy (eds) *Understanding health: a determinants approach*. Oxford University Press, Melbourne.

Martin J 1978 *The migrant presence*. Allen & Unwin, Sydney.

Martyr P 2002 *Paradise of quacks: an alternative history of medicine in Australia*. Macleay Press, Sydney.

Masi C, Suarez-Balcazar Y, Cassey M, Kinney L, Piotrowski H 2003 Internet access and empowerment. *Journal of General Internal Medicine* 18:525–30.

Maslin-Prothero S 2001 *Bailliere's study skills for nurses*. Bailliere Tindall, London.

Maslin-Prothero S, Owen S 2001 Enhancing your clinical links and credibility: the role of nurse lecturers and teachers in clinical practice. *Nurse Education in Practice* 1(4):189–95.

Mathers C, Vos T, Stevenson C 1999 *The burden of disease and injury in Australia*. Catalogue No. PHE 17. AIHW, Canberra.

Mayer R, Goodchild F 1995 *The critical thinker*, 2nd edn. Brown & Benchmark Publishers, Madison.

Mays R M, De Leon Siantz M, Viehweg S A 2002 Assessing cultural competence of policy organizations. *Journal of Transcultural Nursing* 13(2):139–44.

McClure M L 1991 Technology—a driving force for change. *Journal of Professional Nursing* 7(3):144.

McConnell E A 1990 The impact of machines on the work of critical care nurses. *Critical Care Nursing Quarterly* 12(4):45–52.

McCoppin B, Gardner H 1994 *Tradition and reality: nursing and politics in Australia*. Churchill Livingstone, Melbourne.

McCormack B 2004 Person-centredness in gerontological nursing: an overview of the literature. *International Journal of Older Person Nursing* 13(3a):31–8.

McDonald S, Ahern K 1999 Whistle-blowing: effective and ineffective coping responses. *Nursing Forum* 34(4):5–13.

McGee P, Ashford R 1996 Nurses' perceptions of roles in multidisciplinary teams. *Nursing Standard* 10(45):34–6.

McGrath P, Patterson C, Yates P, Treloar S, Oldenbury B, Loos C 1999 A study of postdiagnosis breast cancer concerns for women living in rural and remote Queensland. Part II: support issues. *Australian Journal of Rural Health* 7: 43–52.

McKeon C M, Fogarty G J, Hegney D G 2003 Organisational factors contributing to violations by rural and remote nurses during medication administration. In M Katsikitis (ed) 'Proceedings of the 38th APS annual conference', pp 128–32. Perth.

McLaren P 1988 Schooling the postmodern body: critical pedagogy and the politics of enfleshment. *Journal of Education* 170(3):53–83.

McMahon R 1996 Individual vs collective activity: a primary nursing paradox. *British Journal of Nursing* 5(12):760–3.

McMillan M, Conway J, FitzGerald M 2004 *Issues in workplace, work practice and workforce: the implications for care models and nursing service delivery.* Final report of a desktop study commissioned by the Department of Human Services, Victoria.

McMurray A 1999 *Community health and wellness: a socioecological approach.* Mosby, Sydney.

——2003 *Community health and wellness: a sociological approach*, 2nd edn. Mosby, Sydney.

——2004 Culturally sensitive evidence-based practice. *Collegian* 11(4):14–18.

McMurray A, St John W, Lucas N, Donovan A, Curry A, Hohnke R 1998 *Advanced nursing practice for rural and remote Australia: report to the National Rural Health Alliance.* Griffith University, Gold Coast.

McNeil B J, Elfrink V L, Bickford C J, Pierce S T 2003 Nursing information technology knowledge, skills and preparation of student nurses, nursing faculty and clinicians: A US survey. *Journal of Nursing Education* 42(8):341.

McQueen A C H 2004 Emotional intelligence in nursing work. *Journal of Advanced Nursing* 47(1):101–8.

McVicar A 2003 Workplace stress in nursing: a literature review. *Journal of Advanced Nursing* 44(6):633–42.

Meadows G 2002 Nursing informatics: an evolving specialty. *Nursing Economist* 20(6):300–1.

Meadus R J 2000 Men in nursing: barriers to recruitment. *Nursing Forum* 35(3):515.

Medic to Medic 2004 *Map of medicine.* NHS, London.

Meleis A 1997 *Theoretical nursing: development and progress.* Lippincott, Philadelphia.

Melia K 1987 *Learning and working.* Tavistock, London.

Mercer N 2003 *Redevelopment of the AIHW Knowledgebase—Stage 1: scope and issues paper.* AIHW, Canberra.

Mezirow J 1985 A critical theory of self directed learning. *New Directions for Continuing Education* 25:17–30.

Miles M B, Huberman A M 1994 *Qualitative data analysis*, 2nd edn. Sage, Thousand Oakes, California.

Miller G A 1985 *Psychology: the science of mental life.* Penguin, London.

Miller M, Babcock D 1996 *Critical thinking applied to nursing.* Mosby, St Louis.

Mitchell G D 1987 *A new dictionary of sociology.* Routledge & Kegan Paul, London.

Mok E, Pui Chi Chiu 2004 Nurse–patient relationships in palliative care. *Journal of Advanced Nursing* 48(5):475–83.

Monahan B B 1996 The nurses' media handbook: a reference for nurses planning to meet the media. *Massachusetts Nurse* 66(5):2, 6, 12.

Moore T 1991 *Cry of the damaged man.* Picador, Sydney.

Morgan H 2001 *Bullwinkel, Vivian.* Australian Science and Technology History Centre. Available from: http://www.asap.unimelb.edu.au/bsparcs/biogs/P003351b.htm.

Morin K H 1999 Mothers: responses to care given by male nursing students during and after birth. *Image: Journal of Nursing Scholarship* 31(1):83–7.

Morse J, Solberg S, Neander W, Bottorf J, Johnson J 1990 Concepts of caring and caring as a concept. *Advances in Nursing Science* 13(1):1–14.

Muff J 1982 Handmaiden, battle-ax, whore: an exploration into the fantasies, myths and stereotypes about nurses. In J Muff (ed) *Socialization, sexism, and stereotyping: women's issues in nursing*. Mosby, St Louis.

Muff J 1988 Of images and ideals: a look at socialization and sexism in nursing. In A Jones (ed) *Images of nurses: perspectives from history, art and literature*. University of Pennsylvania Press, Philadelphia.

Muir Gray J A 2001 *Evidenced-based healthcare*. Churchill Livingstone, London.

Mulhall A 1995 Nursing research: what difference does it make? *Journal of Advanced Nursing* 21:576–83.

Munhall P L 1982 Nursing philosophy and nursing research: in apposition or opposition? *Nursing Research* 31:176–7, 181.

Munhall P L, Oiler Boyd C 1993 *Nursing research: a qualitative perspective*. National League for Nursing Press, New York.

Myerson D E 2000 If emotions were honoured: a cultural analysis. In S Fineman *Emotion in organizations*, 2nd edn. Sage, London.

National Advisory Council on Nurse Education and Practice 1997 *Report to the secretary of the Department of Health and Human Services: a national informatics agenda for nursing education and practice*. NACNEP, Washington DC.

National Archives of Australia 2000 *Reverend John Flynn and the Australian Inland Mission*. Available from: http://www.naa.gov.au/Publications/fact_sheets/FS159.html.

National Health and Medical Research Council 1997 *Joint NHMRC/AVCC statement and guidelines on research practice*. NHMRC, Canberra.

——1999 *A guide to the development, implementation and evaluation of clinical practice guidelines*. NHMRC, Canberra.

——2000 *How to use the evidence: assessment and application of scientific evidence*. NHMRC, Canberra.

National Health Information Management Advisory Council 2001 *Health online: a health information action plan for Australia*, 2nd edn. Commonwealth of Australia, Canberra.

National Health Information Management Group 2002 *Health information development priorities*. NHIMG, Canberra.

National Health Service Modernisation Agency 2005 *Changing workforce programme: new ways of working in health care*. Accessed 27 January 2005. Available from: http://www.modernnhs.nhs.uk/scripts/default.asp?site_id=65.

National Multicultural Advisory Council 1999 *Australian multiculturalism for a new century: towards inclusiveness*. Commonwealth of Australia, Canberra.

Neill J, Taylor K 2002 Undergraduate nursing students' clinical experiences in rural and remote areas: recruitment implications. *Australian Journal of Rural Health* 10:239–43.

Nelson S 1995 Humanism in nursing: the emergence of light. *Nursing Inquiry* 2(1):36–43.

——1997 Reading nursing history. *Nursing Inquiry* 4:229–36.

——1999 Entering a professional domain: the making of the modern nurse in 17th-century France. *Nursing History Review* 7:171–81.

——2000 *A genealogy of the care of the sick: nursing, holism and pious practice*. Nursing Praxis International, Hants, England.

Nelson S, Rabach J 2002 Military experience—the new age of Australian nursing and other failures. *Health and History* 4(1):79–86.

Neuhaus W, Piroth C, Kiencke P, Gohring U J, Mallman P 2002 A psychosocial analysis of women planning birth outside hospital. *Journal of Obstetrics and Gynaecology* 22(2):143–9.

Neuman B 1995 *The Neuman systems model: application to nursing education and practice*. Appleton Century Crofts, New York.

Neuman C E 1999 Taking charge: nursing, suffrage and feminism in America, 1973–1920 (review). *Journal of Women's History* 10(4):228–35.

New South Wales Health 1998 *Rural and remote nursing summit report*. NSW Health, Sydney.

——2004. Accessed 1 December 2004. Available from: http://www.health.nsw.gov.au/nursing/scholar.html.

New South Wales Health Department 2001 *Palliative care framework. A guide for the provision of palliative care in NSW*. NSW Health Department, Sydney.

——2002 *Women's health outcomes framework*. NSW Health Department, Sydney.

Newman M A 1983 The continuing revolution: a history of nursing science. In N L Chaska (ed) *The nursing profession: a time to speak*, pp 385–93. McGraw Hill, New York.

Nicolson P 1996 *Gender, power and organisation: a psychological perspective*. Routledge, London.

Nieswiadomy R 2002 ed *Foundations of nursing research*, 4th edn. Prentice Hall, New Jersey.

Nightingale F 1859–1946 *Notes on nursing*. Harrison Book Company, London.

——1969 *Notes on nursing: in what it is, and what it is not*. Dover Publications, New York.

Nixon J A, Wakeley C 1948 *Text-book for nurses: anatomy, physiology, surgery and medicine*. Oxford University Press, London.

Northern Territory Government 2004. Accessed 1 December 2004. Available from: http://www.nt.gov.au/health/careers/studies_assistance.shtml.

Nursing Council of New Zealand 2004 *Competencies for the registered nurse scope of practice*. Nursing Council of New Zealand, Wellington.

O'Tool M ed 1997 *Miller–Kearne encyclopedia and dictionary of medicine, nursing and allied health*. W B Saunders, Philadelphia.

Office of Multicultural Affairs 1989 *National agenda for a multicultural Australia . . . sharing our future*. Department of the Prime Minister and Cabinet, AGPS, Canberra.

Offredy M 2000 Advanced nursing practice: the case of nurse practitioners in three Australian states. *Journal of Advanced Nursing* 31:274–81.

Oleni M, Johansson P, Fridlund B 2004 Nursing care at night: an evaluation using the Night Nursing Care Instrument. *Journal of Advanced Nursing* 47(1):25–32.

Omeri A 1996 Transcultural nursing care values, beliefs and practices of Iranian immigrants in NSW, Australia. Unpublished PhD thesis. Faculty of Nursing, University of Sydney, Sydney.

——1997 Culture care of Iranian immigrants in NSW, Australia: sharing transcultural nursing care knowledge. *Journal of Transcultural Nursing* 8(2):5–16.

——2000 Where is Australia going in transcultural nursing in the new millennium? Reflections. Paper presented at the 26th 'Annual transcultural nursing research conference', Gold Coast.

——2003 Assuring culturally competent nursing care: Whose responsibility? *Nursing Review* September:5.

Omeri A, Ahern M 1999 Utilizing culturally congruent strategies to enhance recruitment and retention of Australian indigenous nursing students. *Journal of Transcultural Nursing* 10(2):150–5.

Omeri A, Lennings C, Raymond L 2004 Hardiness and transformational coping in asylum seekers: the Afghan experience. *Journal of Diversity in Health and Social Care in Community* 1(1):21–30.

Omeri A, Malcolm P, Ahern M, Wellington B 2002 Meeting the challenges of cultural diversity in the academic setting. *Nurse Education in Practice* 3:5–22.

Ong B 2002 Leveraging on information technology to enhance patient care: a doctor's perspective of implementation in a Singapore academic hospital. *Ann Acad Med Singapore* 31(6):707–11.

Orem D 1991 *Nursing: concepts of practice*. Mosby, St Louis.

Owens J, Francis D, Usher K, Tollefson J 1997 *Risks and rewards of reflective thinking*. James Cook University, Townsville.

Pacey A 1999 *Meaning in technology*. MIT Press, Cambridge.

Paley J 2001 An archaeology of caring knowledge. *Journal of Advanced Nursing* 26(2):188–98.

——2002 Caring as a slave morality: Nietzschean themes in nursing ethics. *Journal of Advanced Nursing* 40(1):25–35.

Pape T M 2003 Evidence based nursing practice: to infinity and beyond. *Journal of Continuing Education in Nursing* 34(4):154–61.

Parker B, McFarland J 1991 Feminist theory and nursing: an empowerment model for research. *Advances in Nursing Science* 13(3):59–67.

Parker J 1990 Professional nursing education in the university context. Meredith Memorial Lecture, La Trobe University, Melbourne.

——1995 Searching for the body in nursing. In G Gray & R Pratt (eds) *Scholarship in the discipline of nursing*. Churchill Livingstone, Melbourne.

——2001 The implications of international health policy trends on nursing education: an Australian perspective. *Policy, Politics, & Nursing Practice* 2(2):142–8.

——2002 Evidence based nursing: a defence (editorial). *Nursing Inquiry* 9(3): 139–40.

——2004 Nursing on the medical ward. *Nursing Inquiry* 11(4):210–17.

Parker J, Gibbs M 1998 Truth, virtue and beauty: midwifery and philosophy. *Nursing Inquiry* 5(3):146–53.

Parker J, Johnston L, Faulkner R 2000 Evidence-based nursing: integrating research into practice. In J Greenwood (ed) *Nursing theory in Australia: development and application*, 2nd edn, pp 396–412. Prentice Hall, Sydney.

Parker J, Rickard G 1999 Nursing town and nursing gown: time, space and the reinvention of nursing through collaboration. *Clinical Excellence for Nurse Practitioners* 3(1):36–42.

Parker R 1990 Nurses stories: the search for a relational ethic of care. *Advances in Nursing Science* 13(1):31–40.

Parker S, Clare J 2000 Becoming a critical thinker. In J Daly, S Speedy & D Jackson (eds) *Contexts of nursing: an introduction*, pp 249–64. MacLennan & Petty, Sydney.

Parse R R 1987 ed *Nursing science: major paradigms, theories and critiques*. W B Saunders, Philadelphia.

——2001 *Qualitative inquiry: the path of sciencing*. Jones & Bartlett, Boston.

Patel K R M 2002 *Health care policy in an age of new technologies*. M E Sharpe, New York.

Paul R 1993 *Critical thinking: how to prepare students for a rapidly changing world*. Foundation for Critical Thinking, Santa Rosa, California.

Peach H G, Pearce D C, Farish S J 1998 Age-standardised mortality and proportional mortality analysis of Aboriginal and non-Aboriginal deaths in metropolitan, rural and remote areas. *Australian Journal of Rural Health* 16:36–41.

Peacock J W, Nolan P W 2000 Care under threat in the modern world. *Journal of Advanced Nursing* 32(5):1066–70.

REFERENCES

Pearson A 1989 *Primary nursing: nursing in the Burford and Oxford Nursing Development Units*. Chapman & Hall, London.

——1991 Taking up the challenge: the future for therapeutic nursing. In R McMahon & A Pearson (eds) *Nursing as therapy*. Chapman & Hall, London.

——1992 Knowing nursing: emerging paradigms in nursing. In K Robinson & B Vaughan (eds) *Knowledge for nursing practice*, pp 213–26. Butterworth Heinemann, Oxford.

Pearson A, Baker H 1992 Quality of care: Do contemporary nursing approaches make a difference? Deakin Institute of Nursing Research, Research Paper No. 5. Deakin University, Geelong.

Pearson A, Vaughan B, FitzGerald M eds 2005 *Nursing models for practice*, 3rd edn. Butterworth Heinemann, London.

Pelletier D 1989 Health care technology: sharpening the definition and establishing aspects of the social context. *Australian Health Review* 12(3):56–64.

Pepin J 1992 Family caring and caring in nursing. *Image: Journal of Nursing Scholarship* 24(2):127–31.

Peplau H E 1987 The art and science of nursing: similarities, differences, and relations. *Nursing Science Quarterly* 1:8–15.

Peter E 2004 Nursing resistance as ethical action: literature review. *Journal of Advanced Nursing* 46(4):403–16.

Peter E, Lunardi A L, Macfarlane A 2004 Nursing resistance as ethical action: literature review. *Journal of Advanced Nursing* 46(4):403–16.

Phaneuf M 1976 *The nursing audit*. Appleton Century Crofts, New York.

Pillar B, Jacox A K, Redman B K 1990 Technology, its assessment and nursing. *Nursing Outlook* 38(1):16–19.

Poggi G 2001 *Forms of power*. Polity Press, Cambridge.

Poliafico J K 1998 Nursing's gender gap. *RN* 61(10):39–43.

Polit D F, Beck C T, Hungler B P 2001 *Essentials of nursing research: methods, appraisal and utilisation*, 5th edn. Lippincott, Philadelphia.

Potter T B, Palmer R G 2003 360-degree assessment in a multidisciplinary team setting. *Rheumatology* 42(11):1404–7.

Pratt R, Russell R L 2002 *A voice to be heard: the first fifty years of the New South Wales College of Nursing*. Allen & Unwin, Sydney.

Procter N G 2004a Beyond asylum: the significance of supportive counseling in the process of seeking asylum. *Nursing Review* March:5.

——2004b Retraumatization, fear and suicidal thinking: a case study of 'boatpeople' to Australia. *Migration Letters: An International Journal of Migration* 1(1):42–9.

——2004c Support for temporary protection visa holders: partnering individual mental health support and migration law consultation. *Psychiatry, Psychology and Law* 11:110–12.

Pryce A 2004 'Only odd people wore suede shoes': careers and sexual identities of men attending a sexual health clinic. *Nursing Inquiry* 11(4):258–70.

Pryor L 2005 Add a little optimism to reconnect with the young ones. Comment in *Sydney Morning Herald*, Monday, 24 January 2005, p 11.

Queensland Health 2004. Accessed 1 December 2004. Available from: http://www.health.qld.gov.au/orh/qhrss/default.asp.

Radcliffe M 2001 A short history of PREParation. *Nursing Times* 97(14):22–4.

Ralston Saul J 2001 *On equilibrium*. Penguin Books, Sydney.

Ramjan L M 2004 Nurses and the 'therapeutic relationship': caring for adolescents with anorexia nervosa. *Journal of Advanced Nursing* 45(5):495–503.

Rancine L 2003 Implementing a postcolonial feminist perspective in nursing research related to non-Western populations. *Nursing Inquiry* 10(2):91–102.

Rawls J 1971 *A theory of justice*. Oxford University Press, Oxford.

Rawnsley M 1990 Of human bonding: the context of nursing as caring. *Advances in Nursing Science* 13(1):41–8.

Rawson M 2004 *Poverty and health education.* Accessed 22 December 2004. Available from: http://www.studentbmj.com/back_issues/0601/educatin/180.html.

Ray M 1987 Technological caring: a new model in critical care. *Dimensions in Critical Care Nursing* 6(3):173–9.

——1989 The theory of bureaucratic caring for nursing practice in the organizational structure. *Nursing Science Quarterly* 13(2):31–42.

Reed R G 1998 Breaking through a breakdown in nursing logic. *Nursing Science Quarterly* 11:146–8.

Refugee Council of Australia 2000 *Refugee settlement in Australia: views from the community sector.* RCOA, Glebe.

——2002 *Refugee Council of Australia.* Accessed 22 May 2002. Available from: http://www/refugeecouncil.org.au.

Reich W 1994 The word 'bioethics': its birth and the legacies of those who shaped its meaning. *Kennedy Institute of Ethics Journal* 4:319–35.

Reich W ed 1995a *The encyclopedia of bioethics,* revised edition. Simon & Schuster Macmillan/Simon & Schuster and Prentice Hall International, New York.

——1995b The word 'bioethics': the struggle over its earliest meanings. *Kennedy Institute of Ethics Journal* 5:19–34.

Reid R, Page C, Pounds R 1999 *Just wanted to be there: Australian Service Nurses 1899–1999.* Commonwealth Department of Veteran's Affairs, Canberra.

Reinhardt A C 2004 Discourse on the transformational leader metanarrative or finding the right person for the job. *Advances in Nursing Science* 27(1):21–32.

Reiser S 1981 Valuing the patient's views: a problem for public policy. *Annals of the New York Academy of Sciences* 368(12):17–22.

Reiser S J 1978 *Medicine and the reign of technology.* Cambridge University Press, Cambridge.

——1993 Technology and the use of the senses in twentieth century medicine. In W F Bynum & R Porter (eds) *Medicine and the five senses,* pp 262–73, 322–3. Cambridge University Press, New York.

Reverby S M 1987 *Ordered to care: the dilemma of American nursing, 1850–1945.* Cambridge University Press, New York.

Rinard R 1996 Technology, deskilling, and nurses: the impact of the technologically changing environment. *Advances in Nursing Science* 18(4):60–70.

Roberts K, Taylor B 1998 *Nursing research processes: an Australian perspective.* Nelson ITP, Melbourne.

Roberts S J 2000 Development of a positive professional identity: liberating oneself from the oppressor within. *Advances in Nursing Science* 22(4):71–83.

Robinson-Walker C 1999 *Women in leadership and health care: the journey to authenticity and power.* Jossey-Bass, San Francisco.

Rogers C 1980 *A way of being.* Houghton Mifflin, Boston.

Rogers M 1970 *Theoretical basis of nursing.* F A Davis, Philadelphia.

Rolfe G 1993 Closing the theory–practice gap: a model of nursing praxis. *Journal of Clinical Nursing* 2:173–7.

——2001 Reflective practice: where now? *Nurse Education in Practice* 2(21):21–9.

Rolfe G, Freshwater D, Jasper M 2001 *Critical reflection for nursing and the helping professions: a user's guide.* Palgrave, New York.

Rolley F, Humphreys J S 1993 Rural welfare—the human face of Australia's countryside. In T Sorensen & R Epps (eds) *Prospects and policies for rural Australia,* pp 241–57. Longman Cheshire, Melbourne.

Roper N, Logan W, Tierney A 1990 *The elements of nursing,* 3rd edn. Churchill Livingstone, Edinburgh.

Rosenberg C E 1987 *The care of strangers: the rise of America's hospital system*. John Hopkins University Press, Baltimore.

Roy C 1980 The Roy adaptation model. In J Riehl & C Roy (eds) *Conceptual models for nursing practice*. Appleton Century Crofts, New York.

Roy C, Andrews H A 1999 *The Roy adaptation model*, 2nd edn. Appleton & Lange, Stamford.

Royal College of Nursing Australia 1998 *Continuing professional education position statement*. Available from: http://www.rcna.org.au/content/.

——2003 *Position statement: nursing research*. Available from: http://www.rcna.org.au/content/.

——2004 *Issues paper: poverty profile of Australia*. Accessed 20 January 2004. Available from: http://www.rcna.org.

Rudan V 2003 The best of both worlds: a consideration of gender in team building. *Journal of Nursing Administration* 33(3):179–86.

Rudge T 1999 Situating wound management: technoscience, dressings and 'other' skins. *Nursing Inquiry* 6:167–77.

Ruggiero V 1998 *The art of thinking: a guide to critical and creative thought*, 5th edn. Longman, New York.

Rule J 1995 Nurses may live to regret the 'angel' image era has ended. *Nursing Management* 2(6):5.

Russell R L 2000 Milestones in Australian nursing. In J Daly, S Speedy & D Jackson (eds) *Contexts of nursing: an introduction*. MacLennan & Petty, Sydney.

Ryan S, Porter S 1993 Men in nursing: a cautionary critique. *Nursing Outlook* 41(6):262–7.

Sackett D L, Wennberg J E 1997 Choosing the best research design for each question: it's time to stop squabbling over the 'best' methods (editorial). *British Medical Journal* 317(7123):1636.

Salvage J 1982 Angles, not angels. *The Health Services* 31:12–13.

——1983 Distorted images. *Nursing Times* 79:13–15.

——1990 The theory and practice of the 'new' nursing. *Nursing Times* 86(4):42–5.

Salvation Army Archives, Melbourne. Appendix 1, unpublished SOC BEV BK000825.2.

Sandelowski M 1988 A case of conflicting paradigms: nursing and reproductive technology. *Advances in Nursing Science* 10(3):35–45.

——1996 Tools of the trade: analysing technology as object in nursing. *Scholarly Inquiry for Nursing Practice: An International Journal* 10(1):5–16.

——1997a (Ir)reconcilable differences? The debate concerning nursing and technology. *Image: Journal of Nursing Scholarship* 29(2):169–74.

——1997b Making the best of things: technology in American nursing 1870–1940. *Nursing History Review* 5:3–22.

——1999a Culture, conceptive technology, and nursing. *International Journal of Nursing Studies* 36:13–20.

——1999b Venous envy: the post-World War II debate over IV nursing. *Advances in Nursing Science* 22(1):52–62.

——2000 *Devices and desires: gender, technology and American nursing*. University of North Carolina, Chapel Hill.

Sands and McDougall directories (1862–1881). Sands & McDougall, Melbourne.

Sarantakos S 1993 *Social research*. Macmillan, Melbourne.

——2005 *Social research*, 3rd edn. Palgrave Macmillan, London.

Saul J 1997 *The unconscious civilization*. Penguin, Melbourne.

Schick T, Vaughn L 1995 *How to think about weird things: critical thinking for a new age*. Mayfield Publishing Company, Mountain View, California.

Schneider Z 2003 Strategies for conducting a critical review. In Z Schneider, D Elliott,

REFERENCES

G LoBiondo-Wood & J Haber (eds) *Nursing research: methods, critical appraisal and utilisation*, 2nd edn, pp 52–72. Mosby, Sydney.

Schneider Z, Elliott D, LoBiondo-Wood G, Haber J eds 2003 *Nursing research: methods, critical appraisal and utilisation*, 2nd edn. Mosby, Sydney.

Schön D A 1983 *The reflective practitioner: how practitioners think in action*. Basic Books, New York.

——1987 *Educating the reflective practitioner: towards a new design for teaching and learning in the professions*. Jossey-Bass, San Francisco.

Schrader T 2004 Poverty and health in Australia. *New Doctor* 80:17–19.

Schutz A 1962–73 *Collected papers Volume II: studies in social theory*. The Hague, Netherlands.

Scott D 1992 The ecology of the family and family functions. In A Clements (ed) *Infant and family health in Australia*. Churchill Livingstone, Melbourne.

Scott J 2001 *Power*. Polity Press, Cambridge.

Selzer R 1993 *Raising the dead: a doctor's encounter with his own mortality*. Penguin, Harmondsworth.

Senate Community Affairs References Committee 2002 *The patient profession: time for action*. Australian Government, Canberra.

——2004 *A hand up not a hand out: renewing the fight against poverty. Report on poverty and financial hardship*. Commonwealth of Australia, Canberra. Accessed 20 January 2004. Available from: http://www.aph.gov.au/senate/committee/clac_ctte/poverty/report/index.htm.

Severinsson E I 2001 Confirmation, meaning and self-awareness as core concepts of the nursing supervision model. *Nursing Ethics* 8(1):36–44.

Shakespeare P 2003 Nurses' bodywork: is there a body of work? *Nursing Inquiry* 10(1):47–56.

Sharman E 1998 The glass elevator: how men overtake women in the nursing higher education workforce in Australia. Unpublished PhD thesis, University of New South Wales, Sydney.

Sharman E, Short S, Black D 1996 Why so many? The masculine mystique and men in the nursing higher education workforce in Australia. In conference proceedings of the 'Changing society for women's health conference', Australian National University, Canberra.

Shell R 2001 Bargaining styles and negotiation: the Thomas–Killman conflict model instrument in negotiation training. *Negotiation Journal* 17(1):155–174.

Shildrick M 1997 *Leaky bodies and boundaries: feminism, postmodernism and (bio) ethics*. Routledge, London.

Siegloff L, Hegney D 1996 Recognition for their role—the nurse practitioner project, Wilcannia, New South Wales. In proceedings of 'The windmills, wisdom and wonderment conference'. Association for Australian Rural Nurses Inc, Roseworthy.

Silove D, Steel Z, McGorry P et al 1998 Trauma exposure, postmigration stressors and symptoms of anxiety, depression and posttraumatic stress in Tamil asylum seekers: comparisons with refugees and immigrants. *Acta Psychiatr Scand* 97: 175–81.

Silverman H J 1994 *Textualities: between hermeneutics and deconstruction*. Routledge, New York.

Simpson E, Courtney M 2002 Critical thinking in nursing education: a literature review. *International Journal of Nursing Practice* 8:89–98.

Simpson R 2001 Compassion meets the computer age. *Nursing Management* 32(1):13–14.

Simpson R L, Brown L N 1990 How to survive the next decade. *Nursing Management* 21(12):24–5.

REFERENCES

Sinclair M, Gardner J 2001 Midwives' perceptions of the use of technology in assisting childbirth in Northern Ireland. *Journal of Advanced Nursing* 36(2):229–36.

Singer P 1993 *How are we to live? Ethics in an age of self-interest*. Text Publishing, Melbourne.

Smith F B 1982 *Florence Nightingale, reputation and power*. Croom Helm, London.

Smith J 1992 Enhancing aesthetic knowing: a teaching strategy. *Advances in Nursing Science* 14(3):52–9.

Snellgrove S, Hughes D 2000 Interprofessional relations between doctors and nurses: perspectives from South Wales. *Journal of Advanced Nursing* 31(3):661–7.

Snow C P 1964 *The two cultures: and a second look*. New American Library, New York.

Sorensen T, Epps R 1993 eds *Prospects and policies for rural Australia*, pp 1–6. Longman, Melbourne.

Speedy S 1999 The therapeutic alliance. In M Clinton & S Nelson (eds) *Advanced practice in mental health nursing*. Blackwell Science, Oxford.

Speedy S, Jackson D 2004 Power, politics and gender: issues for nurse leaders and managers. In J Daly, S Speedy & D Jackson (eds) *Nursing leadership*, pp 55–67. Elsevier Australia, Sydney.

Staggers N, Thompson C 2002 The evolution of definitions for nursing informatics: a critical analysis. *Journal of the American Medical Informatics Association* 9(3):255–61.

Standards Australia 2003 *Health concept terminology data base. Draft standard AS5021*. Standards Australia, Sydney.

Stanhope M, Lancaster J 2002 *Foundations of community health nursing*, p 183. Mosby, St Louis.

Stanley F 2002 A new research alliance for children and youth in Australia. Our kids: our present and our future. Conference on 'The importance of the early years of life'. Tasmanian Department of Health and Human Services, Hobart.

Stanley F, Sanson A, McMichael T 2002 New causal pathways thinking for public health. In A Sanson (ed) *Children's health and development: new research and directions for Australia*. Australian Institute of Family Studies, Melbourne.

State Government of Victoria 2004. Accessed 1 December 2004. Available from: http://nursing.vic.gov.au/futhering/postgrad.htm.

State Library of South Australia 2001 Lowitja O'Donoghue—Elder of our nation. In *Women and politics in South Australia: the Aboriginal voice*. Accessed 20 February 2005. Available from: http://www.slsa.sa.gov.au/women_and_politics/abor1.htm.

Steel Z, Sil D M 2001 The mental health implications of detaining asylum seekers. *Medical Journal of Australia* 175:596–604.

Stevens S Y 1995 Sale of the century: images of nursing in the movietowns during World War II [correction] [published erratum appears in *Journal of Military Nursing Research* 1995, 1(4):4] *Journal of Military Nursing Research* 1(3):36.

Stockdale M, Warelow P 2000 Is the complexity of care a paradox? *Journal of Advanced Nursing* 31(5):1258–64.

Strachan G 2001 Present at the birth: 'handywomen' and neighbours in rural New South Wales 1850–1900. *Labour History* 81:13–27.

Strasen L 1992 *The image of professional nursing: strategies for action*. Lippincott, Philadelphia.

Street A 1992 *Inside nursing*. State University Press, New York.

——1995 *Nursing replay: researching nursing culture together*. Churchill Livingstone, Melbourne.

Strong K, Trickett P, Titulaer I, Bhatia K 1998 *Health in rural and remote Australia: the first report of the Australian Institute of Health and Welfare on rural health*. AIHW, Canberra.

Sullivan E J 2004 *Becoming influential: a guide for nurses*. Pearson Prentice Hall, New Jersey.

Sullivan J, Deane D 1994 Caring: reappropriating our tradition. *Nursing Forum* 29(2):5–9.

Sultan A, O'Sullivan K 2001 Psychological disturbances in asylum seekers. *Medical Journal of Australia* 175:593–6.

Summerfield D 2000 Childhood war refugeedom and trauma: three core questions for mental health professionals. *Transcultural Psychiatry* 37:417–33.

Summers A 1989 The mysterious demise of Sarah Gamp: the domiciliary nurse and her detractors c.1830–1860. *Victorian Studies* 32:365–86.

——1997 Sairey Gamp: generating fact from fiction. *Nursing Inquiry* 4:14–18.

Swanson K 1993 Nursing as informed caring for the well-being of others. *Image: Journal of Nursing Scholarship* 25(4):352–7.

Takase M, Kershaw E, Burt L 2001 Nurse–environment misfit and nursing practice. *Journal of Advanced Nursing* 35(6):819–26.

Taylor B J 2000 *Reflective practice: a guide for nurses and midwives*. Allen & Unwin, Sydney.

Teasdale K 1998 *Advocacy in health care*. Blackwell Science, Oxford.

Teekman B 2000 Exploring reflective thinking in nursing practice. *Journal of Advanced Nursing* 31(5):1125–35.

The Argus newspaper (28 July 1848).

Thomson J A, Thomson M 1911 The position of woman: biologically considered. In H E Cuff & W T Gordon Pugh (eds) *The position of woman: actual and ideal*, pp 1–28. William Blackwood, Edinburgh.

Thorne S E, Hayes V E eds 1997 *Nursing praxis: knowledge and action*. Sage, Thousand Oaks, California.

Tisdale S 1986 Swept away by technology. *American Journal of Nursing* 86(4): 429–30.

Tomey A, Alligood M R 1998 *Nursing theorists and their work*, 4th edn. Mosby, St Louis.

Tosh J 2002 *The pursuit of history: aims, methods and new directions in the study of modern history*, revised 3rd edn. Longman, Harlow, England

Touger-Decker R 2002 Developing a continuum for lifelong learning in dietetics. *Topics in Clinical Nutrition* 17(3):1–9.

Townsend J 1994 Challenge models for learning and knowing. In M McMillan & J Townsend (eds) *Reflections on contemporary nursing practice*. Butterworth, Sydney.

Traynor M 1996 Looking at discourse in a literature review of nursing texts. *Journal of Advanced Nursing* 23(2):1155–61.

Treacy M P 1989 Gender prescription in nurse training: its effects on health provision. In L K Hardy & J Randell (eds) *Recent advances in nursing: issues in women's health*. Churchill Livingstone, Edinburgh.

Trembath R, Hellier D 1987 *All care and responsibility: a history of nursing in Victoria 1850–1934*. Florence Nightingale Committee, Trembath City, Melbourne.

Tronto J C 1999 Caring: gender-sensitive ethics. *Hypatia* 14(1):112–20.

Tuckman B W, Jensen M 1993 Stages of small group development revisited. In J M Ivancevich & M T Matteson (eds) *Organisational behaviour and management*. Irwin, Boston.

Turner C 1991 *The ethics of authenticity*. Harvard University Press, Cambridge, Massachusetts.

Turner T 1990 Crushed by the system? *Nursing Times* 86(49):19.

——1992 The indomitable Mr Pink. *Nursing Times* 88(24):26–9.

REFERENCES

Turrell G, Mathers C D 2000 Socio-economic status and health in Australia. *Medical Journal of Australia* 179(9):434–8.

——2001 Socio-economic inequalities in all-cause and specific-cause mortality in Australia: 1985–1987 and 1995–1997. *International Journal of Epidemiology* 30:231–9.

Ulrich L T 2002 *The age of homespun: objects and stories in the creation of an American myth*. Random House, New York.

Umiker W 1998 Collaborative conflict resolution. In E C Hein (ed) *Contemporary leadership behaviour. Selected readings*. Lippincott, New York.

United Nations 1948 *Universal Declaration of Human Rights 1948 Article 25*. United Nations, New York.

United Nations Development Programme 2002–2003 *Human development report*. Accessed 20 December 2004. Available from: www.hdr.undp.org/does/publications/background_papers/2004/HDR2004_Will_Kamolica.Pd8.

Usher K, Francis D, Owens J, Tollefson J 1999 Reflective writing: a strategy to foster critical inquiry in undergraduate nursing students. *Australian Journal of Advanced Nursing* 17(1):7–12.

Usher K, Tollefson J, Francis D 2001 Moving from technical to critical reflection in journaling: an investigation of students' ability to incorporate three levels of reflective writing. *Australian Journal of Advanced Nursing* 19(1):15–19.

Valentine P E B 2001 A gender perspective on conflict management strategies of nurses. *Journal of Nursing Scholarship* 33(1):69–79.

van Manen M 1990 *Researching lived experience*. State University of New York Press, New York.

Victorian Government Health Services 2004 *Enterprise bargaining proposal for registered nurses*. Accessed 12 December 2004. Available from: www.nursing.vic. gov.au.

Vuorinen R, Tarkka M, Meretoja R 2000 Peer evaluation in nurses' professional development: a pilot study to investigate the issues. *Journal of Clinical Nursing* 9:273–81.

Wagner M 1992 Appropriate birth care in industrialised countries. Paper presented at the 'Future birth conference', Sydney.

——1994 *Pursuing the birth machine*. Ace Graphics, Sydney.

Wakerman J, Field P 1998 Remote area health service delivery in central Australia: primary health care and participatory management. *Australian Journal of Rural Health* 6:27–31.

Walker K 1993 On what it might mean to be a nurse: a discursive ethnography. Unpublished doctoral dissertation. La Trobe University, Melbourne.

——1995 Courting competency: nursing and the politics of performance in practice. *Nursing Inquiry* 2(2):90–9.

——1997 Dangerous liaisons: thinking, doing, nursing. *The Collegian* 4(2):4–14.

——2000 Why philosophy? Nursing and the problem of truth. In J Daly, S Speedy & D Jackson (eds) *Contexts of nursing: an introduction*. MacLennan & Petty, Sydney.

Walker L, Avant K 1983 *Strategies for theory construction in nursing*. Appleton Century Crofts, Norwalk, Connecticut.

Walker S, Frean I, Scott P, Conrick M 2003 *Classifications and terminologies in residential aged care: an information paper*. Department of Health and Ageing, Canberra.

Walkowitz J R 1992 *City of dreadful delight: narratives of sexual danger in late-Victorian London*. Virago, London.

Walmsley D J 1993 The policy environment. In T Sorensen & R Epps (eds) *Prospects and policies for rural Australia*, pp 32–56. Longman Cheshire, Melbourne.

REFERENCES

Walmsley D, Sorensen A D 1988 *Contemporary Australia*. Longman Cheshire, Melbourne.

Walters A J 1994 An interpretative study of the clinical practice of critical care nurses. *Contemporary Nurse* 3:21–5.

——1995a A Heideggerian hermeneutic study of the practice of critical care nurses. *Journal of Advanced Nursing* 21:492–7.

——1995b Technology and the lifeworld of critical care nursing. *Journal of Advanced Nursing* 22:338–46.

Warelow P J 1996 Nurse–doctor relationships in multidisciplinary teams: ideal or real? *International Journal of Nursing Practice* 2(1):33–9.

Watson J 1985a *Nursing: human science and human care*. Appleton Century Crofts, Norwalk, Connecticut.

——1985b *Nursing: the philosophy and science of caring*. Colorado Associated University Press, Boulder, Colorado.

——1988 *Nursing: human science and human care. A theory of nursing*. National League for Nursing, New York.

——1999 *Postmodern nursing and beyond*. Churchill Livingstone, London.

Watson J K 1908 *A handbook for nurses*. Scientific Press, London.

Watson J, Foster R 2003 The Attending Nurse Caring Model: integrating theory, evidence and advanced caring—healing therapeutics for transforming professional practice. *Journal of Clinical Nursing* 12(3):360–5.

Watson J, Jackson D, Borbasi S 2005 Contemplating caring: issues, concerns, debates. In J Daly, S Speedy, D Jackson, V Lambert & C Lambert (eds) *Professional nursing: concepts, issues and challenges*. Springer Publishing, New York.

Webb C 1996 Caring, curing, coping: towards an integrated model. *Journal of Advanced Nursing* 23:960–8.

Weedon C 1997 *Feminist practice and poststructuralist theory*. Blackwell Publishers, Oxford.

Wenger A F Z 1999 Cultural openness: intrinsic to human care. *Journal of Transcultural Nursing* 10(1):10.

West M A, Borill C S, Dawson J F, Brodbeck F, Shapiro D A, Haward B 2002 *Leadership clarity and team innovation in health care*. Available from: http://www/modern.nhs.uk/115/23713/25415/Leadership%20Clarity.pdf.

Whittaker R 1998 Re-framing the representation of women in advertisements for hormone replacement therapy. *Nursing Inquiry* 5(2):77–86.

Whittaker S, Carson W, Smolenski M 2000 Assuring continued competence—policy questions and approaches: How should the profession respond? *Online Journal of Issues in Nursing*, 30 June 2000. Accessed 29 January 2003. Available from: http://www.nursingworld.org/ojin/topic10/tpc10_4.htm.

Whittemore R 1999 Natural science and nursing science: Where do the horizons fuse? *Journal of Advanced Nursing* 30(5):1027–33.

Wichowski H C 1994 Professional uncertainty: nurses in the technologically intense arena. *Journal of Advanced Nursing* 19:1162–7.

Wilkin K, Slevin E 2004 The meaning of caring to nurses: an investigation into the nature of caring work in an intensive care unit. *Journal of Clinical Nursing* 13(1):50–9.

Wilkinson R, Marmot M 2003 *Social determinants of health: the solid facts*, 2nd edn. WHO Regional Office for Europe, Copenhagen. Available from: www.euro.who.int/document/e81384.pdf.

Williams C 1992 The glass escalator: hidden advantages for men in the 'female' professions. *Social Problems* 39(3):253–67.

Williams S 1997 Caring in patient-focused care: the relationship of patients' perceptions of holistic nurse care to their levels of anxiety. *Holistic Nursing Practice* 11(3):61–8.

Wilson G 1991 Technology and stress. *Nursing & Health Care* 4(32):31.

Winch J 1989 Why is health care for Aborigines so ineffective? In G Gray & R Pratt (eds) *Issues in Australian nursing 2*. Churchill Livingstone, Melbourne.

Winch S 2005 Ethics, government and sexual health: insights from Foucault. *Nursing Ethics* 12(2):177–86.

Winner L 1977 *Autonomous technology*. MIT Press, Boston, Massachusetts.

Winters J, Ballou K A 2004 The idea of nursing science. *Journal of Advanced Nursing* 45(5):533–5.

Wolf Z R 1986 The caring concept and nurse identified caring behaviours. *Topics in Clinical Nursing* 8(2):84–93.

Wolf Z, Giardino E, Osborne P, Ambrose M 1994 Dimensions of nurse caring. *Image: Journal of Nursing Scholarship* 26(2):107–11.

Women's Hospital Ladies Committee of Management Minutes, 1 October 1909. Royal Women's Hospital Archive, accession number 1991/6/26.

World Bank 1999 *Inequality: trends and prospects*. World Bank Group, Washington DC.

——2000 *World development report 2000–2001—Attacking poverty: opportunity empowerment and security*. World Bank Group, Washington DC.

World Health Organization 1947 *Consultation on the World Health Organization*. WHO, Geneva.

——1986 *Ottawa Charter for Health Promotion*. WHO Health Promotion, Geneva. Available from: http://www.euro.who.int/AboutWHO/Policy/20010827_2.

——1997 *Poverty and health: an overview of the basic linkages and public policy measures*. Health Economics Technical Briefing Note, WHO, Geneva.

——1998 *Health promotion glossary*. WHO, Geneva. Available from: http://www.wpro.who.int.hpr/docs/glossary.pdf.

——2002 *Strategic directions for strengthening nursing and midwifery services*. WHO, Geneva.

——2003 *Phase IV (2003–2007) of the WHO Healthy Cities network in Europe: goals and requirements*. WHO Regional Office for Europe, Copenhagen. Available from: http://www.euro.who.int/healthy-cities.

Wuest J 1997 Illuminating environmental influences on women's caring. *Journal of Advanced Nursing* 26(1):49–58.

Yeatman A 1991 Postmodern critical theorising: introduction. *Social Analysis* 30:3–9.

Zebroski S A 2001 The gender lens: caring and gender. *Journal of Comparative Family Studies* 32(2):322–3.

Zust B L, Moline K 2003 Identifying underserved ethnic populations within a community: the first step in eliminating disparities among racial and ethnic minorities. *Journal of Transcultural Nursing* 14(1):66–74.

GLOSSARY

Acceptability: The test applied to a premise or reason. In order to have a sound argument, a premise must be acceptable to the person evaluating the argument.

Aesthetic: A term defined in the *Australian concise Oxford dictionary* (1987) as 'belonging to the appreciation of the beautiful; having such appreciation; in accordance with principles of good taste . . . philosophy of the beautiful or of art . . . set of principles of good taste and appreciation of beauty'. An abstract notion used in discussing the artistic aspect of nursing (and its creative expression). In this context, it relates broadly to theoretical and practical aspects of nursing art.

Affective: 'Pertaining to the affections . . . being affected, mental state, emotions . . . mental disposition, good will, kindly feeling, love' (*Australian concise Oxford dictionary* 1987).

Altruism: 'Regard for others as a principle for action; unselfishness' (*Australian concise Oxford dictionary* 1987).

Argument: A conclusion that is supported by a set of reasons intended to provide grounds for the acceptability of the conclusion.

Autonomy: 'Personal freedom; freedom of the will' (*Australian concise Oxford dictionary* 1987). Right to self-determination.

Binary: Comprised of two parts. See also dichotomy.

Bioethics: An interdisciplinary field of inquiry characterised by a systematic and critical examination of the moral dimensions of healthcare and other associated fields (e.g. the life sciences) from the standpoint of various ethical perspectives.

Biologism: A particular form of essentialism (see below) in which (women's essence) is defined in terms of their biological capacities.

Community assessment: 'Process of critically thinking about the community and getting to know and understand the community as a client. Assessments help identify community needs, clarify problems, and identify strengths and resources' (Stanhope & Lancaster 2002:183).

Conceptual framework: A developing theoretical model that has little empirical support.

Congruency: 'Agreement or consistency' (*Australian concise Oxford dictionary* 1987). For example, in examining two or more theoretical views one may find that there are areas of agreement across the same ground; hence, there is evidence of congruency.

Construct: 'A type of highly abstract and complex concept whose reality base can only be inferred. Constructs are formed from multiple less abstract or more empirical concepts' (Chinn & Jacobs 1983:200).

Critical friend: A trusted colleague who provides feedback on your journal entries.

Critical incident analysis: The use of clinical or personal incidents as a reflective tool.

Critical thinking: The development of a questioning attitude to that which is normally taken for granted.

Deductive reasoning: The process of inferring particulars from general laws or principles.

Dialectic: Defined in the *Australian concise Oxford dictionary* (1987) as the 'art of investigating the truth of opinions, testing of truth by discussion [or] logical disputation or criticism dealing with metaphysical contradictions and their solutions; existence or action of opposing forces'.

Dialectical: A process or perspective involving a dialectic. For example, in theory development using a dialectical approach to generation of knowledge, the process could involve debate with presentation of an argument (thesis), which is considered critically and challenged by a counterargument (antithesis), which is considered critically in relation to the thesis and other knowledge, possibly leading to new areas of agreement and understanding (synthesis).

Dichotomy: 'A division (especially sharply defined) into two; result of such division; binary classification', according to the *Australian concise Oxford dictionary* (1987). The term can be used to indicate a divide between two theoretical positions, which are polarised or incompatible.

Discourse: An abstract notion used to label a collection of theoretical perspectives within an academic discipline. This may be composed of theses or arguments representing knowledge in the discipline, including areas of agreement and disagreement, fundamental assumptions, values and beliefs, expressed in disciplinary language and symbols. The notion reflects the idea of a conversation using language within these boundaries.

Early intervention: Intervening early through working with parent(s) during pregnancy and infancy, or intervening early during a key transition point or pathway in an individual's life (Edgecombe 2004:143).

Empiricist/logical positivist model: An approach grounded in the belief that the world can be viewed as a machine and that the task of science is to discover the laws by which the machine operated; emphasis on predictability, measurement, and the quantification of observable data.

Epistemology: The theory of knowledge; the origins, nature, methods and limits of human knowledge.

Essentialism: The attribution of a fixed essence to women; that there are given, universal characteristics of women, including biological, psychological and social characteristics, which are not readily amenable to change.

Ethical principalism: The view that moral decisions are best guided by appealing to sound universal moral principles, such as the principles of autonomy, beneficence, nonmaleficence and justice; ethical principalism is one of the most popular approaches used to examine ethical issues in healthcare.

Ethical universalism: The view that there exists one set of universal values/standards that is applicable to all people throughout space and time, regardless of their histories and/or cultural backgrounds (contexts).

Ethics: A branch of philosophic inquiry concerned with understanding and examining the moral life. It seeks rational clarification and justification of basic assumptions and beliefs that people hold about what constitutes right or wrong/ good or bad conduct. Can also be defined as a system of action guiding rules and principles that function by specifying that certain types of conduct are required, prohibited or permitted. The term ethics/ethical may be used interchangeably with the term morality/moral.

Etiquette: A set of behavioural action guides concerned with the maintenance of style and decorum in social settings; often, although mistakenly, confused with ethics/morality.

Feminisms: The variety of theoretical approaches to the advocacy of equal rights for women, accompanied by a commitment to improve the position of women in society; includes liberal feminism, socialist feminism, radical feminism, postmodern feminism, and so on.

Gender: A social construction that expresses the many areas of social life, as distinguished from biological sex; the socially learned behaviours and expectations that are associated with the two sexes.

Generic: A characteristic which is 'general, not specific or special' (*Australian concise Oxford dictionary* 1987).

Grounded theory: A research process designed to lead to generation of theory through study of a particular human situation or context.

Grounds: The degree to which a set of reasons supports a conclusion.

Health policies: 'The strategies and courses of action adopted as being advantageous and expedient to provide within the resources available from a health system that at least maintains, and preferably improves, health' (Hennessy & Spurgeon 2000:6).

Health promotion: 'Health promotion is a broad field of activity ranging from actions that are essentially medically focused and individual (such as individual risk-factor assessment and counselling) to actions aimed at helping people to change their behaviour, and further along to actions that seek to create supportive environments and settings that address a broad range of social and environmental determinants of health' (Marshall 2004:185).

Healthy communities: 'A healthy city [community] is one that is continually creating and improving those physical and social environments and expanding those community resources which enable people to mutually support each other in performing all the functions of life and in developing to their maximum potential' (World Health Organization 1998:13).

Hermeneutics: A process of interpretive analysis, which is concerned with uncovering meaning and a technique for interrogating text. Van Manen states that 'hermeneutics is the theory and practice of interpretation. The word derives from the Greek god Hermes whose task it was to communicate messages from Zeus and other gods to the ordinary mortals' (van Manen 1990:179). Hermeneutics was originally a technique used to interpret religious text, which has made a transition into research activity in the social sciences and humanities. Hermeneutical refers to a process or perspective involving hermeneutics.

Holism: A perspective in which people are seen as made up of biological, psychological, social and spiritual components, which are indivisible.

Hypotheses: Tentative statements of relationships between two or more variables, which have little empirical support. The repeated confirmation of hypotheses changes their status to empirical generalisations (statements with moderate empirical support) and thence to law (statements with overwhelming empirical support).

Iconography: 'Illustration of subject by drawings or figures; book whose essence is pictures; treatise on pictures or statuary; study of portraits esp. of an individual' (*Australian concise Oxford dictionary* 1987).

Inductive reasoning: The process of inferring a general law or principle from the observation of particular instances.

Journalling: The technique of recording thoughts and feeling after reflecting on an event.

Masculinist: Pertaining to the masculine; the male gender characteristics derived from social construction and expectation.

Meta: A prefix commonly encountered in theoretical literature. In this context it means 'beyond or higher order' (*Australian concise Oxford dictionary* 1987). A meta-paradigm of any discipline is a statement or group of statements identifying the relevant phenomena to the discipline (Fawcett 1984).

Model: A schematic representation of some aspect of reality, which may be empirical or theoretical. Empirical models are replicas of observed realities (e.g. a plastic model of the ear). Theoretical models represent the world in language or mathematical symbols (e.g. nursing's 'grand theories').

Moral/morality: See ethics above.

Moral duty: An act that a person is bound to perform for moral reasons.

Moral obligation: An act that a person is bound to perform for moral reasons; is generally regarded as being weaker than a moral duty and may be overridden by stronger moral duties.

Moral principles: General standards of conduct that make up an ethical system of action guides and which carry particular imperatives (e.g. 'Do no harm').

Moral right: A special interest that a person has and which ought to be protected for moral reasons (e.g. the right to life) (contrast with legal right; e.g. a special interest that a person has and which ought to be protected for legal reasons); moral rights generally entail correlative rights.

Moral rules: Derived from principles and prescribed particular standards of conduct (e.g. 'Always tell the truth'). Rules have less scope than principles; they also do not have the same force and can be overridden by principles.

Naturalism: A form of essentialism in which a fixed nature is assumed for women, not readily amenable to change.

Nursing ethics: The examination of all kinds of ethical and bioethical issues from the perspective of nursing theory and practice which, in turn, rest on the agreed core concepts of nursing: person, culture, care, health, healing, environment and nursing itself.

Occam's Razor: The principle that the simplest explanation is most likely to be the right one.

Paradigm: A paradigm is a term used to describe accepted practices and techniques through which a discipline accumulates and refines its knowledge base.

Patriarchy: The social system in which men dominate, oppress and exploit women, within the spheres of reproduction, sexuality, work, culture and the state.

Phenomenology: Is a philosophy and descriptive research method designed to uncover the essence and meaning of lived experiences—for example, suffering or grieving (Parse 2001). In a phenomenological research study, the focus is on the meaning of the phenomenon under investigation for the research participants who participate in the study.

Philanthropic: 'Loving one's fellow men, benevolent, humane' (*Australian concise Oxford dictionary* 1987).

Philosophy (alternative view): 'A way of reflecting not so much on what is true and false but on our relationship to the truth' (Foucault, cited in Lotringer 1989).

Philosophy/philosophic inquiry (conventional view): An argumentative intellectual discipline concerned with the discovery of 'truth' and meaning. Unlike science, which seeks answers to questions that can only be answered by empirical evidence, philosophy seeks answers to questions that cannot be answered by empirical evidence.

Postmodernism: Relates to the critique of modern, capitalist, industrialised society; new political and social strategies, which embrace pluralism and diversity of cultures and values.

Poststructuralism: Refers to a range of theoretical positions in which the mode of knowledge production uses particular theories of language, subjectivity, social processes and institutions to understand existing power relations and to identify areas and strategies for change.

Praxis: Praxis can be seen as the link between reflection and action. Friere (1972) defines praxis as 'reflection and action upon the world in order to transform it' (Cox et al 1991:385).

Premise: A reason offered in support of a conclusion.

Pre-reflection: Preparatory reflection that occurs before the experience.

Preventive ethics: The study and practice of ethics (including ethic education) aimed at preventing (as opposed to remedying) moral problems.

Public health: 'The science and art of promoting health, preventing disease, and prolonging life through the organised efforts of society' (World Health Organization 1998:3).

Rationalism: A philosophical position that argues that the only way to truth is through the deliberations of the rational human mind.

Reductive: From reduction 'in reducing or being reduced; amount by which prices etc are reduced, reduced copy of picture, map etc . . . to absurdity . . . so reductive' (*Australian concise Oxford dictionary* 1987).

Reflection, also **Reflection-on-action:** Reflection that occurs after the experience.

Reflective practice: The incorporation of reflection into practice.

Regulatory authorities: Those organisations responsible for the registration of nurses (e.g. the QNC or N&MRB of NSW).

Relevance: A test applied to a premise or reason. If a premise or reason is relevant, it helps to support the conclusion of the argument.

Social capital: 'Social capital represents the degree of social cohesion which exists in communities. It refers to the processes between people which establish networks, norms, and social trust, and facilitate co-ordination and co-operation for mutual benefit' (World Health Organization 1998:19).

Social support: 'That assistance available to individuals and groups from within communities which can provide a buffer against adverse life events and living conditions, and can provide a positive resource for enhancing the quality of life' (World Health Organization 1998:20).

Sound: An argument is *sound* when the premises are acceptable and provide adequate grounds for accepting the conclusion.

Theory: A logically consistent set of propositions, which presents a systematic view of some aspect of reality.

GLOSSARY

Universalism: Refers to the attributions of functions, social categories and activities to which women of all cultures are assigned; asserts what is shared in common by all women.

Validity: An argument is *valid* when the premises that are offered provide adequate grounds for acceptance of the conclusion.

INDEX